ATTACHMENT THEORY AND CLOSE RELATIONSHIPS

Attachment Theory and ,
Close Relationships

Editors
JEFFRY A. SIMPSON
W. STEVEN RHOLES

THE GUILFORD PRESS
New York   London

© 1998 The Guilford Press
A Division of Guilford Publications, Inc.
72 Spring Street, New York, NY 10012
http://www.guilford.com

Printed in the United States of America

This book is printed on acid-free paper.

Last digit is print number: 9 8 7 6 5 4 3 2

Library of Congress Cataloging-in-Publication Data

Attachment theory and close relationships / Jeffry A. Simpson, W.
Steven Rholes, editors.
     p.   cm.
Includes bibliographical references and index.
ISBN 1-57230-102-3
   1. Attachment behavior. 2. Interpersonal relations. 3. Intimacy
(Psychology) I. Simpson, Jeffry A. II. Rholes, W. Steven (William
Steven)
BF575.A86A8   1998
158.2—dc21   97–37552
                                                      CIP

This book is dedicated to

Cindy, Chris, and Natalie (JAS)
and
Ted and Eric (WSR)

Contributors

Kim Bartholomew, PhD, Department of Psychology, Simon Fraser University, Burnaby, British Columbia, Canada

Kelly A. Brennan, PhD, Department of Psychology, State University of New York at Stony Brook, Stony Brook, New York

Catherine L. Clark, PhD, Department of Psychology, University of California at Davis, Davis, California

Keith E. Davis, PhD, Department of Psychology, University of South Carolina, Columbia, South Carolina

Mary Dozier, PhD, Department of Psychology, University of Delaware, Newark, Delaware

Judith A. Feeney, PhD, Department of Psychology, University of Queensland, St. Lucia, Queensland, Australia

Victor Florian, PhD, Department of Psychology, Bar-Ilan University, Ramat Gan, Israel

R. Chris Fraley, MA, Department of Psychology, University of California at Davis, Davis, California

Jami Grich Stevens, MA, Department of Psychology, Texas A&M University, College Station, Texas

Kate Henry, BSc, Department of Psychology, University of Waterloo, Waterloo, Ontario, Canada

John G. Holmes, PhD, Department of Psychology, University of Waterloo, Waterloo, Ontario, Canada

Oliver P. John, PhD, Department of Psychology, University of California at Berkeley, Berkeley, California

Lee A. Kirkpatrick, PhD, Department of Psychology, College of William and Mary, Williamsburg, Virginia

Eva C. Klohnen, PhD, Department of Psychology, University of California at Berkeley, Berkeley, California

Jennifer Loev, BA, Department of Psychology, University of Texas, Austin, Texas

Mario Mikulincer, PhD, Department of Psychology, Bar-Ilan University, Ramat Gan, Israel

Patricia Noller, PhD, Department of Psychology, University of Queensland, St. Lucia, Queensland, Australia

W. Steven Rholes, PhD, Department of Psychology, Texas A&M University, College Station, Texas

Nigel Roberts, BA(Hons), Department of Psychology, University of Queensland, St. Lucia, Queensland, Australia

Phillip R. Shaver, PhD, Department of Psychology, University of California at Davis, Davis, California

Jeffry A. Simpson, PhD, Department of Psychology, Texas A&M University, College Station, Texas

Christine Tyrrell, MA, Department of Psychology, University of Delaware, Newark, Delaware

Niels G. Waller, PhD, Department of Psychology, University of California at Davis, Davis, California

Shey Wu, MBA, MA, Department of Psychology, University of Texas, Austin, Texas

Contents

PART I

Introduction

1

Attachment in Adulthood

JEFFRY A. SIMPSON
W. STEVEN RHOLES

In the last decade, no single area of research in personality/social psychology has attracted more interest than the application of attachment theory to the study of adult relationships. Although Bowlby (1979) stated that attachment processes affect human beings "from the cradle to the grave" (p. 129) and wrote extensively about attachment phenomena in adulthood (see Bowlby, 1969, 1973, 1980), research on adult attachment did not flourish until the mid-1980s. The purpose of this volume is twofold: (1) to integrate and consolidate important theoretical and empirical advances that have taken place in the area of adult attachment during the last decade, and (2) to suggest promising directions for future research.

In this chapter, we provide a brief historical overview of attachment theory and research as it applies to adults. We begin by discussing the two major "traditions" from which nearly all research on adult attachment emanates: (1) research dealing with attachment in nuclear families, which has relied on attachment interviews to assess adults' memories of childhood experiences with their parents (e.g., the Adult Attachment Interview; George, Kaplan, & Main, 1985), and (2) research focusing on attachments to contemporary peers, which tends to use self-report attachment measures to gauge perceptions of current relationship experiences with peers or romantic partners (e.g., the categorically based romantic attachment scales created by Hazan & Shaver, 1987, and the continuously distributed scales developed by Collins & Read, 1990; Simpson, Rholes, & Nelligan, 1992; and others). After commenting on the theoretical and empirical origins that both traditions share, we discuss how they differ and the types of relationships to which each tradition may be most applicable.

We then review some of the major studies and articles that have appreciably advanced theory and research on adult attachment, after which we briefly describe each chapter in the present volume. The chapters are organized into sections that deal with central or rapidly emerging areas of research: measurement issues, affect regulation, clinical applications, and theoretical and empirical extensions of the basic theory. Finally, we conclude by highlighting a few important avenues for future research.

THE TWO TRADITIONS

Attachment theory is much broader and more pervasive in its scope than many people realize. The theory has two principal components: (1) a *normative* component, which attempts to explain modal, species-typical patterns of behavior and stages of development through which nearly all human beings pass, and (2) an *individual difference* component, which attempts to explain stable, systematic deviations from the modal behavioral patterns and stages (see Hazan & Shaver, 1994; Simpson, in press, for more in-depth discussions). Due to the success of Mary Ainsworth's pioneering research on patterns of attachment in young children (see Ainsworth, Blehar, Waters, & Wall, 1978), most empirical work to date has focused on individual differences in attachment instead of normative features. As the chapters in this volume attest, this preferential focus on individual differences has been true not only of research with children, but of research with adults as well.

As shown in Figure 1.1, both of the "traditions" from which virtually all research on adult attachment stems have their foundations in Bowlby's attachment theory and in Ainsworth's Strange Situation (see Bartholomew & Shaver, Chapter 2, this volume). Indeed, the first and most widely used interview measure of adult attachment—the Adult Attachment Interview (AAI; George et al., 1985)—was developed expressly to *predict* the Strange Situation behavior of respondents' infants. The AAI classifies adults into one of four attachment categories: secure–autonomous, preoccupied, dismissing–avoidant, and disorganized–disoriented. AAI classifications do, in fact, predict patterns of infant attachment, especially for mother–infant dyads (see van IJzendoorn, 1995). In general, adults who are secure–autonomous on the AAI have infants who are rated as secure in the Strange Situation, adults who score as dismissing–avoidant

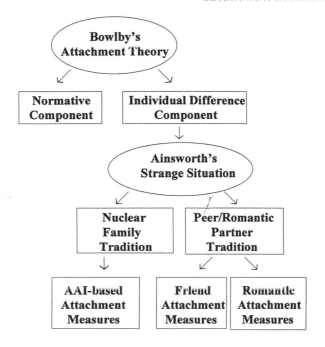

FIGURE 1.1. Origins of the two research traditions in adult attachment.

on the AAI have infants who are anxious–avoidant, and adults who are preoccupied on the AAI have anxious–ambivalent infants.

The AAI assesses patterns of attachment in parent–children relationships within nuclear families. In particular, it is designed to elicit distal memories, beliefs, and feelings of past relationships with one's parents or primary caregivers. One principal focus of the AAI is to determine how information about past attachment figures is structured, organized, and stored. Instead of focusing directly on the content of the information gleaned from the interview (e.g., whether or not an individual reports positive or negative memories of childhood), the AAI assesses various "states of mind" that presumably reflect the operation of deeper, more "unconscious" internal working models stemming from childhood.

In developing the AAI coding categories, Main and her colleagues initially relied on attachment theory for clues about which patterns or styles of adult discourse should be associated with specific attachment patterns in infants. As the development of the AAI progressed, however, it became clear that some patterns of discourse that were highly predictive of attachment classifications in children were *not* anticipated by attachment theory (e.g., "passive speech" exhibited by adults classified as preoccupied on the AAI). Thus, while most of the AAI coding criteria were foreseen by Bowlby (e.g., "coherence of mind," characteristic of securely attached adults; "idealization" of parents, displayed by dismissing–avoidant adults), some important criteria were not. A deeper under-standing of how and why these unexpected styles or patterns of speech are associated with specific patterns of attachment in respondents' young children is likely to extend attachment theory in new and exciting direc-tions.

The peer/romantic partner research tradition also has solid roots in both attachment theory and the Strange Situation, but from a different angle. In developing the first adult attachment vignettes (which measured secure, avoidant, and anxious–ambivalent attachment styles in romantic relationships), Hazan and Shaver (1987) first canvassed attachment theory for insights about how adults with different attachment histories ought to think, feel, and behave in close relationships. They then summarized the prototypical emotional and behavioral attributes of secure, avoidant, and anxious–ambivalent infants in the Strange Situation. Acknowledging that adult romantic relationships differ from infant–caregiver relationships in some significant ways (see Shaver, Hazan, & Bradshaw, 1988), Hazan and Shaver nevertheless theorized that romantic love is fundamentally an attachment process through which affectional bonds are formed. They reasoned that the three patterns of attachment that Ainsworth et al. documented in young children might be "translated" into three primary styles of adult romantic attachment over the course of development. In the last decade, a great deal of research using romantic attachment scales derived from the Hazan and Shaver vignettes has tested and confirmed fundamental predictions of attachment theory. Hence, both the initial categorically based self-report measures of adult romantic attachment (e.g., Hazan & Shaver, 1987) as well as the more recent continuously distributed attachment measures (e.g., Brennan, Clark, & Shaver, Chapter 3, this volume; Collins & Read, 1990; Feeney, Noller, & Callan, 1994; Simpson et al., 1992) contain the direct influence of both Bowlby's theory and Ainsworth et al.'s pioneering empirical work.

Although both traditions have direct ties to Bowlby and Ainsworth, the two traditions should be relevant to different components of individu-als' internal working models at different levels of consciousness. Indeed, studies in which both the AAI and the self-report romantic attachment measures have been administered have found little correspondence be-tween them (see Bartholomew & Shaver, Chapter 2, this volume). This should not be too surprising given that the two traditions focus on—and, therefore, should be relevant to—different life tasks. In fact, Kirkpatrick (Chapter 13, this volume) contends that the two traditions should provide unique information about an individual's attachment history in different kinds of relationships experienced at different points of development.

The AAI has two major advantages over self-report measures. First, because many respondents have not thought deeply about questions on the AAI, it can "surprise" the unconscious. By doing so, the AAI may be able to bypass defenses that could bias self-report attachment styles, especially among dismissing–avoidant people. Second, given the personal and increasingly emotional nature of the questions on the AAI (e.g., questions at the end of the interview that inquire about abuse and loss), respondents are more likely to become aroused—and, therefore, their attachment systems are more likely to be activated—when taking the AAI than when answering questionnaire items dealing with general perceptions of their contemporary attachment figures and relationships. In some situations, researchers might be more interested in assessing adult attachment styles when the attachment system is fully activated than when it is relatively quiescent.

The AAI was developed to *predict* the Strange Situation behavior of respondents' children explicitly. Hence, it should tap working models relevant to parenting and caregiving more directly than working models pertinent to other life tasks (e.g., mating; see Kirkpatrick, Chapter 13, this volume). The peer/romantic partner tradition, on the other hand, focuses on contemporary views and perceptions of peers or romantic partners, which usually are assessed by face-valid self-report scales. Compared to the AAI, the self-report scales measure the explicit *content* of the perceptions and views that individuals currently have about themselves and others in close relationships. Consequently, the self-report inventories probably reflect the nature and operation of internal working models that are more "conscious," accessible, and open to direct inspection.

Self-report measures have some advantages over attachment interviews. First, they are easy to administer and score. Second, they directly assess views that adults have about contemporary attachment figures (usually romantic/sexual partners). Accordingly, self-report attachment scales should be better suited to assess working models that guide social behavior in peer and romantic relationships, but poorer at indexing working models that govern parenting and caregiving. In all likelihood, the two traditions assess different components of working models that are embedded in large, complex, and interrelated mental networks (see Collins & Read, 1994). Different components may represent different types of relationships (e.g., parent–child, romantic, friendship), with components formed earlier in development (i.e., those concerning one's parents and caregiving) possibly affecting components formed later (i.e., those relevant to peers or romantic partners). Within each type of relationship, components are likely to have different levels of abstraction, ranging from general "if–then" beliefs, assumptions, or expectancies about what certain types of relationships are like (or should be like), to specific beliefs, assumptions, or expectancies about how certain people are likely to think, feel, and behave in specific situations.

Nearly all of the research in the nuclear family tradition has focused on how working models of one's parents are tied to patterns of attachment displayed by one's own infant in the Strange Situation. Within the peer/romantic partner tradition, however, separate attachment measures have been developed to assess patterns of attachment to friends (e.g., Bartholomew & Horowitz, 1991) and to romantic partners (e.g., Collins & Read, 1990; Hazan & Shaver, 1987; Simpson et al., 1992). While most of the attachment measures in the peer/romantic partner tradition rely on self-reports, some investigators have used interviews in which respondents' discuss their contemporary relationships with friends and/or romantic partners (e.g., Bartholomew & Horowitz, 1991).

ADVANCES IN ADULT ATTACHMENT

There have been several noteworthy advances in adult attachment during the past decade. In this section, we trace the empirical and theoretical development of the field, highlighting some (but by no means all) of the significant milestones. This short review is intended to provide common historical background and context for the chapters that follow. We begin with a review of research in the nuclear family tradition, after which we review research in the self-report tradition.

The Nuclear Family Tradition

In 1985, Main, Kaplan, and Cassidy published the first article directly structured around assessing the content and organization of internal working models in adults. In doing so, they launched the nuclear family tradition of adult attachment. Main et al. documented that the way in which adults discussed their past relationships with their own parents was systematically linked to the attachment classification of their own infants in the Strange Situation. For example, adults who idealized their own parents yet could not provide clear, episodic memories that supported these glowing assessments (i.e., dismissing–avoidant adults) had children who generally were avoidant in the Strange Situation. Adults who displayed intense, unresolved anger toward their parents or who strayed from the AAI questions (i.e., preoccupied adults) tended to have children classified as anxious–ambivalent. And adults who produced credible, clear, and coherent accounts of their relationship with their parents—even if their experiences were negative or painful—(i.e., secure adults) usually had children who were secure in the Strange Situation.

In 1990, Main and Solomon identified a fourth attachment category in children: disorganized–disoriented. These infants do not have a clear, consistent strategy for handling stress in the Strange Situation. Their behavior includes strange stereotypical movements, unusual motions, or "freezed" postures accompanied by dazed facial expressions. Main and Solomon hypothesized that disorganization might result from certain patterns of parenting behavior. Parents who remain unresolved about traumatic events in their past may display frightening, confused, or bizarre behaviors that produce disorganization in their young children (Main & Hesse, 1990).

Research in the early 1990s addressed both the long-term stability of attachment patterns across the life span as well as the role that sensitive care plays in the formation of attachment bonds. Reporting initial findings from the Minnesota longitudinal project, Elicker, Englund, and Sroufe (1992) revealed that assessments of attachment taken in the Strange Situation during infancy successfully predict specific patterns of social behavior in adolescence, just as Bowlby anticipated. Both correlational research (e.g., Isabella, 1993; Isabella & Belsky, 1991; Smith & Pederson, 1988) and experimental research (e.g., van IJzendoorn, Juffer, & Duyvesteyn, 1995) confirmed that parental sensitivity and responsiveness affect the development of attachment patterns in young children. Parents who provide sensitive, responsive, and situationally contingent care have infants who tend to be classified as secure in the Strange Situation. Conversely, parents who provide insensitive or unpredictable care have anxious–ambivalent infants, whereas those who are cold, unresponsive, and rejecting have avoidant infants. In fact, Ward and Carlson (1995) have found that young mothers with secure attachment orientations (assessed by the AAI *before* the birth of their child) are more sensitive to their infants during play interactions than are insecure mothers.

Examining later points in the life span, Crowell and Feldman (1988) documented that secure mothers are more helpful and supportive of their children while engaging in laboratory teaching tasks (see Rholes, Simpson, & Blakely, 1995, for a conceptual replication using self-report adult attachment measures). Similarly, mothers and fathers who are securely attached on the AAI are warmer and provide more structure for their preschool children in laboratory play sessions relative to insecure parents (Cohn, Cowan, Cowan, & Pearson, 1992; Pearson, Cohn, Cowan, & Cowan, 1994). Focusing on marital conflict, Kobak and Hazan (1991) found that spouses with secure working models regulate their emotions more constructively during problem-solving discussions involving their marital partner and exhibit better marital adjustment.

In 1991, Main published an important theoretical article on metacognitive knowledge, metacognitive monitoring, and the development of singular (coherent) versus multiple (incoherent) working models of attachment. Main hypothesized that the difficulties some children have with the "appearance–reality" distinction could generate multiple, conflicting models of attachment figures and/or attachment experiences. In adulthood, these conflicting models should produce less "coherence" in AAI interviews, which is a defining feature of adult insecurity. With this article, Main moved research on adult attachment deeper into the cognitive realm.

During the mid-1990s, research focused on validating the AAI. Bakersman-Kranenburg and van IJzendoorn (1993) provided some of the first independent validation evidence for the instrument. They found that AAI classifications were stable over 2 months and that AAI scores were *not* highly correlated with measures of IQ, the quality of autobiographical memories involving nonattachment issues, and social desirability. Two years later, van IJzendoorn (1995) conducted a meta-analysis to examine the predictive validity of the AAI, based on 18 available studies. While parents' AAI classifications strongly predicted the Strange Situation classifications of their infants, the results suggested that little is known about precisely how the working models harbored by parents are transmitted to their children. Recently, Crowell et al. (1996) have provided additional validation evidence for the AAI, confirming that it correlates modestly with measures of IQ and social adjustment, but negligibly with general discourse style and social desirability.

The Peer/Romantic Partner Tradition

In 1987, Hazan and Shaver published their seminal article on adult attachment, ushering in the peer/romantic partner tradition. In addition to introducing the first self-report measure of adult attachment, Hazan and Shaver proposed that attachment theory and the three adult attachment styles explained many of the "lovestyles" documented by previous researchers (e.g., Lee, 1973; Tennov, 1979). Following Ainsworth's lead, Hazan and Shaver suggested that the three adult attachment styles should be measured as discrete categories.

The use of categorical measures rather than continuously distributed scales proved to be problematic for conceptual, data-analytic, and logistical reasons. From a conceptual standpoint, there was no compelling reason to believe that, at a *latent* level, attachment styles were really discrete categories (see Fraley & Waller, Chapter 4, this volume, for evidence arguing against the taxonicity of the self-report adult attachment styles). From a data-analytic perspective, the use of categorical measures limited investigators to using analysis of variance statistical techniques. From a logistical standpoint, the categorical measures did not indicate the extent to which each attachment category was characteristic of a given individual.

Foreseeing these problems, Collins and Read (1990) and Simpson (1990) introduced continuous adult attachment scales, which were based on ratings of phrases or sentences contained in Hazan and Shaver's (1987) three original attachment vignettes. Along with work by Levy and Davis (1988), Feeney and Noller (1990), Kobak and Sceery (1988), Pistole (1989), and others, research in the late 1980s and early 1990s revealed how each adult attachment style correlated with important relationship constructs, including commitment, satisfaction, trust, and long-term stability in romantic relationships.

At the same time that psychometric advances were beginning to occur, Bartholomew (1990; Bartholomew & Horowitz, 1991) introduced a major theoretical breakthrough. Returning to Bowlby (1973), she tested and confirmed that two continuously distributed dimensions—views of the self in relationships (positive vs. negative) and views of significant others (positive vs. negative)—defined four (rather than three) principal attachment styles in adults. Retaining the secure and preoccupied styles, Bartholomew (1990) distinguished two forms of avoidance: fearful-avoidance and dismissing-avoidance. According to this model, secure people have positive views of themselves and others, preoccupied people have negative self-views and positive (yet apprehensive) views of others, fearful–avoidant people have negative views of both the self and others, and dismissing–avoidants have positive self-views but negative views of others. Bartholomew's two-dimensional model remains one of the most important theoretical advances in adult attachment.

In 1992, Simpson, Rholes, and Nelligan published one of the first videotaped social interaction studies in the adult attachment area. They documented that women with more secure romantic attachment styles regulate their emotions by turning to their dating partners for reassurance and support when they are upset, whereas more avoidant women withdraw from their partners. In a parallel fashion, more secure men give their partners greater emotional support and reassurance if their partners are distressed, while avoidant men actually become less supportive. Several other studies have been based on the premise that adult attachment styles primarily reflect different ways of regulating, controlling, and mitigating negative affect in interpersonal contexts (e.g., Brennan & Shaver, 1995; Feeney, 1995; Kobak, Cole, Ferenz-Gillies, Fleming, & Gamble, 1993; Mikulincer, Florian, & Tolmacz, 1990; Mikulincer, Florian, & Weller, 1993; Simpson, Rholes, & Phillips, 1996). Indeed, one section of this volume is devoted to affect regulation processes (see Mikulincer & Florian, Chapter 6; Rholes, Simpson, & Grich Stevens, Chapter 7; and Feeney, Chapter 8, this volume).

In 1994, several influential articles appeared. After examining the factor structure of the most widely used self-report romantic attachment scales, Griffin and Bartholomew (1994) concluded that all of the major scales contain two factors that map onto the self and other dimensions reasonably well. Kirkpatrick and Davis (1994) reported the results of a 3-year longitudinal study which indicated that attachment styles are *not* randomly paired in dating couples and that attachment styles predict long-term relationship stability and status in theoretically meaningful ways even when constructs such as commitment and length of relationship are partialed out. Scharfe and Bartholomew (1994) provided some of the first evidence that adult romantic attachment styles remain fairly stable over several months (although see Baldwin & Fehr, 1995; Baldwin, Keelan, Fehr, Enns, & Koh-Rangarajoo, 1996, for an alternate view). Hazan and Shaver (1994) completed the first comprehensive and integrative review of the adult attachment field, highlighting the fact that the normative component of attachment theory needed more attention. In the same year, Bartholomew and Perlman (1994) produced an important edited book devoted entirely to attachment processes in adulthood.

Recently, research has begun to further clarify the nature, structure, and operation of internal working models (see Shaver, Collins, & Clark, 1996, for a review). Mikulincer (1995), for example, has shown that secure individuals have more balanced, complex, and coherent views of themselves than do insecure individuals. Collins (1996) has found that, compared to people with secure working models, people with ambivalent models explain events in more negative ways and report greater emotional distress, whereas people with avoidant models explain events in more negative ways but do not experience severe emotional distress.

THE PRESENT VOLUME

The chapters in this volume are organized into four sections: measurement issues, affect regulation, clinical applications, and conceptual and empirical extensions. Measurement issues are addressed first because, from our perspective, questions concerning how to measure and interpret adult attachment styles represent some of the most vexing, unresolved, and enigmatic issues in the field. The adult attachment area *must* gain a better understanding of which specific nodes or components of interrelated working models are best assessed by which kinds of attachment measures (e.g., those focusing on nuclear family members vs. contemporary peers or romantic partners). Furthermore, given a specific type of relationship, we must develop a better understanding of how various measures fit in the context of Bartholomew's two-dimensional model.

Measurement Issues

In Chapter 2, Bartholomew and Shaver examine whether or not different methods of assessing adult attachment orientations "converge" in classifying adult attachment patterns. After reviewing the two traditions and noting some problems with comparing them, they attempt to anchor measures from the two traditions within Bartholomew's two-dimensional model of attachment. Their results indicate that a single representational system might underlie responses to different attachment measures, but an individual's specific pattern of attachment can vary according to the specific type of relationship under investigation.

In Chapter 3, Brennan, Clark, and Shaver present the results of a large-scale study designed to develop more reliable self-report scales of adult attachment styles based on items from several existing self-report scales. Corroborating previous research (e.g., Griffin & Bartholomew, 1994; Simpson et al., 1992), they find that two primary dimensions underlie responses to these self-report items: Avoidance and Anxiety. They suggest that future research using self-report attachment measures should assess these two dimensions.

In Chapter 4, Fraley and Waller test a long-standing and basic question in the attachment literature: Are adult romantic attachment styles best conceptualized as continuously distributed at a latent level, or do they reflect latent "types"? Applying state-of-the-art taxometric analytical methods, Fraley and Waller find that adult attachment styles are not "typological" variables. Instead, they are continuously distributed at a latent level, suggesting that people differ in the degree to which they possess different attachment styles.

Klohnen and John conclude the section on measurement by summarizing, in Chapter 5, their recent research on expert-based prototypes, which has interesting implications for the assessment of working models in adulthood. They present evidence for the validity of these working model prototypes, along with information about their temporal consistency and malleability in a 25-year longitudinal study. The authors reveal that people with different attachment styles tend to have distinct working models that remain fairly stable across time. Moreover, as people grow older, their working models gradually decrease in resemblance to the preoccupied prototype and increase in resemblance to the secure prototype.

Affect Regulation

The second section of the volume centers on working models and affect regulation. Guided by the theoretical work of Sroufe and Waters (1977), a considerable amount of research has addressed this important topic in the last decade. Chapter 6, by Mikulincer and Florian, introduces this section by reviewing and consolidating the existing research on affect regulation in adults. The authors integrate studies dealing with a wide range of stress-inducing experiences, including the prospect of death, war-related stress, interpersonal loss, personal failures, parenthood, and chronic pain. After reviewing this vast literature, they conclude that, across a gamut of difficult life events, adult attachment styles seem to influence how well individuals adapt to stress in their daily lives.

Rholes, Simpson, and Grich Stevens, in Chapter 7, review and theoretically integrate the results of two laboratory-based behavioral observation studies that used different experimental paradigms to induce distress: fear induction (Simpson et al., 1992) and conflict resolution (Simpson et al., 1996). They describe how each paradigm should differentially affect people with different kinds of working models. Rholes et al. then discuss the implications that this research has for how therapeutic effectiveness can be maximized for people with different attachment histories.

In Chapter 8, Feeney addresses relationship-centered anxiety, focusing primarily on how people react when their attachment figures create physical and/or emotional distance. She presents new research showing that securely attached people are less likely to respond to physical separation with feelings of insecurity, more likely to use viable coping strategies when dealing with separation, and more inclined to confront problems directly by negotiating with their partner. The net effect is that secure people have more positive perceptions of their relationships following separations. In line with previous research (e.g., Kobak et al., 1993; Simpson et al., 1992), Feeney also finds that people with different attachment styles are more likely to behave differently in stressful situations, especially when their relationships are threatened. Greater security, however, tends to buffer individuals' positive perceptions of their relationships.

Clinical Applications

The third section of the volume focuses on clinical applications of adult attachment. In Chapter 9, Dozier and Tyrrell examine the role of attachment in therapeutic relationships. They contend that a primary task for therapists is to provide a secure base that fosters safe exploration by the client. After presenting a model of therapeutic change, Dozier and Tyrrell review research suggesting that securely attached clients are better collaborators in treatment, whereas avoidantly attached clients maintain greater emotional distance from their therapists. The authors also review work indicating that clinicians who use "secure strategies" in therapy are better able to provide clients with experiences that effectively challenge their maladaptive working models.

Chapter 10, by Fraley, Davis, and Shaver, addresses the defensive organization of the dismissing–avoidant attachment orientation. The authors begin by noting striking similarities between avoidant children and dismissing–avoidant adults in how they regulate their behavior and emotions in situations that, for most people, generate considerable anxiety or despair (e.g., separation or relationship loss). They argue that, despite phenotypic similarities, different mechanisms may be responsible for producing avoidance in children and adults. Fraley et al. then attempt to answer three questions: (1) How does the mind need to be structured to suppress attachment-related thoughts and feelings? (2) What kinds of social and cognitive processes are necessary to sustain a defensive psychological orientation? (3) What are some plausible developmental pathways through which avoidance in adulthood might emerge?

Henry and Holmes, in Chapter 11, present the results of an investigation that examines how the working models and social perceptions of adults whose parents divorced differ from adults whose parents were unhappy yet remained married. They propose that witnessing the erosion of trust and love in disintegrating parental relationships should tarnish the working models of adults whose parents divorced, placing them at greater risk for developing negative working models of their own romantic partners and relationships. Henry and Holmes conclude that both adults whose parents divorced and adults whose parents had difficult marriages but did *not* divorce harbor negative beliefs about relationships in general. However, both groups have relatively positive working models about their current romantic partners/relationships. Possible reasons for this "duality" are discussed.

In Chapter 12, Roberts and Noller focus on attachment and violence in heterosexual relationships. After reviewing some of the domestic violence literature, they indicate how attachment theory can offer theoretical insights into who is likely to become abusive, who is likely to be the target of abuse, and the circumstances in which violence is most likely to occur. The authors review research on how different attachment styles are associated with communication skills, withdrawal, and the expression of hostility during conflict episodes. They then report a study that addresses (1) whether relationship satisfaction mediates the link between adult attachment styles and the use of violent tactics in close relationships, and (2) whether attachment styles moderate the relation between partners' use of violence. Roberts and Noller find that anxiety about abandonment tends to be a stronger predictor of violence than discomfort with closeness, although the occurrence of violence also depends on the specific configuration of both partners' attachment styles.

Conceptual and Empirical Extensions

The final section of the book showcases theoretical and empirical extensions. In Chapter 13, Kirkpatrick presents a reconceptualization of adult attachment styles, suggesting that they may reflect different evolutionarily based reproductive strategies. He adopts the position that the attachment "system" in children serves different functions than the "system" witnessed in adults. Kirkpatrick claims that the emotion of love was coopted by evolutionary forces to maintain pair-bonds, and that humans evolved to use both short-term and long-term reproductive strategies. He then reviews evidence consistent with the notion that different romantic attachment styles might reflect long-term versus short-term strategies, and he discusses implications of this revised view of adult attachment styles for our understanding of mating and attachment phenomena in adulthood.

Finally, Chapter 14, by Brennan, Wu, and Loev, deals with attachment styles and individual differences in attitudes toward physical contact in close relationships. Given how important touch is in regulating arousal in mother–infant dyads, the authors contend that touch also should be important for understanding the nature of affectional bonds in adulthood. After documenting the centrality of physical contact within each of the three behavioral systems that comprise romantic love (i.e., attachment, caregiving, and sexuality), Brennan et al. comment on the surprising paucity of research concerning how physical contact affects the formation and maintenance of adult pair-bonds. They then report on the development of self-report scales that assess different empirically derived dimensions of touch: desiring touch, affectionate proximity, sexual touch, touch aversion, discomfort with public touch, coercive control, and safe haven touch.

DIRECTIONS FOR FUTURE WORK

The work described in this volume suggests several directions for future research. In the final part of the introduction, we note some of the most promising empirical and conceptual avenues for future work.

Many unresolved questions center on the nature and measurement of the different types of internal working models that individuals develop. Bowlby, for instance, hypothesized that many people harbor two distinct models of early parental relationships that operate at different levels of awareness. One model is more complex and open to direct consciousness, while the other is more primitive and largely sealed off from awareness. How well do the various adult attachment measures assess these two models? Can we document that the AAI taps the primitive and unconscious parental model more directly, whereas the self-report attachment scales measure the complex and open model more adequately, as we have suggested? Moreover, how do models relevant to different types of relationships (e.g., parents, friends, romantic partners) influence and interact with one another in guiding social perceptions and behavior? For example, if an individual has insecure working models about parents but secure models about close adolescent friends, how do these contrasting models impact the individual's views of romantic partners? To answer these questions, we must discover what kinds of childhood and adolescent experiences generate different romantic attachment styles in adulthood.

Several important yet unanswered questions also remain about the role of affect regulation in adult relationships. Although indirect evidence abounds, there is little direct empirical data demonstrating that the *primary* function of adult attachment styles is to control and mitigate negative affect in interpersonal contexts. From an evolutionary perspective, one possible function of adult attachment styles might be to buffer individuals from distracting, anxiety-producing stressors so they can remain focused on goals central to the two primary tasks in adulthood that affect reproductive fitness: successful mating and parenting. In light of an individual's attachment history, different patterns of affect regulation might reflect the "best available" solution the individual has found to regulate and contain negative affect successfully. Furthermore, little is known about what specific kinds of behavioral, cognitive, and emotional strategies adults with different attachment orientations use to regulate affect. This information is vital to advancing our understanding of affect regulation in adulthood.

With regard to clinical applications of attachment theory, numerous fundamental questions remain unanswered. For example, how is greater security produced in therapy? What are the specific processes, stages, or steps through which an individual must navigate to become more secure? How does "earned" security (i.e., security that is achieved after insecurity has been successfully overcome) differ from "continuous" security? More specifically, how do the adult relationships of individuals classified as earned secure differ from those of individuals who have been secure their entire lives? When major life difficulties arise, are earned secure individuals more capable of fending off and constructively dealing with experiences that would lead most people—including perhaps continuously secure individuals—toward insecurity?

Finally, what *are* the primary functions and purposes of adult romantic attachment styles? Are they merely manifestations of different mating strategies, or do they serve other important evolutionary functions as well? If, as Kirkpatrick (Chapter 13, this volume) suggests, childhood patterns of attachment are closely tied to working models associated with parenting and caregiving, whereas adult attachment styles are more relevant to working models of mating and reproduction, why do adult romantic attachment styles correlate only modestly with measures of mating orientations (e.g., sociosexuality; see Brennan & Shaver, 1995; Simpson & Gangestad, 1991).

These questions, however, are for the future. For now, we hope that readers will derive as much pleasure, interest, and insight from the chapters that follow as we have.

ACKNOWLEDGMENTS

The writing of this chapter was partially supported by National Institute of Mental Health Grant No. MH49599. The authors contributed equally to the writing of this chapter. We thank Jami Grich Stevens for her helpful comments on an earlier draft.

REFERENCES

Ainsworth, M. D. S., Blehar, M. C., Waters, E., & Wall, S. (1978). *Patterns of attachment: A psychological study of the Strange Situation.* Hillsdale, NJ: Erlbaum.

Bakersman-Kranenburg, M. J., & van IJzendoorn, M. H. (1993). A psychometric study of the Adult Attachment Interview: Reliability and discriminant validity. *Developmental Psychology, 29,* 870–880.

Baldwin, M. W., & Fehr, B. (1995). On the instability of attachment style ratings. *Personal Relationships, 2,* 247–261.

Baldwin, M. W., Keelan, J. P. R., Fehr, B., Enns, V., & Koh-Rangarajoo, E. (1996). Social-cognitive conceptualization of attachment working models: Availability and accessibility effects. *Journal of Personality and Social Psychology, 71,* 94–109.

Bartholomew, K. (1990). Avoidance of intimacy: An attachment perspective. *Journal of Social and Personal Relationships, 7,* 147–178.

Bartholomew, K., & Horowitz, L. M. (1991). Attachment styles among young adults: A test of a four-category model. *Journal of Personality and Social Psychology, 61,* 226–244.

Bartholomew, K., & Perlman, D. (Eds.). (1994). *Attachment processes in adulthood.* London: Jessica Kingsley.

Bowlby, J. (1969). *Attachment and loss: Vol. 1. Attachment.* New York: Basic Books.

Bowlby, J. (1973). *Attachment and loss: Vol. 2. Separation: Anxiety and anger.* New York: Basic Books.

Bowlby, J. (1979). *The making and breaking of affectional bonds.* London: Tavistock.

Bowlby, J. (1980). *Attachment and loss: Vol. 3. Loss.* New York: Basic Books.

Brennan, K. A., & Shaver, P. R. (1995). Dimensions of adult attachment, affect regulation, and romantic relationship functioning. *Personality and Social Psychology Bulletin, 21,* 267–283.

Cohn, D. A., Cowan, P. A., Cowan, C. P., & Pearson, J. (1992). Mothers' and fathers' working models of childhood attachment relationships, parenting styles, and child behavior. *Development and Psychopathology, 4,* 417–431.

Collins, N. L. (1996). Working models of attachment: Implications for explanation, emotion, and behavior. *Journal of Personality and Social Psychology, 71,* 810–832.

Collins, N. L., & Read, S. J. (1990). Adult attachment, working models, and relationship quality in dating couples. *Journal of Personality and Social Psychology, 58,* 644–663.

Collins, N. L., & Read, S. J. (1994). Cognitive representations of attachment: The structure and function of working models. In K. Bartholomew & D. Perlman (Eds.), *Attachment processes in adulthood* (pp. 53–90). London: Jessica Kingsley.

Crowell, J. A., & Feldman, S. S. (1988). Mothers' internal models of relationships and children's behavioral and developmental status: A study of mother–child interaction. *Child Development, 59,* 1273–1285.

Crowell, J. A., Waters, E., Treboux, D., O'Connor, E., Colon-Downs, C., Feider, O., Golby, B., & Posada, G. (1996). Discriminant validity of the Adult Attachment Interview. *Child Development, 67,* 2584–2599.

Elicker, J., Englund, M., & Sroufe, L. A. (1992). Predicting peer competence and peer relationships in childhood from early parent–child relationships. In R.

Parke & G. Ladd (Eds.), *Family–peer relationships: Modes of linkage* (pp. 77–106). Hillsdale, NJ: Erlbaum.

Feeney, J. A. (1995). Adult attachment and emotional control. *Personal Relationships, 2*, 143–159.

Feeney, J. A., & Noller, P. (1990). Attachment style as a predictor of adult romantic relationships. *Journal of Personality and Social Psychology, 58*, 281–291.

Feeney, J. A., Noller, P., & Callan, V. J. (1994). Attachment style, communication and satisfaction in the early years of marriage. In K. Bartholomew & D. Perlman (Eds.), *Attachment processes in adulthood* (pp. 269–308). London: Jessica Kingsley.

George, C., Kaplan, N., & Main, M. (1985). *An Adult Attachment Interview: Interview protocol*. Unpublished manuscript, Department of Psychology, University of California, Berkeley.

Griffin, D., & Bartholomew, K. (1994). Models of the self and other: Fundamental dimensions underlying measures of adult attachment. *Journal of Personality and Social Psychology, 67*, 430–445.

Hazan, C., & Shaver, P. (1987). Romantic love conceptualized as an attachment process. *Journal of Personality and Social Psychology, 52*, 511–524.

Hazan, C., & Shaver, P. (1994). Attachment as an organizational framework for research on close relationships. *Psychological Inquiry, 5*, 1–22.

Isabella, R. A. (1993). Origins of attachment: Maternal interactive behavior across the first year. *Child Development, 64*, 605–621.

Isabella, R. A., & Belsky, J. (1991). Interactional synchrony and the origins of infant–mother attachment: A replication study. *Child Development, 62*, 373–384.

Kirkpatrick, L. A., & Davis, K. E. (1994). Attachment style, gender, and relationship stability: A longitudinal analysis. *Journal of Personality and Social Psychology, 66*, 502–512.

Kobak, R. R., Cole, H. E., Ferenz-Gillies, R., Fleming, W. S., & Gamble, W. (1993). Attachment and emotion regulation during mother–teen problem solving: A control theory analysis. *Child Development, 64*, 231–245.

Kobak, R. R., & Hazan, C. (1991). Attachment in marriage: Effects of security and accuracy of working models. *Journal of Personality and Social Psychology, 60*, 861–869.

Kobak, R. R., & Sceery, A. (1988). Attachment in late adolescence: Working models, affect regulation, and representations of self and others. *Child Development, 59*, 135–146.

Lee, J. A. (1973). *The colors of love: An exploration of the ways of loving*. Don Mills, Ontario, Canada: New Press.

Levy, M. B., & Davis, K. E. (1988). Lovestyles and attachment styles compared: Their relations to each other and to various relationship characteristics. *Journal of Social and Personal Relationships, 5*, 439–471.

Main, M. (1991). Metacognitive knowledge, metacognitive monitoring, and singular (coherent) vs. multiple (incoherent) models of attachment. In C. M. Parkes, J. Stevenson-Hinde, & P. Marris (Eds.), *Attachment across the life cycle* (pp. 127–159). London: Tavistock.

Main, M., & Hesse, E. (1990). Parents' unresolved traumatic experiences are related to infant disorganized attachment status: Is frightened and/or frightening parental behavior the linking mechanism? In M. T. Greenberg, D.

Cicchetti, & E. M. Cummings (Eds.), *Attachment in preschool years: Theory, research, and intervention* (pp. 161–184). Chicago: University of Chicago Press.

Main, M., Kaplan, N., & Cassidy, J. (1985). Security in infancy, childhood, and adulthood: A move to the level of representation. In I. Bretherton & E. Waters (Eds.), Growing points in attachment theory and research. *Monographs of the Society for Research in Child Development, 50,* 66–104.

Main, M., & Solomon, J. (1990). Procedures for identifying infants as disorganized/disoriented during the Ainsworth Strange Situation. In M. T. Greenberg, D. Cicchetti, & E. M. Cummings (Eds.), *Attachment in preschool years: Theory, research, and intervention* (pp. 121–160). Chicago: University of Chicago Press.

Mikulincer, M. (1995). Attachment style and the mental representation of the self. *Journal of Personality and Social Psychology, 69,* 1203–1215.

Mikulincer, M., Florian, V., & Tolmacz, R. (1990). Attachment styles and fear of personal death: A case study of affect regulation. *Journal of Personality and Social Psychology, 58,* 273–280.

Mikulincer, M., Florian, V., & Weller, A. (1993). Attachment styles, coping strategies, and post-traumatic psychological distress: The impact of the Gulf War in Israel. *Journal of Personality and Social Psychology, 64,* 817–826.

Pearson, J. L., Cohn, D. A., Cowan, P. A., & Cowan, C. P. (1994). Earned and continuous security in adult attachment: Relations to depressive symptomatology and parenting style. *Development and Psychopathology, 6,* 359–373.

Pistole, M. C. (1989). Attachment in adult romantic relationships: Style of conflict resolution and relationship satisfaction. *Journal of Social and Personal Relationships, 6,* 505–510.

Rholes, W. S., Simpson, J. A., & Blakely, B. S. (1995). Adult attachment styles and mothers' relationships with their young children. *Personal Relationships, 2,* 35–54.

Scharfe, E., & Bartholomew, K. (1994). Reliability and stability of adult attachment patterns. *Personal Relationships, 1,* 23–43.

Shaver, P. R., Collins, N., & Clark, C. L. (1996). Attachment styles and internal working models of self and relationship partners. In G. J. O. Fletcher & J. Fitness (Eds.), *Knowledge structures in close relationships: A social psychological approach* (pp. 25–61). Mahwah, NJ: Erlbaum.

Shaver, P., Hazan, C., & Bradshaw, D. (1988). Love as attachment: The integration of three behavioral systems. In R. J. Sternberg & M. L. Barnes (Eds.), *The psychology of love* (pp. 68–99). New Haven, CT: Yale University Press.

Simpson, J. A. (1990). Influence of attachment styles on romantic relationships. *Journal of Personality and Social Psychology, 59,* 971–980.

Simpson, J. A. (in press). Attachment theory in a modern evolutionary perspective. In J. Cassidy & P. R. Shaver (Eds.), *Handbook of attachment theory and research.* New York: Guilford Press.

Simpson, J. A., & Gangestad, S. W. (1991). Individual differences in sociosexuality: Evidence for convergent and discriminant validity. *Journal of Personality and Social Psychology, 60,* 870–883.

Simpson, J. A., Rholes, W. S., & Nelligan, J. S. (1992). Support seeking and support giving within couples in an anxiety-provoking situation: The role of attachment styles. *Journal of Personality and Social Psychology, 62,* 434–446.

Simpson, J. A., Rholes, W. S., & Phillips, D. (1996). Conflict in close relationships: An attachment perspective. *Journal of Personality and Social Psychology, 71,* 899–914.

Smith, P. B., & Pederson, D. R. (1988). Maternal sensitivity and patterns of infant–mother attachment. *Child Development, 59,* 1097–1101.

Sroufe, A. L., & Waters, E. (1977). Attachment as an organizational construct. *Child Development, 48,* 1184–1199.

Tennov, D. (1979). *Love and limerence: The experience of being in love.* New York: Stein & Day.

van IJzendoorn, M. H. (1995). Adult attachment representations, parental responsiveness, and infant attachment: A meta-analysis of the predictive validity of the Adult Attachment Interview. *Psychological Bulletin, 117,* 387–403.

van IJzendoorn, M. H., Juffer, F., & Duyvesteyn, M. G. C. (1995). Breaking the intergeneration cycle of insecure attachment: A review of the effects of attachment-based interventions on maternal sensitivity and infant security. *Journal of Child Psychology and Psychiatry, 36,* 225–248.

Ward, M. J., & Carlson, E. A. (1995). Associations among adult attachment representations, maternal sensitivity, and infant–mother attachment in a sample of adolescent mothers. *Child Development, 66,* 69–79.

PART II

Measurement Issues

2

Methods of Assessing
Adult Attachment

Do They Converge?

KIM BARTHOLOMEW
PHILLIP R. SHAVER

In recent years, several streams of research have emerged from Bowlby's (1988) and Ainsworth's (1982) attachment theory. Originally, the theory was aimed at explaining child and adult psychopathology in terms of nonoptimal relationships between children and their caregivers, or "attachment figures." According to attachment theory, the long-term effects of early experiences with caregivers are due to the persistence of "internal working models"—cognitive/affective schemas, or representations, of the self in relation to close relationship partners (Bartholomew, 1990; Shaver, Collins, & Clark, 1996). Theoretically, these representations influence a person's expectations, emotions, defenses, and relational behavior in all close relationships. Although the theory does not assume or require that internal working models persist without change across the life span, both theory and empirical evidence from longitudinal studies have led researchers to suspect that the effects of childhood attachment relationships extend into adulthood, where they can be seen in the domains of parenting and close peer relationships, including romantic relationships (e.g., Bartholomew, 1990, 1993; Main, Kaplan, & Cassidy, 1985; Shaver, Hazan, & Bradshaw, 1988; Weiss, 1982).

TWO TRADITIONS OF ADULT ATTACHMENT RESEARCH

In the 1980s, two distinct programs of research were initiated to investigate patterns of attachment in adulthood. In one line of research, Main and her colleagues focused on the possibility that adult "states of mind with respect to attachment" (i.e., adults' current representations of their childhood relationships with parents) affected parenting behavior, which in turn influenced the attachment patterns of the parents' young children. Members of Main's research group interviewed parents about their childhood family relationships and then searched for scorable features of the interview transcripts that could "postdict" their infants' already known attachment classifications in the Ainsworth Strange Situation (Ainsworth, Blehar, Waters, & Wall, 1978). In subsequent predictive studies using this Adult Attachment Interview (AAI; George, Kaplan, & Main, 1985) procedure, the research group confirmed that parents' interview codes were associated with independent assessments of their infants' attachment classifications (a connection that has since been replicated many times; see van IJzendoorn, 1995, for a review). Infants classified as "avoidant" in the Strange Situation had primary caregivers who themselves were dismissing of attachment-related memories and feelings; infants classified as "anxious" had primary caregivers who were anxiously preoccupied with attachment-related issues; and infants classified as "secure" had caregivers who were "free and autonomous" with respect to attachment. In subsequent work, a fourth infant pattern, "disorganized," was found to be associated with caregivers who were "unresolved" with respect to losses and traumas in their attachment history.

In the second, completely independent line of research, Hazan and Shaver (1987), who had been studying adolescent and adult loneliness, followed up Weiss's (1982) idea that chronic loneliness is associated with insecure attachment. Reasoning that most chronically lonely young adults were unsuccessfully seeking a secure romantic attachment, and that orientations to romantic relationships might be an outgrowth of previous attachment experiences, Hazan and Shaver devised a simple self-report questionnaire for adults based on Ainsworth's three patterns of childhood attachment: secure, avoidant, and anxious. The measure asked people to think back across their most important romantic relationships and decide which of the three types was most self-descriptive. In subsequent studies, this measure and several variants of it have been related to a host of theoretically relevant personality variables, behaviors, and experiences in close relationships (for reviews, see Shaver & Clark, 1994; Shaver & Hazan, 1993). Although a few studies have correlated this measure with retrospective reports of childhood experiences with parents, the bulk of research in this tradition has focused on the influence of attachment patterns on personal adjustment and adult relationships.

These two streams of adult attachment research—one focused on parenting and the other focused on romantic relationships—derive from different disciplinary subcultures. Bowlby was primarily a child psychiatrist, and Ainsworth was a child clinical and developmental psychologist. Many of the current attachment researchers in the first "subculture" (e.g., Bretherton, Cassidy, Crittenden, Kobak, Main, and Waters) were students of Ainsworth's. Researchers in this group tend to think psychodynamically, be interested in clinical problems, prefer interview measures and behavioral observations over questionnaires, study relatively small groups of subjects, and focus their attention on parent–child relationships. Hazan and Shaver were personality / social psychologists, and their work was quickly assimilated by other such psychologists, who tend to think in terms of personality traits and social interactions, be interested in normal subject populations, prefer simple questionnaire measures, study relatively large samples, and focus on adult social relationships, including friendships, dating relationships, and marriages. Not surprisingly, the members of these two research subcultures tend to speak past each other, or to concentrate their energies on activities within their own subdiscipline without paying much attention to activities and developments within the other subdiscipline.

Because both lines of research are grounded in Bowlby's and Ainsworth's attachment theory, and both focus on individual differences and classify people into categories parallel to Ainsworth's infant attachment typology, it was inevitable that some researchers would assume that the two adult classification systems, Main's and Hazan and Shaver's, must be highly related. In other words, since both the AAI and Hazan and Shaver's questionnaire place people into categories roughly designated as secure, avoidant, and anxious or preoccupied, it is often assumed that the two assessment procedures are more or less interchangeable.

In 1990, Bartholomew reviewed the adult attachment research in both traditions and came to the conclusion that the two approaches to assessing attachment differed in a number of ways. First, she noted that the dismissing–avoidant individuals identified by the AAI denied experiencing subjective distress and downplayed the importance of attachment needs, whereas avoidant subjects identified by Hazan and Shaver's self-report measure reported relatively high levels of subjective distress and fears of becoming close to others. She argued that two distinct forms of avoidance were evident, one pattern motivated by a defensive maintenance of self-sufficiency (labeled "dismissing") and the other motivated by a conscious fear of anticipated rejection by others (labeled "fearful"). Second, she noted that the two approaches focused on different domains, one on retrospective descriptions of parent–child relationships and the other on more recent experiences in adult love relationships, and that the equivalence of representations in the two domains should not be assumed, but rather was a question for empirical study. Third, she pointed out that the use of interviews and the use of self-reports reflected differing conceptualizations of adult attachment. The AAI focuses on dynamics of internal working models that are revealed indirectly by the way a person talks about childhood relationships; the measure is not based on the assumption that people are conscious of these dynamics. In contrast, the self-report measure focuses on feelings and behaviors in close relationships of which a person is aware and which the person can describe fairly accurately. Building on both traditions, Bartholomew proposed an expanded model of adult attachment that included two forms of avoidance. To assess this model, she used a self-report measure of experiences in close relationships in general (by revising Hazan and Shaver's measure) as well as two interviews, one focusing on childhood experiences (along the lines of the AAI) and the other focusing on peer relationships, including friendships and romantic relationships (Bartholomew & Horowitz, 1991).

Problems in Comparing Measures from the Two Traditions

In recent years, papers have begun to appear (e.g., Borman & Cole, 1993; Crowell, Treboux, & Waters, 1993) that report comparisons between adult attachment measures from the two research traditions we have outlined. Typically, the authors of such papers conclude that the two kinds of measures fail to correspond, in which case the authors usually question the validity of the self-report measure. These kinds of studies are typically conducted by researchers from the clinical/developmental subculture, because, with the exception of Bartholomew and her colleagues, researchers in the personality/social subculture have not taken the time to master the interview techniques. It is easy for interview researchers to add a simple self-report measure to their studies, but difficult for questionnaire researchers to learn to conduct and code what are essentially intensive clinical interviews. Thus, comparisons between different kinds of attachment measures have been made largely by researchers who concentrate on parent–child relationships and take Ainsworth's Strange Situation and the AAI as benchmarks.

To the extent that conclusions about attachment measures affect researchers' understanding of attachment processes or lead them to have little confidence in particular bodies of research, the question of measure convergence is important. Some of the authors who have found little convergence between self-report and interview measures have concluded that self-report measures are especially prone to measurement error and unlikely to be related to behavior. They fail to consider studies such as those by Shaver and Brennan (1992), Feeney and Noller (1991), Kirkpatrick and Davis (1994), Kobak and Hazan (1991), Mikulincer and Nachshon (1991), and Simpson, Rholes, and Nelligan (1992), which show that self-report measures of adult attachment patterns *do* relate significantly to the ways in which a person discusses close relationships, to observations of marital communication, to relationship breakups, to patterns of self-disclosure, and to seeking and providing social support under stressful conditions. Within the personality/social research subculture, to consider the flip side of the coin for a moment, there is a danger of overlooking discoveries made with interview procedures that cannot be duplicated with simple self-report measures. These include insights and research ideas that arise when an investigator hears what people actually say when interviewed in depth about important relationships. Many researchers relying on self-report measures of attachment have also failed to seriously consider the possibility that there are aspects of attachment patterns that are inaccessible to conscious awareness and, therefore, cannot be assessed by self-report methods (cf. Crowell & Treboux, 1995).

Given the significance of the measure convergence issue, it is essential that comparisons between measures be thoughtful and statistically appropriate. Most of the existing comparisons involve cross-tabulations of AAI categories and Hazan–Shaver categories, a strategy which implicitly assumes that the two measures are assessing parallel attachment classifications. Some (e.g., Borman & Cole, 1993) even label the Hazan–Shaver avoidant category "dismissing" (a term never used by Hazan and Shaver), as if the designers of the two measures all had dismissing qualities in mind. This conflation ignores Bartholomew's (1990) distinction between two kinds of avoidance, which indicates that the AAI dismissing category and the Hazan–Shaver (fearful) avoidant category are *not* the same. Other studies include the "unresolved" AAI category, which has no match in the self-report measure, and/or a "cannot classify" interview coding category, which also has no match in the self-report measure. These differences make it unlikely that the two kinds of measures will converge strongly.

Some authors who compare attachment measures also overlook or misinterpret the domain differences between the AAI, which focuses on adults' characterizations of their childhood relationships with parents, and the Hazan–Shaver measure, which focuses on experiences in romantic relationships. Although the AAI has sometimes been conceptualized as assessing generalized attachment representations, the Hazan–Shaver measure was specifically designed to measure attachment patterns in the domain of romantic relationships. Of course, even if the two measures had been intended to measure precisely the same construct, method variance would be expected to reduce the degree of association between them. Self-report measures focus on conscious, potentially inaccurate summaries by a person of his or her own experiences and behaviors. The AAI focuses primarily on the way a person talks about childhood attachment experiences, with the major distinctions having to do with what might be called defensive style (e.g., denial, repression, compulsive self-reliance, and dismissal of attachment needs, on the one hand, versus vigilance, sensitization, enmeshment in relationships, and preoccupation with attachment needs, on the other). These differences in communicational behavior and defensive style are not necessarily noticed or acknowledged by the people who exhibit them. Given all of these differences, a moderate association, at best, would be expected between the AAI and Hazan and Shaver's self-report measure.

Also problematic is the fact that comparers of measures often fail to conduct power analyses (Cohen, 1988) before performing statistical tests. Consequently, they tend to perform insufficiently powerful tests and then conclude that two measures are unrelated (i.e., the null hypothesis is supported) because a test statistic fails to reach conventional levels of significance. Insufficient power (a reflection of sample size and expected effect size) is especially disconcerting when investigators are inclined to accept the null hypothesis, and sufficient power is especially difficult to attain when categorical variables are under investigation. Researchers have also failed to consider that unreliability in both measures will always attenuate the observed degree of correspondence. Single-item measures are particularly likely to be unreliable. Given the systematic differences between the AAI and self-report romantic attachment measures, the low power of the tests used to test the associations between them, and the relatively low reliability of some attachment measures, it is hardly surprising that previous studies have failed to show convergence.

In the remainder of this chapter we compare various measures of attachment based on Bartholomew's typology. Because Bartholomew has created both interview measures of parental and peer attachment and a self-report measure of peer attachment, similar in many respects to the Hazan–Shaver measure but including two avoidant categories, it is possible to compare assessment methods without confounding them with different conceptual schemes. In addition, continuous prototype ratings of the four attachment patterns allow for adequate power to test for moderate associations in relatively small samples. In two separate samples, the associations between three measures of attachment were assessed—a self-report measure of general orientation to close relationships, an interview measure focusing on early family relationships, and a second interview focusing on peer relationships.

BARTHOLOMEW'S TWO-DIMENSIONAL FOUR-CATEGORY SCHEME

Bartholomew has systematized Bowlby's (1973) conception of internal working models in a four-category classification scheme (Bartholomew, 1990; Bartholomew & Horowitz, 1991) (see Figure 2.1). Four prototypical attachment patterns are defined in terms of two dimensions: positivity of a person's model of self and positivity of a person's model of others. The

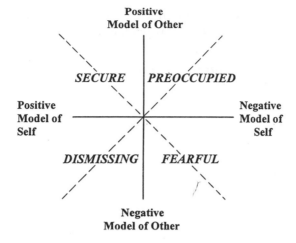

FIGURE 2.1. Two-dimensional four-category model of adult attachment.

positivity of the self model indicates the degree to which a person has internalized a sense of his or her self-worth (versus feeling anxious and uncertain of the self's lovability). The self model is therefore associated with the degree of anxiety and dependency on other's approval in close relationships. The positivity of the other model indicates the degree to which others are generally expected to be available and supportive. The other model is therefore associated with the tendency to seek out or avoid closeness in relationships.

Secure adult attachment is characterized by the combination of a positive self model and a positive model of others. Secure individuals have an internalized sense of self-worth and are comfortable with intimacy in close relationships. *Preoccupied* attachment is characterized by a negative self model and a positive model of others. Preoccupied individuals anxiously seek to gain acceptance and validation from others, seeming to persist in the belief that they could attain safety, or security, if they could only get others to respond properly toward them. *Fearful* attachment is characterized by negative self *and* other models. Fearful individuals, like the preoccupied, are highly dependent on others' acceptance and affirmation; however, because of their negative expectations, they avoid intimacy to avert the pain of loss or rejection. *Dismissing* attachment is characterized by a positive self model and a negative model of others. Dismissing individuals also avoid closeness because of negative expectations; however, they maintain a sense of self-worth by defensively denying the value of close relationships.

As indicated previously, three of these patterns—secure, preoccupied, and dismissing—are conceptually similar to the corresponding AAI categories. And three—secure, preoccupied, and fearful—are similar to Hazan and Shaver's secure, anxious–ambivalent, and avoidant categories.

A Test of Correspondence among Bartholomew's Attachment Measures

The convergence of different approaches to assessing adult attachment was tested in two samples. In Sample 1, participants were 69 college students (see Study 2 in Bartholomew & Horowitz, 1991); in Sample 2, participants were 134 young adults involved in established romantic relationships (for more information on the sample, see Scharfe & Bartholomew, 1994). Participants completed three measures: (1) a brief self-report measure that asked them to rate their degree of fit with each of the four attachment prototypes (the Relationship Questionnaire), (2) an interview focusing on close friendships and past and present romantic relationships (the Peer Attachment Interview), and (3) an interview focusing on representations of childhood experiences in the family (the Family Attachment Interview). Two independent raters coded each interview for interviewee's degree of fit to a prototype for each of the four attachment patterns. Final interview ratings were based on an average of the two coders' ratings. Thus, each participant received a profile of ratings on the four attachment patterns. The highest of the four ratings was also used to define a best fitting categorization for each method.

For each combination of methods, correlations were computed between the continuous ratings of corresponding attachment patterns (see Table 2.1). For both samples, each of the associations between corresponding peer and family interview ratings was significant. In addition, the associations between corresponding ratings were stronger than those between noncorresponding ratings, and none of the noncorresponding ratings were significantly positively associated with each other (not shown in the table), suggesting both convergent and discriminant validity. Associations between corresponding ratings on the peer interview and self-report measure were also significant, and the pattern of correlations again suggested both convergent and discriminant validity. In contrast, associations between corresponding ratings on the family interview and self-report measure were weaker and more variable. In both samples, security and dismissing ratings were positively correlated. However, corresponding fearful ratings were associated only in Sample 1, and preoccupied ratings were not significantly correlated in either sample. In the two other studies we are aware of that included the Relationship Questionnaire and Family Attachment Interview, the obtained associations between corresponding ratings were stronger. In a sample of assaultive men, correlations between self-report and family interview measures ranged from .22 (for the fearful) to .55 (for the preoccupied) (Saunders, 1992). Similarly, in a sample of women undergoing treatment for breast

TABLE 2.1. Correlations between Corresponding Attachment Ratings across Methods

	Secure	Fearful	Preoccupied	Dismissing
Peer interview and family interview				
Sample 1[a]	.39**	.29*	.66**	.41**
Sample 2[b]	.37**	.46**	.42**	.35**
Peer interview and self-report measure				
Sample 1	.27*	.45**	.24*	.36**
Sample 2	.36**	.37**	.35**	.29**
Family interview and self-report measure				
Sample 1	.25*	.35**	.19	.33**
Sample 2	.23*	.00	.08	.17*

Note. Sex was partialed out of the Sample 2 correlations to avoid bias (see Gonzalez & Griffin, 1997). [a]$n = 67$; [b]$n = 134$.
*$p < .05$; **$p < .01$.

cancer, correlations ranged from .22 (for the preoccupied) to .42 (for the fearful) (Bellg, 1995).

Because of inadequate power, it was not possible to test the correspondence between classifications derived from the three different methods, but there was sufficient power to compare the secure and insecure categories across methods. With one exception, the proportion of agreement for the secure–insecure distinction ranged from .63 to .68 and a significant chi-square indicated that the categorizations across methods were not independent. However, the proportion of agreement between the family interview and self-report measure in Sample 2 was .57, which is only marginally significant ($p = .07$).

Finally, factor analyses were performed to examine the convergence of the three measures. Figures 2.2 and 2.3 show the results of principal components factor analyses with varimax rotation of the intercorrelations of the three sets of attachment ratings (with axes rotated to facilitate interpretation). The two factors accounted for 48% of the variance in Sample 1 and 41% of the variance in Sample 2. As can be seen in the figures, the three methods exhibit substantial convergence; the three measures of a particular attachment pattern are always closer to each other than to measures of different patterns. (See Griffin & Bartholomew, 1994, for similar results based on confirmatory factor analyses of different methods of assessing the two dimensions underlying Bartholomew's model.)

The findings indicate a moderate degree of convergence across the three approaches. As might be expected, the correlational results were weakest when both the method (interview vs. self-report) and the content domain (family history vs. current close relationships) differed. The con-

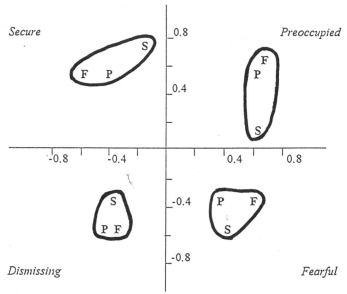

FIGURE 2.2. Factor analysis of Relationship Questionnaire, Peer Attachment Interview, and Family Attachment Interview ratings: Sample 1. P = peer interview; F = family interview; S = self-report.

vergence was greater when both measures were based on interviews or when both measures had to do with the peer relationship domain. The results of the factor analyses also indicate convergence. In sum, when parallel conceptualizations of attachment patterns are used, there is a moderate degree of convergence between interview and self-report measures, and across the family and peer domains. This conclusion agrees with findings obtained by Bellg (1995), O'Hearn and Davis (1997), and Saunders (1992). But it would be easy to miss the convergence if one compared different conceptualizations of attachment (such as three vs. four categories, or systematically differing definitions of avoidance) or relied on insufficiently powerful statistical tests.

ANCHORING BARTHOLOMEW'S MEASURES IN THE TWO TRADITIONS OF ADULT ATTACHMENT RESEARCH

The findings reported in the previous section are relevant to bridging the gap between the two adult attachment subcultures only to the extent that Bartholomew's measures are empirically related to the AAI, on the one side, and Hazan and Shaver's romantic attachment measure, on the other side.

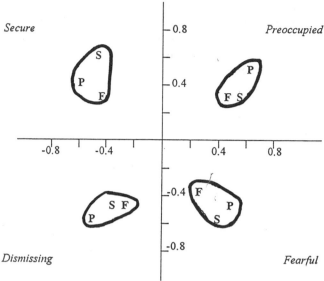

FIGURE 2.3. Factor analysis of Relationship Questionnaire, Peer Attachment Interview, and Family Attachment Interview ratings: Sample 2. P = peer interview; F = family interview; S = self-report.

A Comparison of the AAI and Bartholomew's Interview Coding System

Mardi Horowitz and a group of colleagues at the University of California, San Francisco, gave us access to clinical interviews with 30 bereaved women that had been coded, by well-trained coders, using the AAI and Bartholomew's scoring systems. The interviews focused on the participants' relationship with the deceased and their responses to the loss; they were coded by independent sets of AAI and Bartholomew coders. Both coding systems contain the secure, preoccupied, and dismissing categories. The AAI usually includes an "unresolved loss and trauma" (U) category as well, but in the bereavement study it could not be used because the interviewees were all mourning a loss that had occurred within the previous year. As explained earlier, Bartholomew's coding system includes a fourth, "fearful," category not included in the AAI.

A chi-square analysis indicated that the classifications obtained from the two systems (three AAI categories and four Bartholomew categories) were significantly related, $\chi^2(6) = 24.80$, $p < .001$. Perhaps a more appropriate test of the association between the two measures is one that leaves out the seven interviewees who were classified as fearful in Bartholomew's system. When that analysis was performed, the association was again significant, $\chi^2(4) = 23.93$, $p < .0001$, and the proportion of agreement was .78. Of seven people judged preoccupied by the AAI coders, all seven were also judged preoccupied by the Bartholomew coders. Of eight people judged dismissing by the AAI coders, seven were judged dismissing by the Bartholomew coders. Of eight people judged secure by the AAI coders, four were judged secure by the Bartholomew coders, three were judged dismissing, and one was judged preoccupied. All five disagreements involved the secure category and were mainly a result of the different secure-category base rates for the two sets of coders. The AAI coders more readily labeled people secure. The seven people who were coded fearful in Bartholomew's system (and omitted from the 3×3 analysis) were distributed as follows in the AAI system: four were preoccupied, one was dismissing, and two were secure.

As a more powerful test of the association, we conducted analyses of variance (ANOVAs) in which the AAI categories served as the independent variable and the four continuous prototype ratings from Bartholomew's scoring system served as dependent variables. (See Table 2.2.) The ANOVA for the secure rating was significant, $F(2,27) = 5.29$, $p < .05$, and a follow-up planned comparison indicated that the secure AAI group differed significantly from both insecure groups, $t (27) = 2.96$, $p < .01$. For the preoccupied rating, $F(2,27) = 12.60$, $p < .0001$; the preoccupied AAI group's rating scale mean was significantly greater than the secure and dismissing means $t(27) = 4.74$, $p < .001$. For the dismissing rating, $F(2,27) = 11.45$, $p < .001$; the dismissing AAI group's rating scale mean was significantly greater than the secure and preoccupied means $t(27) = 4.53$, $p < .001$. For the fearful rating, the ANOVA was not significant, $F(2,27) = 1.12$, ns), as could be expected given that the AAI scoring system does not include a fearful category.

Considering that the interview being coded was not primarily an attachment interview (i.e., it was not highly similar to either the AAI or Bartholomew's interviews), that the sample size was small, and that many of the interviewees were still quite upset about their loss, the degree of correspondence between the two classification systems is impressive. The results suggest that strong evidence for convergence (to the extent that the coding systems are parallel) would be obtained from a study of a larger, more representative sample based on appropriate attachment interviews.

TABLE 2.2. Means on Bartholomew's Four Prototype Ratings across AAI Categories

Bartholomew prototype ratings	AAI categories		
	Autonomous ($n = 10$)	Enmeshed ($n = 11$)	Dismissing ($n = 9$)
Secure	4.20	2.45	3.11
Preoccupied	3.40	5.36	2.22
Dismissing	3.20	2.18	5.67
Fearful	3.10	4.00	2.67

A Comparison of Hazan and Shaver's and Bartholomew's Self-Report Measures

In a self-report study of 840 college students, Brennan, Shaver, and Tobey (1991) included both Hazan and Shaver's (1987, 1990) romantic attachment questionnaire and Bartholomew's (Bartholomew & Horowitz, 1991) relationship questionnaire. Participants placed themselves into one of Hazan and Shaver's three categories (secure, anxious, and avoidant) and rated how self-descriptive each of the three prototypes was. They also placed themselves into one of Bartholomew's four categories (secure, preoccupied, fearful, and dismissing) and rated how self-descriptive each of the four prototypes was.

A chi-square analysis indicated that the classifications obtained from the two systems (three Hazan–Shaver categories and four Bartholomew categories) were significantly related, $\chi^2(6) = 370.31$, $p < .001$. Of the people who classified themselves as secure on Bartholomew's measure, 82% were secure on the Hazan–Shaver measure. Of those who classified themselves as preoccupied on Bartholomew's measure, 57% were anxious–ambivalent (the conceptually parallel category) on the Hazan–Shaver measure. Of those who classified themselves as fearful on Bartholomew's measure, 61% called themselves avoidant on the Hazan–Shaver measure. Of those who classified themselves as dismissing on Bartholomew's measure, 43% called themselves avoidant on the Hazan–Shaver measure and 45% called themselves secure. As suggested earlier, there is no category on the Hazan–Shaver measure that is strongly parallel to dismissing, so most dismissing subjects are forced to choose fearful, which acknowledges their avoidant tendencies, or secure, which emphasizes their autonomy and self-esteem.

Because participants in the Brennan et al. (1991) study rated all seven prototypes from the two self-report measures, it was possible to conduct correlational as well as categorical analyses. The correlations for the parallel ratings (secure with secure, etc.) were all highly significant and ranged from .46 (for fearful with avoidant) to .55 (for the two secure ratings). In each case, these correlations were higher than any of the correlations among nonparallel ratings. The dismissing rating was not strongly correlated with any of the Hazan–Shaver ratings, but its correlation with the avoidant rating—the most logical quasi-parallel category— was a highly significant .23. When the seven ratings were submitted to factor analysis, two clear factors emerged. On the first factor, the two secure ratings loaded positively (.78 and .79), the avoidant and fearful ratings loaded negatively (−.77 and −.68), and the other ratings loaded below .35. On the second factor, the anxious–ambivalent and preoccupied ratings loaded positively (.84 and .77), the dismissing rating loaded negatively (−.52), and the other ratings loaded below .20. These factors confirm the convergence between the two measures, and they correspond clearly to the diagonals of Bartholomew's two-dimensional classification scheme shown in Figure 2.1.

THE ARRAY OF MEASURES FROM THE AAI TO HAZAN AND SHAVER'S QUESTIONNAIRE

Our findings indicate that when appropriate comparisons are drawn, one finds considerable evidence for convergence across various measures of adult attachment. The convergence is greatest when similar techniques are used within the same domain—for example, when two self-report measures of peer attachment are used. The convergence is also substantial when the same domain is examined with two conceptually parallel methods—for example, when attachment to peers is measured with Bartholomew's interview and with self-report measures. The least convergence occurs in exactly the situation that other researchers have been inclined to study, where an interview measure in the family domain (e.g., the AAI) is compared with a self-report measure in the peer or romantic domain (e.g., the Hazan–Shaver questionnaire). Even in the latter case, however, there is evidence of modest convergence when conceptually parallel attachment patterns are assessed in the two domains.

Researchers who have compared AAI classifications with Hazan–Shaver classifications have generally ignored Bartholomew's discovery that the "avoidant" categories embodied in these two measures are fundamentally different. The results discussed in the present chapter indicate that Bartholomew's fearful category, as assessed by interview, has no parallel in the AAI classification system, although the corresponding dismissing categories converge well. The dismissing category, in turn, has no clear parallel in the Hazan–Shaver classification system, although that system's avoidant category converges fairly well with Bartholomew's fearful category. Thus, direct comparisons between the AAI and the Hazan–Shaver measure are misleading.

We propose that the different measures of adult attachment—at least those discussed in this chapter—can be systematically arrayed along a rough continuum, ranging, let us say, from the left to the right (see Figure 2.4). On the left end is the AAI, an interview procedure that assesses attachment issues in the family domain and places people into three major and two secondary categories not organized by any particular dimensional scheme. In the next position is Bartholomew's Family Attachment Interview, which also assesses attachment issues in the family domain but rates people on four attachment prototypes defined in terms of two dimensions. In the next position to the right would be Bartholomew's Peer Attachment Interview, which assesses attachment in the peer domain in a way that is conceptually parallel to her family interview ratings. In the next position would be her self-report measure, which conceptually par-

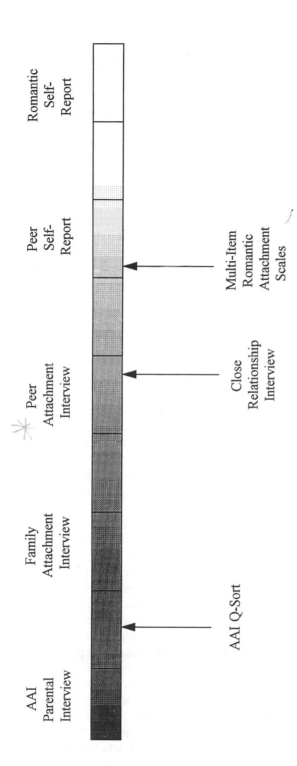

FIGURE 2.4. Hypothetical continuum of adult attachment measures. The examples range, on top of the horizontal band, from the Adult Attachment Interview (AAI; George, Kaplan, & Main, 1985) through Bartholomew's three measures (Family Attachment Interview, Peer Attachment Interview, and Peer Self-Report, all conceptualized in terms of two dimensions; Bartholomew & Horowitz, 1991) to Hazan and Shaver's (1987, 1990) Romantic Self-Report measure. Underneath the horizontal band are hypothesized locations of other adult attachment measures. The AAI Q-Sort (Kobak, Cole, Ferenz-Gillies, Fleming, & Gamble, 1993) uses the AAI interview format but codes the interviews in terms of two dimensions similar to a 45-degree rotation of Bartholomew's two dimensions. The Close Relationship Interview (CRI; Crowell, 1990) was designed to be similar to the AAI in format and coding emphases, but it focuses on romantic/marital relationships. There are several multi-item romantic attachment scales based on phrases and concepts mentioned in Hazan and Shaver's and Bartholomew's measures (e.g., Collins & Read, 1990; Feeney, Noller, & Hanrahan, 1994; Simpson, 1990; Simpson, Rholes, & Nelligan, 1992); all of these reduce to two dimensions similar to those postulated by Bartholomew (1990; see Brennan, Clark, & Shaver, Chapter 3, this volume).

39

allels her interviews. And in the rightmost position would be Hazan and Shaver's measure, which places people into three peer/romantic categories that can be located in Bartholomew's two-dimensional conceptual space.

Other adult attachment measures can be placed along the same continuum. For example, Kobak, Cole, Ferenz-Gillies, Fleming, and Gamble (1993) have devised a two-dimensional Q-sort scoring system for the AAI. Coders characterize a particular interview using a large number of statements based on the AAI scoring system, and then the Q-sort results (averaged across coders) are summarized in terms of a secure–insecure dimension and a deactivating–hyperactivating dimension. These dimensions are very similar conceptually to the diagonals of Figure 2.1 (see also Shaver & Hazan, 1993), with the secure–insecure dimension being similar to the secure–fearful diagonal and the deactivating–hyperactivating dimension being similar to the dismissing–preoccupied diagonal. Because the Kobak et al. measure is based on the AAI but is scored in terms of dimensions similar to Bartholomew's, we would expect it to fall between those two measures on our proposed continuum.

A second pair of examples are the multi-item questionnaire measures devised by Collins and Read (1990) and Simpson et al. (1992). These were created by breaking Hazan and Shaver's three prototypes into 13–18 separate phrases that could be scored as Likert items. When factor analyzed, the items formed two major dimensions that correlated quite highly with Bartholomew's two dimensions (Griffin & Bartholomew, 1994). These measures, we suspect, fall along the continuum between Bartholomew's self-report measure, which is conceptually based on two dimensions, and the Hazan–Shaver measure from which most of the items were drawn. Future self-report dimensional measures may better capture Bartholomew's dismissing style, in which case they may fall somewhere on the continuum between her peer interview and her simple self-report measure. (Both of us are currently testing such dimensional measures, so we have anticipated their location with an additional upward arrow in Figure 2.4.) A third example is the Close Relationship Interview (CRI; Crowell, 1990), which was designed for studies of married couples and is closely related to the AAI in theoretical conception, coding procedures, and ultimate classifications. Because it was based so closely on the AAI and is scored categorically rather than dimensionally, romantic/marital relationships, it is also related to self-report attachment scales (e.g., Treboux, 1997). Thus, we have placed it near the center of our hypothetical continuum and marked it with a third upward arrow in Figure 2.4.

In general, we predict that adult attachment measures that lie near each other on the continuum will relate to each other more strongly than those that lie further apart. The AAI and the Hazan–Shaver measures should be most weakly related because they lie at opposite ends of the continuum. At the very least, a researcher wanting to detect the underlying connection between the constructs assessed by these measures would need a high degree of statistical power.

THEORETICAL AND
METHODOLOGICAL IMPLICATIONS

The results suggest both (1) that there may be a single representational system or set of core relational tendencies underlying responses to the various attachment measures (Griffin & Bartholomew, 1994), and (2) that an individual's domain-specific attachment patterns can be substantially different (Collins & Read, 1994). This interpretation of the results is compatible with the idea, central to attachment theory (e.g., Bowlby, 1988), that adult attachment orientations have their roots in childhood experiences with important attachment figures. Bowlby wrote about "developmental pathways" along which children and adults travel, being moved toward and away from attachment security by events such as the death of important attachment figures, supportive treatment by a therapist, and the quality of a marital relationship. As a person moves along these increasingly differentiated pathways, it is quite possible for internal working models of relationships with parents to diverge from working models of romantic relationships; the person may feel and act one way in one kind of relationship and a different way in another.

If a researcher wished to tap the deepest, most general representation of attachment, it would probably be wise to combine measures to form latent attachment variables (e.g., Griffin & Bartholomew, 1994). Otherwise, the choice of measures should be dependent upon the researcher's conceptualization of attachment. For example, if a researcher wanted to measure individual differences in the quality of romantic attachments, it would be wise to use either a highly reliable (probably multi-item measure) of that specific construct or a latent-variable combination of conceptually compatible but methodologically different measures (e.g., a romantic attachment interview and a reliable self-report romantic attachment questionnaire). In general, except when exploring, or searching for, the most distant possible connections within the attachment domain, attachment measures should be chosen according to the domain of interest. It would not be optimally promising to try to predict, say, the attachment orientation of a parent's infant or the quality of parent–child interaction from the parent's attachment classification on a measure of romantic attachment (nevertheless, see Rholes, Simpson, & Blakely, 1995), nor would it be optimally powerful to predict outcomes of a romantic relationship from a family attachment interview.

The findings presented in this chapter do not address the differential predictive or external validity of various measures of attachment. In order to compare predictive validity, it would be necessary to include multiple methods (such as an interview focusing on childhood relationships and a self-report measure of romantic attachment) and multiple relevant outcomes (such as observations of parenting behaviors and marital communication) in one study. We expect that such studies would indicate stronger relationships between attachment and outcome variables within domain than across domain, and no relationship across domain when the overlapping variance of the attachment measures is controlled for. In other words, we would expect attachment in the family domain to predict outcomes in the marital domain only to the extent that the former had developmentally contributed to the formation of romantic attachment patterns. There is also a continuing need for studies that actually track the divergence of domain-specific developmental pathways over time.

In conclusion, measures of adult attachment differ in terms of *domain* (family, peer, or romantic relationships), *method* (interview, Q-sort, or self-report), *dimensionality* (categories, prototype ratings, or dimensions), and categorization systems. Despite such differences, the measures converge to varying degrees, especially when reliability and statistical power are sufficiently high. Each of the currently used measures is associated with a sizable body of empirical findings inspired by and compatible with Bowlby and Ainsworth's attachment theory. The different measures lie along a continuum of domains, methods, and degree of dimensionalization. When we step back from the details of specific measures and measure-specific findings, the results produced by attachment researchers are all compatible with the possibility that various forms of adult attachment arise from a continuous but branching tree of attachment experiences, beginning in infancy and developing throughout the life course.

ACKNOWLEDGMENTS

Preparation of this chapter was supported by a Social Science and Humanities Research Council of Canada research grant to Kim Bartholomew and a MacArthur Foundation Grant to Mardi Horowitz. We are grateful to Elaine Scharfe for her help in the collection and coding of the data.

REFERENCES

Ainsworth, M. D. S. (1982). Attachment: Retrospect and prospect. In C. M. Parkes & J. Stevenson-Hinde (Eds.), *The place of attachment in human behavior* (pp. 3–30). New York: Basic Books.

Ainsworth, M. S., Blehar, M. C., Waters, E., & Wall, S. (1978). *Patterns of attachment: A psychological study of the Strange Situation.* Hillsdale, NJ: Erlbaum.

Bartholomew, K. (1990). Avoidance of intimacy: An attachment perspective. *Journal of Social and Personal Relationships, 7,* 147–178.

Bartholomew, K. (1993). From childhood to adult relationships: Attachment theory and research. In S. Duck (Ed.), *Understanding relationship processes: Vol. 2. Learning about relationships* (pp. 30–62). Beverly Hills, CA: Sage.

Bartholomew, K., & Horowitz, L. M. (1991). Attachment styles among young adults: A test of a four-category model. *Journal of Personality and Social Psychology, 61*, 226–244.

Bellg, A. J. (1995). *Adult attachment and adjustment to breast cancer.* Unpublished doctoral dissertation, University of Rochester, Rochester, NY.

Borman, E., & Cole, H. (1993, March). *A comparison of three measures of adult attachment.* Poster presented at the meeting of the Society for Research in Child Development, New Orleans.

Bowlby, J. (1973). *Attachment and loss: Vol. 2. Separation: Anxiety and anger.* New York: Basic Books.

Bowlby, J. (1988). *A secure base: Parent–child attachment and healthy human development.* New York: Basic Books.

Brennan, K. A., Shaver, P. R., & Tobey, A. E. (1991). Attachment styles, gender, and parental problem drinking. *Journal of Social and Personal Relationships, 8*, 451–466.

Cohen, J (1988). *Statistical power analysis for the behavioral sciences* (2nd ed.). Hillsdale, NJ: Erlbaum.

Collins, N. L., & Read, S. J. (1990). Adult attachment, working models, and relationship quality in dating couples. *Journal of Personality and Social Psychology, 58*, 644–663.

Collins, N. L., & Read, S. J. (1994). Cognitive representations of attachment: The structure and function of working models. In K. Bartholomew & D. Perlman (Eds.), *Advances in personal relationships* (Vol. 5, pp. 53–90). London: Jessica Kingsley.

Crowell, J. A. (1990). *Current Relationship Interview.* Unpublished manuscript, State University of New York, Stony Brook.

Crowell, J., & Treboux, D. (1995). A review of adult attachment measures: Implications for theory and research. *Social Development, 4*, 294–327.

Crowell, J., Treboux, D., & Waters, E. (1993). *Alternatives to the Adult Attachment Interview: Self-reports of attachment style and relationships with mothers and partners.* Poster presented at the meeting of the Society for Research in Child Development, New Orleans.

Feeney, J. A., & Noller, P. (1991). Attachment style and verbal descriptions of romantic partners. *Journal of Social and Personal Relationships, 8*, 187–215.

Feeney, J. A., Noller, P., & Hanrahan, M. (1994). Assessing adult attachment. In M. B. Sperling & W. H. Berman (Eds.), *Attachment in adults: Clinical and developmental perspectives* (pp. 128–152). New York: Guilford Press.

George, C., Kaplan, N., & Main, M. (1985). *The Berkeley Adult Attachment Interview.* Unpublished protocol, University of California, Berkeley.

Gonzalez, R., & Griffin, D. W. (1997). On the statistics of interdependence: Treating dyadic data with respect. In S. Duck (Ed.), *Handbook of personal relationships* (2nd ed., pp. 271–302). London: Wiley.

Griffin, D., & Bartholomew, K. (1994). Models of the self and other: Fundamental dimensions underlying measures of adult attachment. *Journal of Personality and Social Psychology, 67*, 430–445.

Hazan, C., & Shaver, P. R. (1987). Romantic love conceptualized as an attachment process. *Journal of Personality and Social Psychology, 52,* 511–524.

Hazan, C., & Shaver, P. R. (1990). Love and work: An attachment-theoretical perspective. *Journal of Personality and Social Psychology, 59,* 270–280.

Kirkpatrick, L. A., & Davis, K. E. (1994). Attachment style, gender, and relationship stability: A longitudinal analysis. *Journal of Personality and Social Psychology, 66,* 502–512.

Kobak, R. R., Cole, H. E., Ferenz-Gillies, R., Fleming, W. S., & Gamble, W. (1993). Attachment and emotion regulation during mother–teen problem-solving: A control theory analysis. *Child Development, 64,* 231–245.

Kobak, R. R., & Hazan, C. (1991). Attachment in marriage: The effects of security and accuracy of working models. *Journal of Personality and Social Psychology, 60,* 861–869.

Main, M., Kaplan, N., & Cassidy, J. (1985). Security in infancy, childhood, and adulthood: A move to the level of representation. *Monographs of the Society for Research in Child Development, 50*(1–2), 66–104.

Mikulincer, M., & Nachshon, O. (1991). Attachment styles and patterns of self-disclosure. *Journal of Personality and Social Psychology, 61,* 321–331.

O'Hearn, R. E., & Davis, K. E. (1997). Women's experience of giving and receiving emotional abuse: An attachment perspective. *Journal of Interpersonal Violence, 12*(3), 375–391.

Rholes, W. S., Simpson, J. A., & Blakely, B. S. (1995). Adult attachment styles and mothers' relationships with their young children. *Personal Relationships, 2,* 35–54.

Saunders, K. D. (1992). *The links between patterns of male attachment and the development of wife assault.* Unpublished doctoral dissertation, University of British Columbia, Vancouver.

Scharfe, E., & Bartholomew, K. (1994). Reliability and stability of adult attachment patterns. *Personal Relationships, 1,* 23–43.

Shaver, P. R., & Brennan, K. A. (1992). Attachment styles and the "Big Five" personality traits: Their connections with each other and with romantic relationship outcomes. *Personality and Social Psychology Bulletin, 18,* 536–545.

Shaver, P. R., & Clark, C. L. (1994). The psychodynamics of adult romantic attachment. In J. M. Masling & R. F. Bornstein (Eds.), *Empirical perspectives on object relations theory* (pp. 105–156). Washington, DC: American Psychological Association.

Shaver, P. R., Collins, N. L., & Clark, C. L. (1996). Attachment styles and internal working models of self and relationship partners. In G. J. O. Fletcher & J. Fitness (Eds.), *Knowledge structures in close relationships: A social psychological approach* (pp. 25–61). Mahwah, NJ: Erlbaum.

Shaver, P. R., & Hazan, C. (1993). Adult romantic attachment: Theory and evidence. In D. Perlman & W. H. Jones (Eds.), *Advances in personal relationships* (Vol. 4, pp. 29–70). London: Jessica Kingsley.

Shaver, P. R., Hazan, C., & Bradshaw, D. (1988). Love as attachment: The integration of three behavioral systems. In R. J. Sternberg & M. L. Barnes (Eds.), *The psychology of love* (pp. 68–99). New Haven, CT: Yale University Press.

Simpson, J. A. (1990). The influence of attachment styles on romantic relationships. *Journal of Personality and Social Psychology, 59,* 971–980.

Simpson, J. A., Rholes, W. S., & Nelligan, J. S. (1992). Support seeking and support giving within couples in an anxiety-provoking situation. *Journal of Personality and Social Psychology, 62,* 434–446.

Treboux, D. (1997, April). *Are self-reports reliable measures of secure base behavior?* Paper presented at the meeting of the Society for Research in Child Development, Washington, DC.

van IJzendoorn, M. H. (1995). Adult attachment representations, parental responsiveness, and infant attachment: A meta-analysis on the predictive validity of the Adult Attachment Interview. *Psychological Bulletin, 177,* 387–403.

Weiss, R. S. (1982). Attachment in adult life. In C. M. Parkes & J. Stevenson-Hinde (Eds.), *The place of attachment in human behavior* (pp. 171–184). New York: Basic Books.

3

Self-Report Measurement
of Adult Attachment

An Integrative Overview

KELLY A. BRENNAN
CATHERINE L. CLARK
PHILLIP R. SHAVER

Ever since Hazan and Shaver (1987) showed that it is possible to use a self-report questionnaire to measure adolescent and adult romantic attachment orientations (secure, anxious, and avoidant—the three patterns identified by Ainsworth, Blehar, Waters, & Wall, 1978, in their studies of infant–caregiver attachment), a steady stream of variants and extensions of their questionnaire have been proposed. The resulting diversity often arouses frustration and confusion in newcomers to the field who wonder which of the many measures to use. The three of us are probably typical of attachment researchers in receiving as many as five telephone calls, letters, and E-mail messages a week from researchers who want to know either "Has anything happened since 1987?" or "Which measure is the best?" In the present chapter we attempt to solve this problem by creating an all-purpose reply to future attachment researchers who wish to use self-report measures. Interview measures have also been proposed, but we will say little about them here. Attachment interviews are powerful and perhaps uniquely revealing, but they are also impractical for most researchers. (See Bartholomew & Horowitz, 1991; Bartholomew & Shaver, Chapter 2, this volume; Main, Kaplan, & Cassidy, 1985; Scharfe & Bartholomew, 1994; and van IJzendoorn, 1995, for discussions of attachment interview measures, not all of which measure the same constructs.)

Hazan and Shaver (1987, 1990) asked research participants to indicate which of three attachment-style prototypes (shown here in Table 3.1) best characterized their feelings and behavior in romantic relationships. These authors naively took for granted that Ainsworth et al. (1978) were correct in thinking of attachment patterns (usually called "attachment styles" by social psychologists) as *categories* or *types*. In retrospect, it is evident that Hazan and Shaver should have paid attention to Ainsworth et al.'s (1978) Figure 10 (p. 102), which summarized the results of a discriminant analysis predicting infant attachment type (secure, anxious, or avoidant) from the continuous rating scales used by coders to characterize the infants' behavior in a laboratory "Strange Situation." Our Figure 3.1 reproduces the essential features of the Ainsworth et al. figure and also includes our names for the two discriminant functions: Avoidance and Anxiety.

The coding scales that correlated most highly with the Avoidance dimension (Function 1) were (1) avoiding mother during episodes 5 and 8 of the Strange Situation (the two reunion episodes), (2) not maintaining contact with mother during episode 8, (3) not seeking proximity during episode 8, and (4) engaging in more exploratory behavior and more distance interaction (communication with a stranger while mother was absent) in episode 7 of the Strange Situation. All of these scales indicate avoidance of mother, lack of closeness to mother, and less distress during mother's absence (in the presence of an adult stranger). The coding scales that correlated most highly with the Anxiety dimension (Function 2) were (1) crying (all through episodes 2–8, but especially episode 6, when the infant was left alone for 3 minutes), (2) greater angry resistance to mother during episodes 5 and 8 (the reunions), (3) greater angry resistance to the

---

TABLE 3.1. Hazan and Shaver's (1987, 1990) Three Prototypes

Avoidant. I am somewhat uncomfortable being close to others; I find it difficult to trust them completely, difficult to allow myself to depend on them. I am nervous when anyone gets too close, and often, love partners want me to be more intimate than I feel comfortable being.

Anxious–ambivalent. I find that others are reluctant to get as close as I would like. I often worry that my partner doesn't really love me or won't want to stay with me. I want to get very close to my partner, and this sometimes scares people away.

Secure. I find it relatively easy to get close to others and am comfortable depending on them. I don't often worry about being abandoned or about someone getting too close to me.

stranger during episodes 3, 4, and 7 (when the stranger tried to comfort or play with the infant), and (4) reduced exploration in episode 7, when the solitary infant was joined by a stranger.

Figure 3.1 indicates that, right from the start, Ainsworth's three major attachment "types" could be conceptualized as regions in a two-dimensional space, the dimensions being Avoidance (discomfort with closeness and dependency) and Anxiety (crying, failing to explore confidently in the absence of mother, and angry protest directed at mother during reunions after what was probably experienced as abandonment). When Levy and Davis (1988) first asked adult subjects to rate *how well* each of Hazan and Shaver's (1987) romantic attachment prototypes described them, it was revealed that the three ratings could be reduced to two dimensions, one corresponding to Avoidance (discomfort with closeness and dependency) and the other to Anxiety (about abandonment). In subsequent studies, Simpson (1990) and Collins and Read (1990) broke Hazan and Shaver's multisentence attachment-style prototypes into separate propositions with which subjects could agree or disagree to varying extents. When these Likert-type items were factor analyzed, a two-factor (Simpson) or three-factor (Collins & Read) solu-

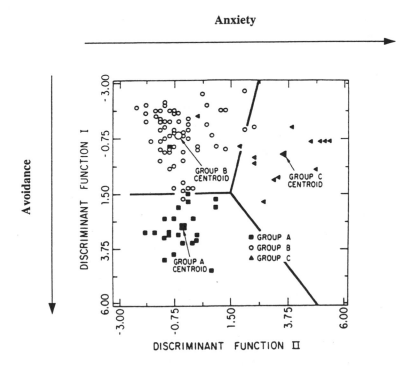

FIGURE 3.1. Ainsworth et al.'s (1978) Figure 10 (p. 102), with our names for the two discriminant functions. Copyright 1978 by Lawrence Erlbaum Associates, Inc. Reprinted by permission.

tion was obtained. In the case of the three-factor solution, two of the factors (Discomfort with Closeness and Discomfort with Dependence on romantic partners) were significantly correlated ($r = .38$). Simpson and his colleagues (e.g., Simpson, Rholes, & Nelligan, 1992) called their two dimensions "Security versus Avoidance" and "Anxiety" (about abandonment). Collins and Read (1990) called their three dimensions "Close," "Depend," and "Anxiety" (about abandonment). If we interpret the close and depend dimensions as "facets" of avoidance (the term facets being borrowed from Costa & McCrae, 1992), all of the early analyses of the structure of Hazan and Shaver's measure are compatible with the interpretation that adult attachment measures, like Ainsworth et al.'s coding scales for the Strange Situation, primarily assess avoidance and attachment-related anxiety.

The two-dimensional empirical and conceptual structure underlying attachment orientations was articulated more completely when researchers who study infant–caregiver attachment and those who study adolescent and adult romantic attachment realized that a two-dimensional space makes room for four, rather than three, quadrants or conceptual patterns. Crittenden (1988) and others who focused on infant–caregiver attachment in abusive and troubled families noted a mixed avoidant–anxious type. Main and Solomon (1990) identified a somewhat similar pattern, called "disorganized, disoriented" attachment. A diagram of the four infant types organized by the Avoidance and Anxiety dimensions is shown in Figure 3.2.

In the area of adult attachment, Bartholomew (1990), who had noticed that Hazan and Shaver's (1987, 1990) avoidant type and Main et al.'s (1985) dismissing (avoidant) type differed in the degree to which they exhibited anxious as well as avoidant qualities, proposed the now-familiar two-dimensional, four-category conceptual scheme shown in Figure 3.3. The parallels between Figures 3.2 and 3.3 are obvious. In both diagrams the upper left-hand quadrant represents securely attached individuals— infants and adults who are neither anxious about abandonment nor avoidant in their behavior. The upper right-hand quadrant of both diagrams represents anxious or preoccupied attachment, defined as a mixture of anxiety and interpersonal approach (nonavoidance). The lower left-hand quadrant represents dismissingly avoidant attachment, a combination of avoidant behavior and apparent lack of anxiety about abandonment. The lower right-hand quadrant represents fearfully avoidant attachment, which combines anxiety about abandonment with avoidant behavior.

In subsequent work, Bartholomew has shown that it is possible to assess the four types and/or the two dimensions in adolescent and adult populations using either questionnaires or coded interviews (e.g., Bartholomew & Horowitz, 1991; Griffin & Bartholomew, 1994a, 1994b; Scharfe & Bartholomew, 1994). As shown in Figure 3.3, Bartholomew labels the two dimensions "Model of Self" and "Model of Other," but she

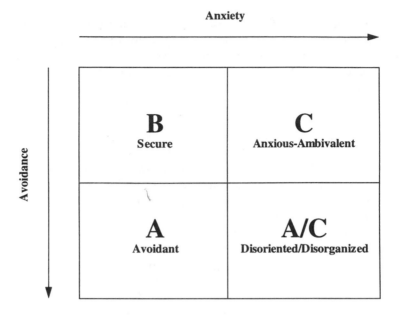

FIGURE 3.2. A diagram of the four infant attachment types.

and her coauthors also sometimes use the terms "Anxiety" and "Avoidance" (e.g., Scharfe, 1996), suggesting that a negative model of self is closely associated with anxiety about abandonment and that a negative model of others is closely associated with avoidant behavior. (Whether particular cognitive models, discussed in the present volume by Klohnen & John, Chapter 5, actually *account for* the anxious and avoidant reactions or get built up around them during cognitive and personality development remains to be determined.)

While the two-dimensional structure underlying adult attachment styles was being revealed, many researchers created their own measures, some in an attempt to tap the two dimensions (e.g., Wagner & Vaux, 1994) or the four styles defined by them (Griffin & Bartholomew, 1994a). Others delineated additional styles (Hatfield, 1993; Latty-Mann & Davis, 1996) or included additional psychological content (e.g., anger; Sperling, Berman, & Fagen, 1992). Still others returned to Bowlby's (e.g., West & Sheldon-Keller, 1994) or Ainsworth's (e.g., Feeney, Noller, & Hanrahan, 1994) more specific constructs, such as compulsive self-reliance and separation protest, from which two or more dimensions might be constructed. Although each of these efforts made sense and yielded interesting results, when first encountered en masse they constitute a bewildering obstacle to researchers who wish to study romantic attachment.

In the remainder of this chapter we will report some of the results of a large-sample study that incorporated most of the extant self-report attachment measures, including some that are rarely referenced by attachment researchers. We began with a thorough search of the literature, including available conference papers, from which we created a pool of 482 items designed to assess 60 named attachment-related constructs. The three of us then independently evaluated the degree of redundancy among similar items, reducing them to a single exemplary item if two or three of us agreed that they were completely or almost completely redundant. (As will be seen, this still left a substantial amount of interitem similarity.) We thus reduced the 482 items to 323, from which all 60 subscale scores could be computed. We then factor-analyzed the 60 subscale scores, producing two essentially independent factors that correspond to the already familiar Avoidance and Anxiety dimensions. When we clustered subjects into four groups based on their scores on the two factors, the groups corresponded conceptually to Bartholomew's four types (see Figure 3.3). But the relations between the clusters and other theoretically appropriate target variables proved to be stronger than the corresponding relations between Bartholomew's self-report measure and

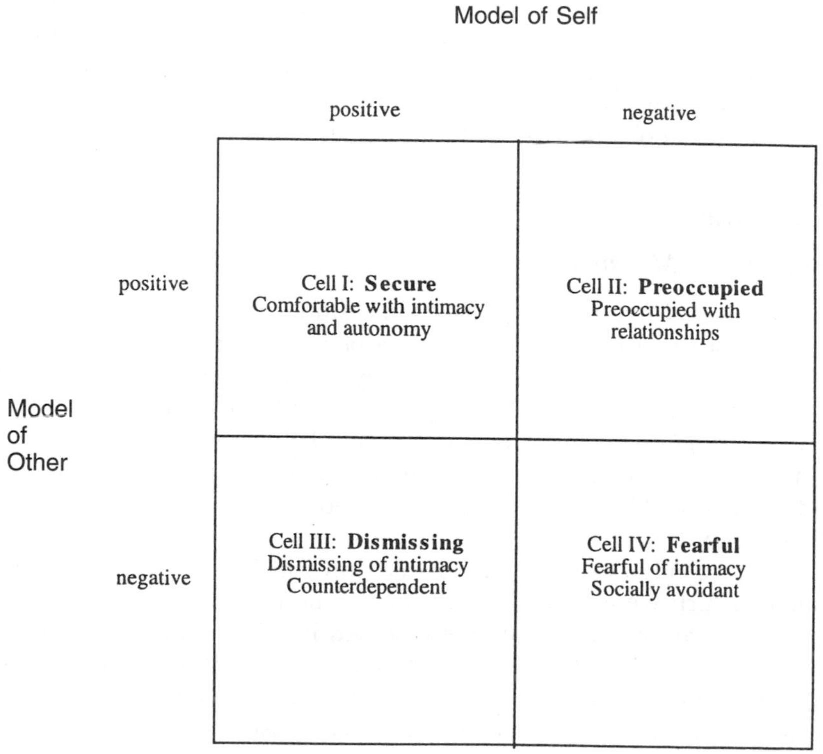

Model of Self

	positive	negative
positive	Cell I: **Secure** Comfortable with intimacy and autonomy	Cell II: **Preoccupied** Preoccupied with relationships
negative	Cell III: **Dismissing** Dismissing of intimacy Counterdependent	Cell IV: **Fearful** Fearful of intimacy Socially avoidant

Model
of
Other

FIGURE 3.3. Bartholomew's (1990) four-category diagram.

those same target variables. We also computed two internally consistent but relatively brief scales to represent the Avoidance and Anxiety factors and used those scales to predict theoretically appropriate target variables. The results were promising and suggest that self-report attachment research might benefit from the use of the two scales. We turn now to a more detailed description of the study.

COMBINING ALL SELF-REPORT ATTACHMENT MEASURES IN A SINGLE QUESTIONNAIRE

Participants and Procedure

In order to perform reliable factor analyses with large numbers of items and constructs, we administered questionnaires to a sizable group of research participants: 1,086 undergraduates (682 women and 403 men) enrolled in psychology courses at the University of Texas at Austin. These students ranged in age from 16 to 50, with a median age of 18. Just under half the sample (487) described themselves as seriously involved in a relationship at the time of testing; the rest were dating casually (220) or not at all (376). Of those in a relationship, median relationship length was 15 months. Students received research credits in their classes for participating in the study, but their answers were completely anonymous. The questionnaire took approximately 2 hours to complete.

Materials

Attachment Measures

The first set of five measures asked the students to classify themselves into one of three or four briefly described attachment-style categories. (The measures were those designed by Hazan & Shaver, 1987, 1990; Bartholomew & Horowitz, 1991; Sperling et al., 1992; and Latty-Mann & Davis, 1996.) For purposes of the present chapter, we will discuss data from only one categorical instrument, an adaptation of the Bartholomew and Horowitz (1991) measure that focused on experiences in romantic relationships.[1]

The second set of attachment measures included every multi-item scale of which we are aware, including some from never-published but useful conference papers. The items varied in content, but all dealt with specific aspects of adolescent and adult attachment. Where necessary, we adapted item wording to emphasize romantic relationships (our own special interest) rather than all close relationships. After eliminating duplicate or very similar items (from different authors' scales), we were left with 323 statements that could be combined into a single questionnaire. The 323 items were printed in a randomly determined order. Space limitations here preclude a detailed discussion of each measure, but in general the following aspects of attachment were addressed: trust, separation protest, ambivalence, caregiving, careseeking, comfort with closeness, communication, commitment, avoidance, perceived partner availability, anxious attachment, alienation, angry withdrawal, loneliness, confidence in self and partner, defensiveness, disclosure, fear of rejection, jealousy/fear of abandonment, feared loss, proximity-seeking, self-reliance, viewing relationships as secondary, and romantic obsession. Participants were asked to rate all 323 items on a 7-point scale ranging from "not at all like me" to "very much like me," a task requiring approximately 60 minutes. The following sources were drawn upon for items: Armsden and Greenberg (1987); Brennan and Shaver (1995); Carnelley, Pietromonaco, and Jaffe (1994); Carver (1994); Collins and Read (1990); Feeney et al. (1994); Griffin and Bartholomew (1994a); Hindy, Schwartz, and Brodsky (1989); Onishi and Gjerde (1994); Rothbard, Roberts, Leonard, and Eiden (1993); Shaver (1995); Simpson (1990); Wagner and Vaux (1994); West and Sheldon-Keller (1994).

Measures of Personality and Social Behavior

Two additional kinds of measures were included in the study so that we could assess relations between self-report attachment constructs and two theoretically associated variables, intimate touch and romantic sexuality. Touch is an issue that has been addressed in studies of infant attachment (e.g., Main, 1990) but until recently not in studies of adult romantic attachment (see Brennan, Wu, & Loev, Chapter 14, this volume). Sexuality was postulated by Shaver, Hazan, and Bradshaw (1988) to be one of three behavioral systems combined to form romantic love (along with attachment and caregiving). Except for a seminal study by Hazan, Zeifman, and Middleton (1994), however, sexuality has not been closely linked empirically with attachment patterns. The touch and sexuality measures used in the present study allowed us to determine how well various attachment measures fit within an interesting and understudied nomological network of other variables. (Actually, we included several additional nodes in the nomological network but do not have space to discuss them here.) Each domain of questions will be described briefly.

Touch Scales

These 51 items assessed individual differences in touch within the context of romantic relationships. Of the seven constructs measured by the items, we will consider only four here: using touch to express affectionate proximity, desiring more physical contact, touch aversion, and using touch to assure a haven of safety. (See Brennan et al., Chapter 14, this volume.)

Sex Questions

Of the 47 items included in this domain (Hazan et al., 1994; Janus & Janus, 1993; Laumann, Gagnon, Michael, & Michaels, 1994), 21 assessed the degree to which participants enjoy various kinds of *sexual behavior* on 7-point scales ranging from "not at all" to "a great deal," and 12 assessed the frequency with which respondents experienced various *emotions* following sexual activities (e.g., feeling loved, sad, wanted/ needed). For purposes of the present chapter, we will ignore the remaining items.

A principal components analysis of the 21 sexual-preference items produced five oblique factors, together accounting for 61.4% of the variance. The first of the resulting five unit-weighted scales assesses preference for "promiscuous" sexual behavior (e.g., one-night stands, alpha = .85). The second scale assesses what might be called "normative" sexual behavior in our sample (e.g., oral or manual stimulation of partners' genitals [two items], partners' oral/manual stimulation of participants' genitals [two items], and vaginal intercourse; alpha = .87). The third scale assesses preference for sadistic or masochistic sexual behavior (alpha = .89). The fourth scale assesses preference for miscellaneous "non-normative" sexual behaviors (e.g., voyeurism, group sex, exhibitionism, attempting sexual contact with a nonconsenting person, anal intercourse; alpha = .71). The fifth scale assesses a preference for romantic/affectionate sexual behavior (cuddling, kissing, gazing; alpha = .66). For purposes of the present chapter we will consider only the three scales most relevant to attachment: promiscuous, normative, and affectionate sexuality.

Based on the same analytic procedures, the items assessing emotions typically experienced after sex produced two factors: a "positive" factor (satisfied, loved, wanted/needed, taken care of, thrilled/excited) and a "negative" factor (scared/afraid, guilty, sad, anxious/worried, disgusted, frustrated/angry, alienated/lonely). The two factors accounted for 60.9% of the variance. Alpha was .87 for both scales.

RESULTS OF THE SURVEY

Underlying Structure of the Attachment Measures

Correlations among 60 Attachment Constructs

We are unable to include the entire 60 × 60 matrix here, but we can summarize it briefly. Correlations among the 60 subscales were highly patterned: 62% were either > .50 (i.e., quite high) or < .20 (i.e., quite low). This pattern of high and low correlations suggested that there were in fact a few underlying factors to be identified, some of which were likely to be independent. Interestingly, the high correlations included ones spanning domains of measurement that have remained segregated in the literature. Table 3.2, for example, shows strong correlations between the subscales of Collins and Read's (1990), Armsden and Greenberg's (1987), and West and Sheldon-Keller's (1994) measures. These correlations are especially impressive given that each measure was developed under a different conceptual rubric and for a different research purpose. Collins and Read's measure was based on Hazan and Shaver's (1987) speculative extension of Ainsworth's infant typology to the realm of romantic love; Armsden and Greenberg's (1987) measure was designed to tap affective and cognitive dimensions of adolescents' attachment to peers; and the subscales from West and Sheldon-Keller's measure were rooted more in Bowlby's clinical constructs than in Ainsworth's observational studies of infants. Notice that West and Sheldon-Keller's scales, which are not much discussed in the literature on romantic relationships, appear highly redundant with scales designed to measure romantic attachment—at least when they are completed with romantic attachment figures in mind. Despite the somewhat different aims and ideas behind these three sets of subscales, some of the correlations across the sets are quite high, indicating the existence of common underlying dimensions.

Principal Components Analysis of the 60 Attachment Scales

A principal components analysis of the 60 subscales produced two major factors, which were rotated using an oblique procedure.[2] Although this

TABLE 3.2. Selected Examples of the Intercorrelations of the 60 Subscales

	Collins & Read's (1990) scales		
	Anxious	Close	Depend
Armsden & Greenberg's (1987) scales			
Alienation	.62	−.39	−.62
Trust	−.50	.49	.66
Communication	−.41	.49	.58
West & Sheldon-Keller's (1994) scales			
Angry withdrawal	.57	−.18	−.51
Availability of partner	−.61	.46	.73
Compulsive caregiving	.08	.32	.18
Compulsive careseeking	.19	.12	.04
Feared loss of partner	.78	−.30	−.54
Proximity-seeking	.18	.21	.06
Compulsive self-reliance	.40	−.77	−.65
Separation protest	.30	.05	−.12
Use partner as secure base	−.30	.57	.58

Note. All coefficients above .11 are statistically significant at $p < .001$.

procedure allowed the factors to correlate with each other to any degree, the correlation between the two major factors was only .12, suggesting that the dimensions underlying attachment styles are essentially orthogonal. Together, the two factors accounted for 62.8% of the variance in the 60 subscales and were easily identifiable as 45-degree rotations of the dimensions obtained in previous work by Brennan, Shaver, and Tobey (1991) and Brennan and Shaver (1995). The two factors are conceptually equivalent to the horizontal and vertical axes of Bartholomew's four-category typology of attachment styles (e.g., Bartholomew & Horowitz, 1991; Griffin & Bartholomew, 1994a, 1994b). (Refer back to Figure 3.3.)

Table 3.3 presents the loadings of each of the 60 attachment subscales on the two higher-order factors. Avoidance of Intimacy (Rothbard et al., 1993), Discomfort with Closeness (Feeney et al., 1994), and Self-Reliance (West & Sheldon-Keller, 1994) emerged as the top three scales representative of the first factor, which we call Avoidance. Preoccupation (Feeney et al., 1994), Jealousy/Fear of Abandonment (Brennan & Shaver, 1995), and Fear of Rejection (Rothbard et al., 1993) emerged as the three scales most representative of the second factor, Anxiety.

TABLE 3.3. Factor Loadings of the 60 Attachment Subscales with Two Higher-Order Factors

Attachment subscale	Factor 1	Factor 2
Avoidance of intimacy (Rothbard et al., 1993)	.91	
Discomfort with closeness (Feeney et al., 1994)	.90	
Self-reliance (West & Sheldon-Keller, 1994)	.88	
Avoidance (Carver, 1994)	.86	
Discomfort with closeness (Carnelley et al., 1994)	.86	
Self-reliance (Carnelley et al., 1994)	.86	
Fearful prototype (Onishi & Gjerde, 1994)	.85	
Discomfort with disclosure (Carnelley et al., 1994)	.85	
Comfort with closeness (Collins & Read, 1990)	−.84	
Security (Simpson, 1990)	−.83	
Proximity-seeking (Brennan & Shaver, 1995)	−.82	
Dismissing prototype (Onishi & Gjerde, 1994)	.82	−.40
Self-reliance (Brennan & Shaver, 1995)	.82	

(continued)

TABLE 3.3. *(cont.)*

Attachment subscale	Factor 1	Factor 2
Secure prototype (Onishi & Gjerde, 1994)	−.82	
Fearfulness (Griffin & Bartholomew, 1994a)	.82	
Avoidance (Simpson, 1990)	.81	
Use partner as secure base (West & Sheldon-Keller, 1994)	−.79	
Comfort depending on others (Collins & Read, 1990)	−.79	
Ambivalence (Brennan & Shaver, 1995)	.76	
Ambivalence (Carnelley et al., 1994)	.75	
Dismissiveness (Shaver, 1995)	.73	
Defensiveness (Carnelley et al., 1994)	.72	
Communication (Armsden & Greenburg, 1987)	−.72	
Trust (Brennan & Shaver, 1995)	−.72	
Trust (Armsden & Greenburg, 1987)	−.72	
Model of others (Wagner & Vaux, 1994)	−.70	−.31
Security (Carver, 1994)	−.70	
Self-confidence (Feeney et al., 1994)	−.70	
Security (Griffin & Bartholomew, 1994a)	−.69	−.30
Distrust (Carnelley et al., 1994)	.68	.39
Availability of partners (West & Sheldon-Keller, 1994)	−.66	−.39
Relationships as secondary (Feeney et al., 1994)	.61	
Frustration with partners (Brennan & Shaver, 1995)	.60	.50
Model of self (Wagner & Vaux, 1994)	−.52	−.35
Dismissiveness (Griffin & Bartholomew, 1994a)	.50	−.42
Compulsive caregiving (West & Sheldon-Keller, 1994)	−.46	.45
Preoccupation (Feeney et al., 1994)		.86
Jealousy/fear of abandonment (Brennan & Shaver, 1995)		.85
Fear of rejection (Rothbard et al., 1993)		.83

(continued)

TABLE 3.3. *(cont.)*

Attachment subscale	Factor 1	Factor 2
Preoccupied prototype	−.39	.82
(Onishi & Gjerde, 1994)		
Jealousy		.80
(Carnelley et al., 1994)		
Preoccupation		.79
(Griffin & Bartholomew, 1994a)		
Anxiety		.77
(Simpson, 1990)		
Worry		.76
(Carver, 1994)		
Anxious-clinging to partners	.33	.76
(Brennan & Shaver, 1995)		
Anxious-clinging to partners		.75
(Carnelley et al., 1994)		
Anxiety	.41	.74
(Collins & Read, 1990)		
Anxious attachment		.72
(Hindy et al., 1989)		
Romantic anxiety	.38	.71
(Hindy et al., 1989)		
Proximity-seeking		.68
(Carnelley et al., 1994)		
Romantic obsession	−.40	.67
(Hindy et al., 1989)		
Desire to merge with partner		.66
(Carver, 1994)		
Dependent self-esteem		.66
(Rothbard et al., 1993)		
Angry withdrawal		.65
(West & Sheldon-Keller, 1994)		
Feared loss of partner	.41	.64
(West & Sheldon-Keller, 1994)		
Need for approval		.62
(Feeney et al., 1994)		
Proximity-seeking	−.36	.59
(West & Sheldon-Keller, 1994)		
Compulsive careseeking		.57
(West & Sheldon-Keller, 1994)		
Alienation	.53	.53
(Armsden & Greenburg, 1987)		
Separation protest		.48
(West & Sheldon-Keller, 1994)		

Note. Loadings lower than .30 were omitted.

Creation of Two Higher-Order Scales

Two 18-item scales were constructed from the 36 items (out of the total pool of 323) with the highest absolute-value correlations with one of the two higher-order factors. Correlations of the two new (unit-weighted) scales, Avoidance and Anxiety, with the 60 major subscales and the four

Bartholomew romantic style self-ratings are listed in Table 3.4. (The two scales, like their parent factors, are almost uncorrelated, $r = .11$, and each correlates very highly with its parent factor, $r = .95$ in both cases.) The correlations in Table 3.4 will allow experienced attachment researchers to see how their favorite scales fit into our two-dimensional scheme, and, we hope, will help novices decide whether or not to use our scales for their particular purposes. Our Avoidance scale correlates highly with several other scales measuring avoidance and discomfort with closeness. The Anxiety scale correlates highly with scales measuring anxiety and preoccupation with attachment, jealousy, and fear of rejection.

Creation of Four Clusters from the Two Higher-Order Scales

The two higher-order factors were used to cluster participants according to guidelines suggested by Hair, Anderson, Tatham, and Black (1995, pp. 137–112). We first used a hierarchical clustering procedure (Ward's method, with squared Euclidean distance) to obtain initial cluster centers. Those centers were then used as a starting point for a second, nonhierarchical cluster analysis (K-Means, with an optimization method of assigning cases to clusters). We chose to conduct two cluster analyses, first hierarchical and then nonhierarchical, because nonhierarchical analyses typically provide more robust solutions. Nonhierarchical analyses allow cases to be switched from their initial cluster to a better-fitting cluster, a process known as optimizing, or "updating," the cluster centers. In hierarchical analyses, once a case has been assigned to a cluster center, it cannot be reassigned in a later iteration when alternative, better-fitting clusters may emerge. Here, the hierarchical cluster analysis was conducted first to provide initial cluster centers without which the nonhierarchical method would have had to use random starting points.

The initial pattern of clusters derived from Ward's hierarchical cluster analysis (in SPSS) revealed four distinct groups whose patterns of scores on the Avoidance and Anxiety factors clearly resembled Bartholomew's descriptions of the secure, fearful, preoccupied, and dismissing categories. Participants in the "secure" cluster scored low on both Avoidance and Anxiety. Those in the "fearful" cluster scored high on both Avoidance and Anxiety. Those in the "preoccupied" cluster appeared low on Avoidance and high on Anxiety, while those in the "dismissing" cluster scored high on Avoidance and low on Anxiety. (The quotation marks are intended to distinguish the four cluster-based styles from the similar styles derived from Bartholomew's measure.) Interestingly, when we instructed the program to find three clusters, the two avoidant clusters were collapsed into one, similar to the way Hazan and Shaver (1987) originally measured romantic attachment. When five clusters were selected, the preoccupied group split into those very low on Avoidance but only moderately high

TABLE 3.4. Correlations of 60 Attachment Subscales with Two Higher-Order Attachment Scales

	Avoidance	Anxiety
Armsden & Greenberg's (1987) scales		
Alienation	.51	.58
Communication	−.68	−.24
Trust	−.65	−.34
Brennan & Shaver's (1995) scales		
Ambivalence	.73	.30
Anxious–clinging to partners	.31	.78
Jealousy/fear of abandonment	.11	.82
Frustration with partners	.54	.56
Proximity-seeking	−.78	.12
Self-reliance	.79	.00
Trust	−.66	−.37
Carnelley et al.'s (1994) scales		
Ambivalence	.75	.26
Anxious–clinging to partners	.02	.75
Defensiveness	.68	.20
Discomfort with closeness	.86	−.02
Discomfort with disclosure	.86	.14
Distrust	.62	.46
Jealousy	.26	.80
Proximity-seeking	−.05	.60
Carver's (1994) scales		
Avoidance	.90	.09
Desire to merge with partners	.16	.70
Security	−.63	.14
Worry	.27	.79
Collins & Read's (1990) scales		
Anxiety	.41	.79
Comfort with closeness	−.87	−.05
Comfort depending on others	−.73	−.39
Feeney et al.'s (1994) scales		
Self-confidence	−.69	−.25
Discomfort with closeness	.88	.22
Need for approval	.24	.63
Preoccupation	.13	.88
Relationships as secondary	.56	.16
Griffin & Bartholomew's (1994a) scales		
Dismissiveness	.39	−.29
Fearfulness	.81	.32
Preoccupation	−.13	.73
Security	−.70	−.46
Hindy et al.'s (1989) scales		
Anxious attachment	.22	.71
Romantic anxiety	.35	.75
Romantic obsession	−.34	.55
Onishi & Gjerde's (1994) scales		
Dismissing prototype	.73	−.22
Fearful prototype	.80	.33
Preoccupied prototype	−.34	.68
Secure prototype	−.79	−.39

(continued)

TABLE 3.4. *(cont.)*

	Avoidance	Anxiety
Rothbard et al.'s (1993) scales		
Avoidance of intimacy	.89	.07
Dependent self-esteem	−.07	.60
Fear of rejection	.29	.88
Shaver's (1995) scale		
Dismissiveness	.64	−.12
Simpson's (1990) scales		
Anxiety	.06	.75
Avoidance	.82	.20
Security	−.84	−.28
Wagner & Vaux's (1994) scales		
Model of self	−.52	.42
Model of others	−.63	−.40
West & Sheldon-Keller's (1994) scales		
Angry withdrawal	.26	.67
Availability of partner	−.61	−.47
Compulsive caregiving	−.36	.30
Compulsive careseeking	−.18	.49
Feared loss of partner	.39	.69
Proximity-seeking	−.28	.48
Compulsive self-reliance	.88	.14
Separation protest	−.02	.48
Use partner as secure base	−.78	−.08

Note. Scales are listed in alphabetical order by author and, within author, by scale name.
All coefficients above .11 are statistically significant at $p < .001$.

on Anxiety and those very high on Anxiety but only moderately low on Avoidance, a distinction not previously made in the romantic attachment literature. (This split may have been encouraged by the larger-than-usual number of items on our scales. As explained later, we do not wish to place much emphasis on any particular number of types because other analyses, reported in the present volume by Fraley and Waller, Chapter 4, indicate that the types are not "real" in any case. Ultimately, only the dimensional scores matter.) For purposes of comparing scale-based clusters with the types generated by Bartholomew's self-report measure, we chose the four-cluster solution, which is justified by the pattern of agglomeration coefficients, the dendrogram, and previous research and theory (cf. Feeney et al., 1994, for similar analyses and a similar conclusion).

The pattern of clusters from the second, nonhierarchical cluster analysis was quite similar to that from the hierarchical analysis. A look at the final cluster centers revealed that the "secure" cluster center was low on both Avoidance (−1.02) and Anxiety (−.67) factors, whereas the "fearful" cluster was high on both Avoidance (.94) and Anxiety (.52). The "preoccupied" cluster was low on Avoidance (−.34) and high on Anxiety (1.10).

The "dismissing" cluster was high on Avoidance (.78) and low on Anxiety (–.91). This cluster-based attachment-style category system will be used in subsequent analyses in this chapter, beginning with a detailed comparison between it and Bartholomew's self-report measure (Bartholomew & Horowitz, 1991, modified to refer to romantic relationships). Readers who wish to use our scales will find the questionnaire in Appendix 3.1 and scoring instructions in Appendix 3.2. It is not necessary to ask us for permission to use the scales.

Comparison of Categorical Attachment Measures

Association with Each Other

Table 3.5 shows the cross-tabulation of attachment style categories assessed with the Bartholomew four-category self-classification measure and our new, cluster-based method. A chi-square test comparing the two assessment schemes was highly significant, indicating substantial similarity. Collapsing across secure and insecure categories allows meaningful comparison of the two measures' rates of secure versus insecure classifications. Just over half (52.8%) of the people classified as secure on Bartholomew's measure were placed in the "secure" category of the new, cluster-based classification. Only a very small minority (11.2%) of those classified as insecure on Bartholomew's measure were classified as "secure" on the new measure. A very large percentage (88.8%) of the sample classified as insecure with Bartholomew's measure were also classified as insecure by the new measure. But nearly half (47.2%) classified as secure on Bartholomew's measure were classified as insecure on the new measure. In other words, participants were more likely to be categorized as insecure and less likely to be categorized as "secure" using our new measure compared with Bartholomew's measure, so the new procedure is more conservative than Bartholomew's in classifying a person as secure.[3] This is probably because our scales discriminate more precisely than Bartholomew's measure among people with different degrees of insecurity. At least in relation to the nomological

TABLE 3.5. Relationship between Bartholomew's and Cluster-Based Attachment-Style Categories

Cluster-based category	Bartholomew's attachment-style category				Row total
	Secure	Fearful	Preoccupied	Dismissing	
Secure	264	21	20	24	329 (30.4%)
Fearful	65	116	38	45	264 (24.4%)
Preoccupied	94	52	112	6	264 (24.4%)
Dismissing	77	60	4	84	225 (20.8%)
Column total:	500	249	174	159	1,082 (100%)
	(46.2%)	(23.0%)	(16.1%)	(14.7%)	

Note. $\chi^2(9) = 497.78$, $p < .0001$; $n = 1,082$.

network we have been exploring in our research, this conservatism about calling a person secure generally leads to statistically stronger results, as illustrated in the next two sections.

Associations between Bartholomew's Measure, Anxiety and Avoidance, and Touch and Sex Subscales

Three multivariate analyses of variance (MANOVAs) were computed on (1) the Anxiety and Avoidance scales, (2) the touch subscales, and (3) the sex subscales as a function of the Bartholomew self-classification measure. The first MANOVA on the two higher-order factor scales was highly significant, as were the MANOVAs on the touch and sex subscales. The means for the two higher-order scales and the touch and sex subscales are listed in Table 3.6, along with the univariate Fs. Follow-up Tukey pairwise comparisons were computed to determine which groups differed significantly.

Both the fearful and dismissing groups, which did not differ from each other, scored higher on the Avoidance scale than either the secure or the preoccupied group; preoccupied individuals scored higher than se-

TABLE 3.6. Two New Attachment-Scale Scores and Touch and Sex Subscale Scores as a Function of Bartholomew's Attachment-Style Category

	Bartholomew's attachment-style category				Univariate F	η^2
	Secure	Fearful	Preoccupied	Dismissing		
New scales						
(df = 3, 1,073)						
Avoidance	2.36_a	3.71_c	2.68_b	3.74_c	151.00^{***}	.30
Anxiety	3.08_a	3.83_b	4.54_c	2.99_a	132.12^{***}	.27
Touch						
(df = 3, 1,051)						
Affectionate proximity	5.79_c	5.47_b	5.86_c	4.98_a	28.49^{***}	.08
Desire for more touch	2.45_a	2.86_b	3.30_c	2.71_b	27.21^{***}	.07
Touch aversion	2.15_a	2.66_b	2.24_a	2.64_b	17.61^{***}	.05
Haven of safety	4.48_b	4.34_b	4.96_c	3.95_a	23.57^{***}	.06
Sexual preferences						
(df = 3, 1,055)						
Promiscuous	1.91_a	2.01_a	2.06_a	2.58_b	9.70^{***}	.03
Normative	5.49_b	5.10_a	$5.40_{a,b}$	5.13_a	5.01^{**}	.01
Affectionate	6.11_c	5.86_b	6.08_c	5.59_a	13.87^{***}	.04
Postcoital emotions						
(df = 3, 698)						
Positive	3.90_a	3.35_b	3.48_b	3.20_b	17.98^{***}	.07
Negative	$.84_a$	1.38_c	$1.22_{b,c}$	1.08_b	15.71^{***}	.06

Note. Numbers in the first four columns are means. Means within each row whose subscripts differ are different at $p < .05$.
$^{**}p < .01$; $^{***}p < .001$ (two-tailed).

cures. Both secure and dismissing individuals scored lower on Anxiety than either fearful or preoccupied individuals; preoccupied individuals scored even higher than fearfuls on the Anxiety scale. These findings suggest, as expected, that Anxiety is similar to Bartholomew's self-model dimension, and Avoidance is similar to her other-model dimension. (See also Griffin & Bartholomew, 1994b; Simpson, Rholes, & Phillips, 1996.)

Bartholomew's secure and preoccupied groups scored similarly on the touch subscales. Both groups scored high on using touch to express affection. Both scored low on the touch aversion scale. The two kinds of avoidants were similarly touch averse. Both avoidant groups reported a moderate amount of touch deficit in their relationships (suggesting that they are not oblivious to such deficits). Preoccupied individuals were most different from Dismissing individuals in using touch to seek care (establish a safe haven) in their relationships. (Dismissing individuals are what Bowlby and many subsequent attachment researchers have called "compulsively self-reliant.") Safe-haven touch was the only scale on which fearful and secure subjects scored similarly—in between preoccupied and dismissing subjects. Finally, preoccupied individuals distinguished themselves by desiring more touch than they were receiving. All of these findings are compatible with previous research and theoretical writings on adult attachment.

In terms of preferences for various sexual behaviors, interesting differences emerged among the four Bartholomew attachment categories. In general, secures, along with preoccupieds, were most likely to endorse romantic/affectionate sexual behaviors. Secures also differed from fearful and dismissing individuals in their preference for "normative" sexual behaviors. Of the four groups, Dismissing individuals were the most likely to endorse promiscuous sexual behavior.

Secures were also more likely than insecures to experience positive emotions, and less likely to experience negative emotions, following sex. Fearful individuals scored highest on the negative emotions scale, followed by preoccupied and then dismissing individuals.

Associations between the New Attachment Categories, Anxiety and Avoidance, and the Touch and Sex Subscales

Three MANOVAs, paralleling the ones just described, were computed on (1) the Anxiety and Avoidance scales, (2) the touch subscales, and (3) the sex subscales as a function of the new cluster-based attachment categories. The first MANOVA on the two higher-order scales was highly significant, as were the MANOVAs on the touch and sex subscales. All of the F values were much higher than the corresponding values based on Bartholomew's categorical self-report measure. The attachment-group means for the two higher-order scales and all of the touch and sex subscales are listed in Table 3.7, along with the univariate Fs. Follow-up Tukey pairwise comparisons were computed to determine which groups differed significantly.

TABLE 3.7. Two New Attachment-Scale Scores and Touch and Sex Subscale Scores as a Function of the Cluster-Based Attachment-Style Category

	Cluster-based attachment-style category					
	Secure	Fearful	Preoccupied	Dismissing	Univariate F	η^2
New scales						
(df = 3, 1,076)						
Avoidance	1.88_a	3.96_c	2.40_b	3.87_c	614.67^{***}	.63
Anxiety	2.64_a	4.06_b	4.60_c	2.60_a	604.41^{***}	.63
Touch						
(df = 3, 1,052)						
Affectionate proximity	6.10_c	5.14_b	6.05_c	4.93_a	104.23^{***}	.23
Desire for more touch	2.07_a	3.34_c	3.16_c	2.43_b	101.70^{***}	.22
Touch aversion	1.80_a	2.86_c	2.17_b	2.78_c	74.42^{***}	.17
Haven of safety	4.67_c	4.22_b	5.00_d	3.72_a	66.95^{***}	.06
Sexual preferences						
(df = 3, 1,055)						
Promiscuous	1.60_a	$2.24_{b,c}$	2.08_b	2.49_c	21.37^{***}	.06
Normative	5.61_b	4.95_a	5.60_b	5.05_a	15.42^{***}	.04
Affectionate	6.25_b	5.75_a	6.11_b	5.66_a	25.17^{***}	.07
Postcoital emotions						
(df = 3, 698)						
Positive	4.16_c	3.08_a	3.57_b	3.29_a	43.80^{***}	.16
Negative	$.68_a$	1.45_c	1.14_b	1.18_b	27.31^{***}	.11

Note. Numbers in the first four columns are means. Means within each row whose subscripts differ are different at $p < .05$.
$^{***}p < .001$ (two-tailed).

The findings for the univariate Avoidance, Anxiety, touch, and sex scales were similar to those obtained with Bartholomew's measure, but the F values were all substantially higher with the new scale-based clusters. (Compare corresponding sections of Tables 3.6 and 3.7—particularly the column showing variance accounted for [η^2].) Also, the pairwise group differences were sharper with the new measure. For example, on the safe-haven touch subscale, all four attachment groups differed using the new measure, whereas secure and fearful groups were indistinguishable when Bartholomew's measure was used.

We also conducted a series of simultaneous regression analyses to examine the ability of the two dimensions, Avoidance and Anxiety, to account for variance in the touch and sex scores. Table 3.8 displays the parameter estimates (η^2s) for predicting the sex and touch scores from the Bartholomew and the new cluster-based measures as well as from the continuous Avoidance and Anxiety scales (R^2s). This time we included the interaction effects produced when each categorical measure was treated as two separate variables—model of self and model of other—as well as the interaction term created by multiplying the Avoidance and Anxiety

TABLE 3.8. Parameter Estimates for the Prediction of Touch and Sex Subscale Scores from Bartholomew's and Cluster-Based Categorical Attachment Measures, and Avoidance and Anxiety Attachment Dimensions

	Bartholomew's measure (η^2)	Cluster-based measure (η^2)	Dimensional measures (R^2)
Touch			
Affectionate proximity	.07	.23	.32
Desire for more touch	.07	.23	.30
Touch aversion	.05	.18	.20
Haven of safety	.06	.16	.26
Sexual preferences			
Promiscuous	.03	.06	.06
Normative	.01	.04	.06
Affectionate	.04	.07	.10
Postcoital emotions			
Positive	.07	.16	.21
Negative	.06	.11	.15
Sum (Σ):	.46	1.24	1.66
Average (M):	.05	.14	.18

Note. Parameter estimates for the categorical measures are η^2s. Parameter estimates for the Avoidance and Anxiety dimensions are R^2s. For the categorical variables, two-way analyses of variance were conducted in which self (positive vs. negative) and other (positive vs. negative) were treated as separate factors. Thus, parameter estimates include variance due to both main effects and the interaction between self and other models. For the dimensional variables, parameter estimates include variance due to both main effects and the interaction between Avoidance and Anxiety.

scores.[4] (The interaction terms for the categorical measures did not generally produce large effects, which is why the overall parameter estimates for the ANOVAs in Table 3.8 are not very different from those reported in Tables 3.6 and 3.7.) Notice in Table 3.8 that the variance accounted for, on average, by the new categorical measure is greater than 2½ times the variance accounted for by Bartholomew's measure. Furthermore, the variance accounted for by the Avoidance and Anxiety scales is over 3½ times as high as that accounted for by Bartholomew's measure, and about one-third higher than that accounted for by the new cluster-based categories. This pattern indicates that the dimensions are more precise than the categories, a conclusion also reached by Fraley and Waller (Chapter 4, this volume).

Finally, we should add that, when factored at the item level, our pool of 323 items produced 12 specific attachment-related dimensions, each with enough high-loading items (viz., 10) to produce reliable unit-weighted scales. Not surprisingly, a higher-order factor analysis of the 12 scales again revealed two underlying dimensions which, when rotated, corresponded to the familiar Avoidance and Anxiety constructs. The 12 scales, which can be viewed as "facets" (Costa & McCrae, 1992) of Avoidance and Anxiety, are as follows: (1) Partner is a Good Attachment Figure; (2) Separation Anxiety; (3) Self-Reliance; (4) Discomfort with Closeness; (5) Attachment-Related Anger at Partners; (6) Uncertainty

About Feelings for Partners; (7) Discomfort with Dependence; (8) Trust; (9) Lovability/Relational Self-Esteem; (10) Desire to Merge with Partners; (11) Tough-Minded Independence; and (12) Fear of Abandonment. These scales are treated in more detail elsewhere (Brennan, Clark, & Shaver, 1996). Here, we mainly want to remind readers that romantic attachment researchers have been measuring a fairly broad array of attachment-related constructs, some of which may be worth highlighting in particular future studies. At a more abstract level, however, these lower-order constructs reduce to the two dimensions of Avoidance and Anxiety.

IMPLICATIONS FOR THE MEASUREMENT OF ADULT ROMANTIC ATTACHMENT

In writing this chapter, we had three purposes in mind. First, we sought to provide a concise overview of issues related to the self-report measurement of adult romantic attachment. Second, we sought to encourage researchers to use a common metric for assessing adult romantic attachment styles. Toward this goal, we offer our two attachment-dimension scales as useful tools for researchers hoping to circumvent the unreliability inherent in single-item response formats. Our scales, Avoidance and Anxiety, have the advantage of being derived from virtually every other extant self-report adult romantic attachment measure. That is, these two dimensions underlie virtually all self-report adult romantic attachment measures and appear crucial for capturing important individual differences in adult romantic attachment. Of course, we are claiming no originality. Our scales are based on other researchers' items (many of them adapted from Hazan & Shaver, 1987), and our conclusions are compatible with those of Simpson (1990), Bartholomew and Horowitz (1991), and others. But our two 18-item scales, having high internal consistency, and being based on a large, comprehensive item pool, may be more precise than previous scales. The two dimensions have the advantage of being analogous to the ones first discovered by Ainsworth and her colleagues (Ainsworth et al., 1978). (As explained earlier in this chapter, Ainsworth et al. were able to distinguish among secure, avoidant, and anxious–ambivalent babies using two discriminant functions, similar to our Avoidance and Anxiety dimensions, formed by the continuous scales used to code infants' behavior in the Strange Situation.)

Third, we sought to define attachment patterns, or styles, in terms of regions in a two-dimensional space. Our two 18-item attachment scales can be used to classify individuals into one of four adult romantic attachment categories. This categorization procedure produces stronger results than Bartholomew's self-classification measure, at least in relation to measures of attachment-related emotions, thoughts, and behaviors regarding touch and sexuality in romantic relationships. We are conducting additional comparisons of the two classification procedures in studies of other topics of interest to attachment researchers—for example, partner abuse, violence in one's family of origin, and relationship-initiation strategies. We want to reiterate, however, that categorization of research participants is unnecessary when dimensional measures are available; and some power and precision are lost when categories rather than continuous scales are used. Given that Fraley and Waller (Chapter 4, this volume) found no evidence for the categorical nature of attachment styles, it is difficult to justify categorical measures except on grounds of convenience.

In this chapter we deliberately side-stepped the issue of self-report versus interview measures of attachment style. Researchers who use interview measures (e.g., Bartholomew & Horowitz, 1991; Main et al., 1985) generally believe that interviews are more powerful and revealing than self-report measures. There are good reasons why they may be correct. Self-report measures are subject to response biases, and they rely on research participants' honesty and self-insight, which are probably limited in any case but especially so when fears and defenses are at issue. It remains to be seen how well the dimensional measures described here stand up in comparisons with interview measures. We think it is possible that the increased precision we have demonstrated in relation to Bartholomew's self-classification measure will make our dimensional measures more similar to interviews. (See Bartholomew & Shaver, Chapter 2, this volume, for a discussion of the importance of precision and statistical power in revealing weak but valid associations.) Further, our longer-than-usual scales may circumvent some of the temptation toward biased responding aroused by simple measures that require people to say fairly directly whether they are or are not secure. It is worth noting that self-report measures of attachment, like interview measures, do not require that people understand or probe into their own dynamics and defenses. Self-report measures require only a modicum of familiarity with one's own feelings, social behavior, and beliefs about relationships and the feedback one has received from relationship partners. It is possible to classify people on these grounds without them understanding their own histories or dynamics.

Looking ahead to the next decade of research on romantic attachment, we are cautiously optimistic. We are cautious because of the field's continuing lack of convergence on a common, reliable method for assessing adult attachment orientations. A common method is necessary if researchers are to communicate clearly with each other about the same constructs, if neophyte researchers are to enter the field relatively easily and quickly, and if all researchers are to move on to substantive issues rather than remaining hung up on psychometric ones. We are optimistic because of the remarkable strides made in the previous decade and because there is more commonality underlying different research procedures than might have been expected. We have shown here, in line with previous work by Simpson, Bartholomew, and their coauthors, that everyone is working with the same two dimensions that Ainsworth and her colleagues identified in 1978: Avoidance and Anxiety. The origins and implications of people's scores on those dimensions are what all attachment researchers deal with, whether knowingly or not.

Appendix 3.1

MULTI-ITEM MEASURE OF ADULT ROMANTIC ATTACHMENT

EXPERIENCES IN CLOSE RELATIONSHIPS

Instructions: The following statements concern how you feel in romantic relationships. We are interested in how you generally experience relationships, not just in what is happening in a current relationship. Respond to each statement by indicating how much you agree or disagree with it. Write the number in the space provided, using the following rating scale:

Disagree strongly			Neutral/mixed			Agree strongly
1	2	3	4	5	6	7

___ 1. I prefer not to show a partner how I feel deep down.
___ 2. I worry about being abandoned.
___ 3. I am very comfortable being close to romantic partners.
___ 4. I worry a lot about my relationships.
___ 5. Just when my partner starts to get close to me I find myself pulling away.
___ 6. I worry that romantic partners won't care about me as much as I care about them.
___ 7. I get uncomfortable when a romantic partner wants to be very close.
___ 8. I worry a fair amount about losing my partner.
___ 9. I don't feel comfortable opening up to romantic partners.
___ 10. I often wish that my partner's feelings for me were as strong as my feelings for him/her.
___ 11. I want to get close to my partner, but I keep pulling back.
___ 12. I often want to merge completely with romantic partners, and this sometimes scares them away.
___ 13. I am nervous when partners get too close to me.
___ 14. I worry about being alone.
___ 15. I feel comfortable sharing my private thoughts and feelings with my partner.
___ 16. My desire to be very close sometimes scares people away.
___ 17. I try to avoid getting too close to my partner.
___ 18. I need a lot of reassurance that I am loved by my partner.
___ 19. I find it relatively easy to get close to my partner.
___ 20. Sometimes I feel that I force my partners to show more feeling, more commitment.

___ 21. I find it difficult to allow myself to depend on romantic partners.
___ 22. I do not often worry about being abandoned.
___ 23. I prefer not to be too close to romantic partners.
___ 24. If I can't get my partner to show interest in me, I get upset or angry.
___ 25. I tell my partner just about everything.
___ 26. I find that my partner(s) don't want to get as close as I would like.
___ 27. I usually discuss my problems and concerns with my partner.
___ 28. When I'm not involved in a relationship, I feel somewhat anxious and insecure.
___ 29. I feel comfortable depending on romantic partners.
___ 30. I get frustrated when my partner is not around as much as I would like.
___ 31. I don't mind asking romantic partners for comfort, advice, or help.
___ 32. I get frustrated if romantic partners are not available when I need them.
___ 33. It helps to turn to my romantic partner in times of need.
___ 34. When romantic partners disapprove of me, I feel really bad about myself.
___ 35. I turn to my partner for many things, including comfort and reassurance.
___ 36. I resent it when my partner spends time away from me.

Appendix 3.2

ATTACHMENT SCALES AND SCORING INSTRUCTIONS FOR TWO HIGHER-ORDER ATTACHMENT DIMENSION SCALES

AVOIDANCE (alpha = .94)

Item#	Item–Total Correlation	Item
1.	.73	I prefer not to show a partner how I feel deep down.
3.	.71	I am very comfortable being close to romantic partners. (R)
5.	.70	Just when my partner starts to get close to me I find myself pulling away.
7.	.70	I get uncomfortable when a romantic partner wants to be very close.
9.	.69	I don't feel comfortable opening up to romantic partners.
11.	.68	I want to get close to my partner, but I keep pulling back.
13.	.68	I am nervous when partners get too close to me.
15.	.68	I feel comfortable sharing my private thoughts and feelings with my partner. (R)
17.	.68	I try to avoid getting too close to my partner.
19.	.67	I find it relatively easy to get close to my partner. (R)
21.	.67	I find it difficult to allow myself to depend on romantic partners.
23.	.65	I prefer not to be too close to romantic partners.

25.	.64	I tell my partner just about everything. (R)
27.	.64	I usually discuss my problems and concerns with my partner. (R)
29.	.64	I feel comfortable depending on romantic partners. (R)
31.	.63	I don't mind asking romantic partners for comfort, advice, or help. (R)
33.	.62	It helps to turn to my romantic partner in times of need. (R)
35.	.60	I turn to my partner for many things, including comfort and reassurance. (R)

ANXIETY (alpha = .91)

Item#	Item–Total Correlation	Item
2.	.67	I worry about being abandoned.
4.	.65	I worry a lot about my relationships.
6.	.65	I worry that romantic partners won't care about me as much as I care about them.
8.	.63	I worry a fair amount about losing my partner.
10.	.62	I often wish that my partner's feelings for me were as strong as my feelings for him/her.
12.	.60	I often want to merge completely with romantic partners, and this sometimes scares them away.
14.	.60	I worry about being alone.
16.	.57	My desire to be very close sometimes scares people away.
18.	.56	I need a lot of reassurance that I am loved by my partner.
20.	.55	Sometimes I feel that I force my partners to show more feeling, more commitment.
22.	.54	I do not often worry about being abandoned. (R)
24.	.52	If I can't get my partner to show interest in me, I get upset or angry.
26.	.52	I find that my partner(s) don't want to get as close as I would like.
28.	.51	When I'm not involved in a relationship, I feel somewhat anxious and insecure.
30.	.51	I get frustrated when my partner is not around as much as I would like.
32.	.51	I get frustrated if romantic partners are not available when I need them.
34.	.50	When romantic partners disapprove of me, I feel really bad about myself.
36.	.50	I resent it when my partner spends time away from me.

SPSS-PC SCORING INSTRUCTIONS

STEP 1: Recode the reversed variables, such that 1 = 7, 2 = 6, and so on. You may want to create temporary variables, which can be reversed without potentially incorrectly transforming the original data. (We computed "temp3" for item number 3, etc., for use in scoring below.)

Compute temp 3 = A3.
Compute temp15 = A15.
Compute temp19 = A19.
Compute temp25 = A25.
Compute temp27 = A27.
Compute temp29 = A29.
Compute temp31 = A31.
Compute temp33 = A33.
Compute temp35 = A35.
Compute temp22 = A22.
Recode temp3 to temp22 (1=7) (2=6) (3=5) (5=3) (6=2) (7=1).

STEP 2: Compute scores for the two dimensions, avoidance and anxiety.

Compute AVOIDANC = mean.14(A1,temp3,A5,A7,A9, A11,A13,temp15,A17, temp19,A21,A23,temp25,temp27,temp29,temp31,temp33,temp35).

Compute ANXIETY = mean.14(A2,A4,A6,A8,A10,A12, A14,A16,A18,A20, temp22,A24,A26,A28,A30,A32,A34,A36).

STEP 3: Compute attachment-style categories from the classification coefficients (Fisher's linear discriminant functions) based on our sample of n = 1,082.

Compute SEC2 = avoidanc*3.2893296 + anxiety*5.4725318 − 11.5307833.
Compute FEAR2 = avoidanc*7.2371075 + anxiety*8.1776446 − 32.3553266.
Compute PRE2 = avoidanc*3.9246754 + anxiety*9.7102446 − 28.4573220.
Compute DIS2 = avoidanc*7.3654621 + anxiety*4.9392039 − 22.2281088.

Variable Labels
   sec2 "coeff secure dimension"
   fear2 "coeff fearful dimension"
   pre2 "coeff preoccupied dimension"
   dis2 "coeff dismissing dimension."

If (sec2 > max(fear2,pre2,dis2)) ATT2 = 1.
If (fear2 > max(sec2,pre2,dis2)) ATT2 = 2.
If (pre2 > max(sec2,fear2,dis2)) ATT2 = 3.
If (dis2 > max(sec2,fear2,pre2)) ATT2 = 4.

Variable labels
   ATT2 "coefficient-based attachment category."

Value labels
   ATT2 1 "secure" 2 "fearful" 3 "preocc" 4 "dismiss"

NOTES

1. We modified the instructions for the Bartholomew and Horowitz (1991) attachment measure to make it refer specifically to *romantic* relationships: "Read each of the four self-descriptions below and place a check mark next to the single alternative that best describes how you usually act and feel in romantic relation-

ships or that comes nearest to describing you." In our close relationship version, the word "romantic" was replaced with "close." Both measures included the following four options: *Secure*: "It is easy for me to become emotionally close to others. I am comfortable depending on others and having others depend on me. I don't worry about being alone or having others not accept me." *Fearful*: "I am uncomfortable getting close to others. I want emotionally close relationships, but I find it difficult to trust others completely, or to depend on them. I worry that I will be hurt if I allow myself to become too close to others." *Preoccupied*: "I want to be completely emotionally intimate with others, but I often find that others are reluctant to get as close as I would like. I am uncomfortable being without close relationships, but I sometimes worry that others don't value me as much as I value them." *Dismissing*: "I am comfortable without close emotional relationships. It is very important to me to feel independent and self-sufficient, and I prefer not to depend on others or have others depend on me." (The romantic and peer measures were highly associated, $\chi^2[9] = 1049.07$, $p < .0001$, as Bartholomew expected when she decided to use one wording to apply to all close relationships with peers, whether romantic or not.)

2. We actually conducted the factor analyses twice, once in each of two halves of the sample. The results were virtually identical (the same two factors, with the same items loading on each factor in almost exactly the same order), so here we present only the results for the sample as a whole.

3. The number of people who are "truly" secure or insecure is something that cannot be stated firmly. The Adult Attachment Interview (Main et al., 1985) tends to place around 65% of adults into the secure category because it was designed to predict the Strange Situation classification of subjects' 12-month-old children. Ainsworth originally said that around 65% of middle-class American infants were secure (based on the scoring criteria she invented). Bartholomew's adaptation of the AAI procedure for assessing adult attachment to peers and romantic partners (Bartholomew & Horowitz, 1991) tends to label around 45% of college students as secure. This is simply a function of how she instructs coders to identify security. Hazan and Shaver's (1987, 1990) simple three-category measure results in around 55% of college students and nonstudent adults calling themselves secure. The cluster analysis reported here, based on scales whose items refer mainly to nuances of insecurity (Anxiety and Avoidance), places relatively few people in the secure category, with good effects on analyses to be reported later. But Fraley and Waller (Chapter 4, this volume) suggest that all such category breaks are somewhat arbitrary, given that there are no clear or natural category boundaries between attachment styles.

4. For each categorical measure, models of self and other were computed as follows. Model of *self* was coded as 1 for individuals with secure or dismissing attachment styles, and coded as 0 for those with fearful or preoccupied attachment styles. Model of *other* was coded as 1 for those with secure or preoccupied attachment styles, and as 0 for those with dismissing or fearful attachment styles. The two resulting variables—self and other—were then treated as grouping variables (with two levels each) in a two-way analysis of variance.

REFERENCES

Ainsworth, M. S., Blehar, M. C., Waters, E., & Wall, S. (1978). *Patterns of attachment: A psychological study of the Strange Situation.* Hillsdale, NJ: Erlbaum.

Armsden, G. C., & Greenberg, M. T. (1987). The inventory of parent and peer attachment: Individual differences and their relationship to psychological well-being in adolescence. *Journal of Youth and Adolescence, 16*, 427–454.

Bartholomew, K. (1990). Avoidance of intimacy: An attachment perspective. *Journal of Social and Personal Relationships, 7*, 147–178.

Bartholomew, K., & Horowitz, L. M. (1991). Attachment styles among young adults: A test of a four-category model. *Journal of Personality and Social Psychology, 61*, 226–244.

Brennan, K. A., Clark, C. L., & Shaver, P. R. (1996, August). *Development of a new multi-item measure of adult romantic attachment: A preliminary report.* Paper presented at the meeting of the International Society for the Study of Personal Relationships, Banff, Alberta, Canada.

Brennan, K. A., & Shaver, P. R. (1995). Dimensions of adult attachment, affect regulation, and romantic relationship functioning. *Personality and Social Psychology Bulletin, 21*, 267–283.

Brennan, K. A., Shaver, P. R., & Tobey, A. E. (1991). Attachment styles, gender, and parental problem drinking. *Journal of Social and Personal Relationships, 8*, 451–466.

Carnelley, K., Pietromonaco, P., & Jaffe, K. (1994). Depression, working models of others, and relationship functioning. *Journal of Personality and Social Psychology, 66*, 127–140.

Carver, C. S. (1994). *Personality and adult attachment.* Unpublished manuscript, University of Miami, Coral Gables, FL.

Collins, N. L., & Read., S. J. (1990). Adult attachment, working models, and relationship quality in dating couples. *Journal of Personality and Social Psychology, 58*, 644–663.

Costa, P. T., Jr., & McCrae, R. (1992). *Revised NEO Personality Inventory: NEO-PI and NEO Five-Factor Inventory* (Professional manual). Odessa, FL: Psychological Assessment Resources.

Crittenden, P. M. (1988). Relationships at risk. In J. Belsky & T. Nezworski (Eds.), *Clinical implications of attachment* (pp. 136–174). Hillsdale, NJ: Erlbaum.

Feeney, J. A., Noller, P., & Hanrahan, M. (1994). Assessing adult attachment. In M. B. Sperling & W. H. Berman (Eds.), *Attachment in adults: Clinical and developmental perspectives* (pp. 128–152). New York: Guilford Press.

Griffin, D., & Bartholomew, K. (1994a). The metaphysics of measurement: The case of adult attachment. In K. Bartholomew & D. Perlman (Eds.), *Advances in personal relationships: Vol. 5. Attachment processes in adulthood* (pp. 17–52). London: Jessica Kingsley.

Griffin, D., & Bartholomew, K. (1994b). Models of the self and other: Fundamental dimensions underlying measures of adult attachment. *Journal of Personality and Social Psychology, 67*, 430–445.

Hair, J. F., Anderson, R. E., Tatham, R. L., & Black, W. C. (1995). *Multivariate data analysis, with readings* (4th ed.). Englewood Cliffs, NJ: Prentice-Hall.

Hatfield, E. (1993, October). *Varieties of romantic attachment.* Paper presented at the annual meeting of the Society of Experimental Social Psychology, Santa Barbara, CA.

Hazan, C., & Shaver, P. (1987). Romantic love conceptualized as an attachment process. *Journal of Personality and Social Psychology, 52*, 511–524.

Hazan, C., & Shaver, P. R. (1990). Love and work: An attachment-theoretical perspective. *Journal of Personality and Social Psychology, 59*, 270–280.

Hazan, C., Zeifman, D., & Middleton, K. (1994, July). *Adult romantic attachment, affection, and sex.* Paper presented at the Seventh International Conference on Personal Relationships, Groningen, The Netherlands.

Hindy, C. G., Schwartz, J. C., & Brodsky, A. (1989). *If this is love, why do I feel so insecure?* New York: Atlantic Monthly Press.

Janus, S. S., & Janus, C. L. (1993). *The Janus report on sexual behavior.* New York: Wiley.

Latty-Mann, H., & Davis, K. E. (1996). Attachment theory and partner choice: Preference and actuality. *Journal of Social and Personal Relationships, 13,* 5–23.

Laumann, E. O., Gagnon, J. H., Michael, R. T., & Michaels, S. (1994). *The social organization of sexuality: Sexual practices in the United States.* Chicago: University of Chicago Press.

Levy, M. B., & Davis, K. E. (1988). Lovestyles and attachment styles compared: Their relations to each other and to various relationship characteristics. *Journal of Social and Personal Relationships, 5,* 439–471.

Main, M. (1990). Parental aversion to infant-initiated contact is correlated with the parent's own rejection during childhood: The effects of experience on signals of security with respect to attachment. In K. E. Barnard & T. B. Brazelton (Eds.), *Touch: The foundation of experience* (pp. 461–495). Madison, CT: International Universities Press.

Main, M., Kaplan, N., & Cassidy, J. (1985). Security in infancy, childhood, and adulthood: A move to the level of representation. In I. Bretherton & E. Waters (Eds.), Growing points in attachment theory and research. *Monographs of the Society for Research in Child Development, 50*(1–2, Serial No. 209), 66–106.

Main, M., & Solomon, J. (1990). Procedures for identifying insecure-disorganized/disoriented infants: Procedures, findings, and implications for the classification of behavior. In M. Greenberg, D. Cicchetti, & M. Cummings (Eds.), *Attachment in the preschool years: Theory, research, and intervention* (pp. 121–160). Chicago, IL: University of Chicago Press.

Onishi, M., & Gjerde, P. F. (1994). *Adult attachment styles: A multi-method examination of personality characteristics.* Paper presented at the biennial meeting of the International Society for the Study of Behavioral Development, Amsterdam, The Netherlands.

Rothbard, J. C., Roberts, L. J., Leonard, K. E., & Eiden, R. D. (1993, August). *Attachment styles and marital interaction behavior.* Paper presented at the annual meeting of the American Psychological Association, Toronto, Ontario.

Scharfe, E. (1996). *A test of Bartholomew's four-category model of attachment in a clinical sample of adolescents.* Unpublished doctoral dissertation, Department of Psychology, Simon Fraser University, Burnaby, British Columbia.

Scharfe, E., & Bartholomew, K. (1994). Reliability and stability of adult attachment patterns. *Personal Relationships, 1,* 23–43.

Shaver, P. R. (1995). *Additional items to measure dismissing avoidance.* Unpublished technical memorandum, Department of Psychology, University of California, Davis.

Shaver, P. R., Hazan, C., & Bradshaw, D. (1988). Love as attachment: The integration of three behavioral systems. In R. J. Sternberg & M. Barnes (Eds.), *The psychology of love* (pp. 68–99). New Haven, CT: Yale University Press.

Simpson, J. A. (1990). Influence of attachment styles on romantic relationships. *Journal of Personality and Social Psychology, 59,* 971–980.

Simpson, J. A., Rholes, W. S., & Nelligan, J. S. (1992). Support-seeking and support-giving within couple members in an anxiety-provoking situation: The role of attachment styles. *Journal of Personality and Social Psychology, 62,* 434–446.

Simpson, J. A., Rholes, W. S., & Phillips, D. (1996). Conflict in close relationships: An attachment perspective. *Journal of Personality and Social Psychology, 71,* 799–914.

Sperling, M. B., Berman, W. H., & Fagen, G. (1992). Classification of adult attachment: An integrative taxonomy from attachment and psychoanalytic theories. *Journal of Personality Assessment, 59,* 239–247.

van IJzendoorn, M. H. (1995). Adult attachment representations, parental responsiveness, and infant attachment: A meta-analysis on the predictive validity of the Adult Attachment Interview. *Psychological Bulletin, 117,* 387–403.

Wagner, L., & Vaux, A. (1994, May). *The Wagner Attachment Scale (WAS): Reliability and validity of a self-report measure of adult attachment.* Paper presented at the annual meeting of the Midwestern Psychological Association, Chicago.

West, M. L., & Sheldon-Keller, A. E. (1994). *Patterns of relating: An adult attachment perspective.* New York: Guilford Press.

4

Adult Attachment Patterns

A Test of the Typological Model

R. CHRIS FRALEY
NIELS G. WALLER

Although attachment researchers have favored typological models when assessing individual differences in infant and adult attachment patterns (Ainsworth, Blehar, Waters, & Wall, 1978; Bartholomew & Horowitz, 1991; George, Kaplan, & Main, 1985; Hazan & Shaver, 1987; Sroufe & Waters, 1977), they have devoted little attention to assessing the validity of the typological approach. When typological models are valid they provide information that cannot be obtained from dimensional models, such as group membership probabilities, latent base rates of types, and indicator specificity and sensitivity rates (Meehl, 1995). When they are not valid, however, unfortunate problems can arise that serve to undermine the research enterprise—such as reductions in statistical power (Cohen, 1988), decreases in scale reliability (Cohen, 1983), the spurious overestimation (Maxwell & Delaney, 1993) and underestimation (Cohen, 1983) of empirical relationships, and the inability to uncover nonlinear relationships with other variables (Tellegen & Lubinski, 1983).

Because attachment theory has the potential to integrate a diverse set of findings in the fields of close relationships and personality (see Hazan & Shaver, 1994), it is important to ensure that the measurement models used by adult attachment researchers are as powerful as possible. Therefore, the primary goal of the present chapter is to determine whether adult attachment patterns are more indicative of latent types or latent dimensions. To achieve this goal, we analyze attachment data from a large sample (n = 639) of young adults using several taxometric procedures (MAMBAC and MAXCOV-HITMAX) that were developed by Paul Meehl and his colleagues (Meehl, 1995; Meehl & Golden, 1982; Meehl & Yonce, 1994; Waller & Meehl, in press). In doing so, we hope to resolve the types versus dimensions debate in adult attachment research and provide recommendations for both the conceptualization and measurement of adult attachment. We begin the chapter by reviewing the status of typological approaches in attachment research and in psychological research more broadly. Next, we review procedures that have traditionally been used to validate categorical models in the social sciences and we discuss limitations of these approaches for corroborating typological or dimensional models. As an alternative to these procedures, we describe taxometric techniques for distinguishing latent types (classes, natural kinds, taxa) from latent continua (dimensions, factors). Next, we review arguments for the taxonic and dimensional models of attachment security. Because both models can be theoretically justified, we apply our taxometric procedures to a large sample of adult attachment data to determine which approach is best supported by the data. Finally, we discuss the implications of our findings for advancing knowledge on adult attachment phenomena.

THE TYPOLOGICAL CONCEPTUALIZATION AND MEASUREMENT OF ATTACHMENT STYLES

Infants and Children

The typological conceptualization and measurement of adult attachment stems from Ainsworth's (Ainsworth & Bell, 1970; Ainsworth, Blehar, Waters, & Wall, 1978) ground-breaking research on infant attachment behavior. In this research, Ainsworth examined the infant's use of its mother as a *secure base* from which to explore the environment (Blatz, 1966; Bowlby, 1969/1982). Ainsworth found that an infant's desire to explore the environment is facilitated by the knowledge that it can return to a secure "home base" if necessary (Ainsworth, 1967). Thus, if exploration results in undue anxiety, secure infants can easily seek a parent for comfort, reassurance, and safety. However, when an infant lacks basic trust in the availability of its attachment figures, it is less likely to venture out into the world, preferring to stay close to its caregivers (Ainsworth, 1967).

Both Ainsworth (1967) and Bowlby (1969/1982, 1973) have argued that an infant's sense of trust regarding the availability and responsiveness of its caregivers is a fairly accurate reflection of the interactions that have occurred between the infant and its caregivers. According to Bowlby (1973), when these interactions are characterized by warmth and support, the child learns that he or she can count on others when needed. Alternatively, when these interactions are characterized by distrust and rejection, the child learns that he or she cannot rely on others. These expectations, or *working models*, are theorized to play a critical role in the strategies and goals adopted by the child to regulate his or her emotions and social behaviors.

In an influential study providing empirical support for Bowlby's arguments, Ainsworth and her colleagues (1978) demonstrated an association between the sensitivity of maternal behavior in an infant's first year of life and the subsequent organization of the infant's attachment behavior at 12 months of age. Using the Strange Situation, a procedure developed to examine the interplay between attachment and exploration in a controlled laboratory setting (Ainsworth et al., 1978; Ainsworth & Wittig, 1969), Ainsworth and her colleagues proposed three primary patterns of attachment organization: insecure–avoidant (Group A), secure (Group B), and insecure–resistant or anxious–ambivalent (Group C). In this study, infants who were classified as secure (Group B) were confident in their exploration of the laboratory environment and sought the comfort of their mothers when distressed. In general, these infants had mothers who had been rated as more sensitive and responsive in home observations in the year before the laboratory visit. Infants who were classified as insecure–avoidant (Group A) generally did not seek the comfort of their mothers when distressed. Instead, they tended to look away from their mothers—that is, to avoid them—and they failed to respond to their mother's attempts to reestablish communication. Infants who were classified as anxious–ambivalent (Group C) were less comfortable exploring the laboratory and tended to maintain a high degree of proximity to their mothers. Furthermore, these infants exhibited a mixture of anger and contact-seeking when their mothers attempted to comfort them. Home observations prior to the laboratory visit suggested that the mothers of these infants were often unresponsive or inconsistently available.

Ainsworth et al. (1978, pp. 55–64) argued that these disparate behavioral patterns constituted qualitatively different classes of attachment organization.[1] As evidence for the validity of this approach, Ainsworth et al. (1978, pp. 95–115) presented the results of a multiple discriminant function analysis to show that the qualitative infant attachment classifications could be accurately predicted from two linear composites of quantitative behavioral codes (see also Brennan, Clark, & Shaver, Chapter 3, this volume). Although Ainsworth and her colleagues extensively explored the quantitative dimensions, which were derived from the protocols and the discriminant function analysis, they decided to retain the classification system in their major conceptual and statistical analyses for three reasons. First, they felt that the "classificatory groups [help] retain the picture of patterns of behavior, which tend to become lost in—or at least difficult to retrieve from—the quantification process" (p. 57). Second, they suggested that it "would be foolish to believe that the dimensions that we have so far subjected to quantification take into account all the behaviors that are important components to the patterning of individual differences. . . . To abandon the classificatory system in favor of our present set of component behavioral scores . . . would freeze our knowledge in its present state" (p. 57). Third, they felt that "the patternings described and differentiated within a classificatory system keep [the issue of developmental origins] to the forefront rather than burying it in a welter of refined statistics" (p. 57).

Consistent with this theoretical orientation, Ainsworth and her colleagues adopted and advocated a threefold typological model of attachment. This three-category model has subsequently become the standard for researchers investigating attachment in infancy and early childhood (Sroufe, 1990). Efforts to extend this model have, for the most part, involved adding categories (such as Crittenden's [1988] *A-C type* or Main & Solomon's [1986] *D* or *disorganized-disoriented type*) rather than testing the validity of the typological approach. Moreover, when dimensional measures have been used to assess attachment patterns (e.g., Cummings, 1990; Waters & Deane, 1985), they have sometimes been used to classify individuals into attachment categories (Howes & Hamilton, 1992). Furthermore, attempts to treat attachment patterns as continuously distributed constructs have been met with considerable skepticism (e.g., Colin, 1996).

Adolescents and Adults

The influence of Ainsworth's categorical model has been extensive, as can be seen in any introductory textbook on general, developmental, social, or personality psychology. Accordingly, when Hazan and Shaver (1987; Shaver, Hazan, & Bradshaw, 1988) began their influential work on adult romantic attachment, they adopted Ainsworth's threefold typology as a framework for conceptualizing individual differences in the way adults think, feel, and behave in intimate relationships. In their initial study, Hazan and Shaver (1987) developed paragraph-long descriptions of each of the three attachment types—avoidant, secure, and anxious–ambivalent—to assess working models of attachment in adulthood. These descriptions were subsequently given to participants who were asked to choose the paragraph that best described their approach to romantic relationships.

Many researchers quickly adopted Hazan and Shaver's categorical measure, largely because of its brevity and ease of administration (Baldwin, Fehr, Keedian, Seidel, & Thomson, 1993; Doherty, Hatfield, Thompson, & Choo, 1994; Feeney & Noller, 1990; Kirkpatrick & Davis,

1994; Kirkpatrick & Hazan, 1994; Mikulincer, Florian, & Tolmacz, 1990; Mikulincer, Florian, & Weller, 1993; Mikulincer & Nachshon, 1991; Mikulincer & Orbach, 1995; Pietromonaco & Carnelley, 1994; Sprecher et al., 1994). Nevertheless, a few researchers quickly recognized the limitations of this measure (Collins & Read, 1990; Hazan & Shaver, 1987; Simpson, 1990). For instance, some authors noted that the categorical nature of the instrument (1) assumes that each attachment style is independent of the others, (2) does not allow one to assess the degree to which each style is characteristic of an individual, and (3) does not allow one to estimate measurement error.

To address these issues, attachment researchers soon began to use continuous rating scales in their assessments. For example, in 1988, Levy and Davis asked participants to rate the degree to which each attachment type was characteristic of their relationship experiences and feelings. A few years later, Collins and Read (1990) and Simpson (1990) deconstructed Hazan and Shaver's three paragraph descriptions into multiple items that could be individually rated. More recently, several authors have developed scales to assess dimensions (Brennan & Shaver, 1995; Feeney, Noller, & Hanrahan, 1994; Griffin & Bartholomew, 1994b).

The move from single-item to multi-item rating scales represents an important step in increasing measurement precision. Nevertheless, many of the authors of these scales have explicitly discouraged researchers from abandoning typological models of attachment (Brennan & Shaver, 1995; Collins & Read, 1990; Hazan & Shaver, 1987; Simpson, 1990). In some cases, the continuously scaled scores are only used to validate the categories (Mikulincer, Florian, & Weller, 1993; Mikulincer & Orbach, 1995) or to assign individuals to the categories (Collins & Read, 1990; Feeney & Kirkpatrick, 1996).

Interestingly, in parallel with the childhood attachment literature, recent discussion on individual differences in adult attachment has focused on the *number* of types (Bartholomew & Horowitz, 1991; Feeney et al., 1994; Hazan & Shaver, 1994; Latty-Mann & Davis, 1996; Sperling & Berman, 1994) rather than the validity of the typological approach itself (but, see Griffin and Bartholomew, 1994a, for a notable exception). For example, Latty-Mann and Davis (1996) proposed an *ambivalent* attachment type as an addition to the Hazan and Shaver three-group typology. Sperling, Berman, and Fagen (1992) offered a four-group typology based on their clinical experience. Their model includes *dependent, avoidant, hostile,* and *resistant–ambivalent* attachment styles.

In one of the most influential revisions of the tripartite typology, Bartholomew proposed a four-category model (Bartholomew, 1990; Bartholomew & Horowitz, 1991). According to this model, the four categories—*secure, fearful, preoccupied,* and *dismissing*—are located in a two-dimensional space defined by *anxiety* and *avoidance* (see also Brennan et al., Chapter 3, this volume). Researchers who have adopted Bartholomew's model typically classify individuals into one of these categories (Bartholomew & Horowitz, 1991; Brennan, Shaver, & Tobey, 1991; Shaver et al., 1996) and/or use the continuous ratings to assess the degree to which individuals fit each type (Bartholomew & Horowitz, 1991; Griffin & Bartholomew, 1994b; Shaver et al., 1996).

Bartholomew's model, combined with an emerging consensus that two latent dimensions underlie Hazan and Shaver's (1987) and Bartholomew's (1990) attachment types (see Feeney & Noller, 1996; Griffin & Bartholomew, 1994a, 1994b; Hazan & Shaver, 1994), has encouraged researchers to use continuous measures. Nevertheless, there has yet to be a solid resolution to the types versus dimensions issue. Consequently, the measurement models adopted by attachment researchers are often based on convenience, convention, or fiat, rather than rigorous empirical or psychometric investigation.

THE CONCEPTUALIZATION AND
MEASUREMENT OF TYPES IN PSYCHOLOGY

The typological approach in infant and adult attachment research has enjoyed a lengthy and productive history. The popularity of the categorical model in this domain is somewhat unusual, however, because typological constructs have generally played only a minor or an ambiguous role in American psychology. This is unfortunate because typological models, when appropriately used, can make substantial contributions to psychological knowledge (Meehl, 1995). We believe that the ambiguous role of types in psychology can be attributed to popular misconceptions about the nature of types. These misconceptions, in turn, have led psychologists to use inadequate methods to test taxonic hypotheses. Below, we discuss some common misunderstandings concerning the nature of types and explain why popular methods for testing taxonic hypotheses are insufficient.

Misunderstandings about Types

Meehl (1992, 1995) has argued that much of the bias and confusion regarding types can be attributed to popular misconceptions about types. According to Meehl, many psychologists conceive of categories as arbitrary matters of semantic convenience and not reflections, to borrow from Plato, of nature's true joints. Although it is often the case that categorical designations are used as convenient labels in the social sciences (e.g., *introvert, repressor, intelligent*), being derived from arbitrary cutting procedures (e.g., median-splits, quartile-splits, conventional cut-points), it does not follow that all psychological categories are necessarily arbitrary. *We believe that whether an individual or behavior belongs to a taxon is a question that cannot—and should not—be resolved through social convention or convenience.*

Meehl also cites the nearly ubiquitous and fallacious belief that categorical variables require sharp distinctions or clear-cut boundaries in their manifest indicators (Meehl, 1995, pg. 268–269). *This misunderstanding reflects a common confusion among social scientists between the patterning of manifest indicators and the patterning of the latent constructs they indicate.* The patterning or distribution of the manifest indicators of a latent qualitative variable can be qualitative *or* quantitative. For instance, Down syndrome has a clear qualitative etiology being the result of a specific chromosomal defect (i.e., an extra Chromosome 21). Nevertheless, the distribution of IQ scores in mixed samples of persons with and without Down syndrome is continuous. This illustrates that one would be taking a serious risk by making inferences about the distribution of a latent variable solely on the basis of the distribution of its manifestations.

The important point here is that one should not reject a taxonic hypothesis about a construct because the distribution of its indicators is not bimodal. Similarly, one should not accept a taxonic hypothesis simply because the distribution of indicators is bimodal. Bimodality is a *strong* indication of taxonicity (although see Grayson, 1987); however, it is neither a necessary nor sufficient condition (see Murphy, 1964, for mathematical justification of this point). The data presented in Panel A of Figure 4.1 illustrate this point. These data were generated from a latent taxonic model. Notice that the histograms for the variables labeled x and y are well approximated by the bell-shaped curve that we have superimposed on them. Although the means for the two latent groups are separated by two within-group standard deviations on the manifest indicators, the histograms are not noticeably bimodal. Compare these data with those in Panel B, which were generated from a latent dimensional model. Notice that the histograms and scatterplots in the two panels are highly similar. Even an astute observer will note that the borders between the two classes in the taxonic case (shown in Panel A) are "fuzzy," at best.[2] Clearly, a simple examination of the indicator distributions cannot distinguish the taxonic from the dimensional data.[3]

Measurement Procedures Traditionally Used to Validate Typological Models

As we noted earlier, it is critical to distinguish between manifest, observable behaviors and the latent entities that influence those behaviors. Although the manifest–latent distinction has enjoyed quite a bit of popularity since Freud (e.g., Freud, 1900/1953), modern psychologists often disregard this distinction when discussing and testing typological theories. For instance, the most popular methods for 'validating' categorical or taxonic models in psychology are multiple discriminant function analysis (MDFA; Tatsuoska, 1970) and clustering algorithms (Everitt, 1974). These procedures are called *phenetic methods* because they are used to infer characteristics of manifest

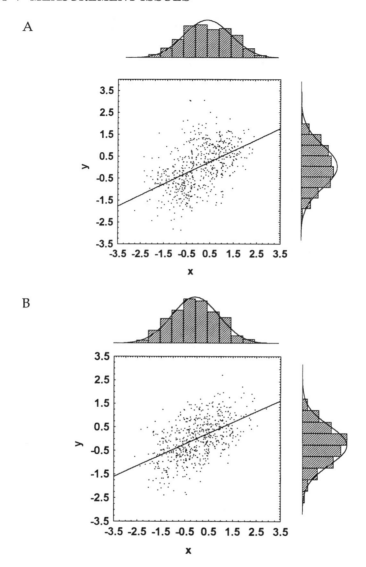

FIGURE 4.1. Panel A represents data that were generated from a latent taxonic model in which the proportion of taxon members, *p*, was .5. Panel B represents data in which the indicators have the same characteristics as those in Panel A (same means and correlations) but were generated from a latent dimensional model. It is noteworthy that a simple examination of the manifest characteristics of each data set does not allow one to determine the latent structure of the construct.

indicators rather than the latent sources of those indicators. Phenetic methods are useful for reducing complex multivariate relations, but they are inappropriate for *testing* taxometric theories.

Specifically, discriminant function analysis and cluster analysis seek to maximize within-group phenetic similarity and between-group phenetic dissimilarity. In the former case, the groups are specified *a priori*. In the latter case, the typological structure is imposed on the data. For instance, cluster algorithms often find easily interpretable clusters—even with dimensional data. Therefore, cluster analysis does not allow researchers to "rigorously" test taxonic conjectures.[4]

By relying on these phenetic methods, attachment researchers have implicitly focused on the patterning of observable behaviors (Ainsworth et al., 1978; Bartholomew & Horowitz, 1991; Collins & Read, 1990; Feeney et al., 1994; Hazan & Shaver, 1987; Mikulincer & Orbach, 1995; Richters, Waters, & Vaughn, 1988; Van Dam & van IJzendoorn, 1988). However, as exemplified by Ainsworth's concern with developmental origins, the conclusions we often want to draw as scientists concern the *sources* of those behavioral patterns rather than the behaviors themselves. To make meaningful inferences about latent sources of manifest patterns, we need methods that go beyond phenetic similarities. Fortunately, procedures have been developed that allow investigators to test the validity of taxonic conjectures. These procedures are called *taxometric techniques* (Meehl, 1995; Waller & Meehl, in press). Because these taxometric procedures are *structure uncovering*, as opposed to *structure imposing*, we will review them in some detail below. We then apply two taxometic procedures to a large adult attachment data set.

DISTINGUISHING BETWEEN LATENT TAXONIC AND DIMENSIONAL STRUCTURES

Explication of Taxonicity

The primary goal of a taxometric analysis is to determine whether a construct represents a "naturally occurring type," a "natural kind," or a "nonarbitrary class" (Meehl, 1992). From this perspective, a true type exists if all group members share a common source of influence upon their manifest characteristics. Because the classic taxonic situation is a dichotomous state of affairs (either a latent entity exists or it does not), discrete entities are most easily thought of as biological agents (e.g., genes or germs). However, as Meehl (1992) notes, many taxa of interest to psychologists are of the "environmental mold" variety, in which exposure to a common culture, history, or belief system results in a tightly knit class of individuals (e.g., Italian speakers, Baptists, bridge players). In such cases the taxonic situation is discrete (e.g., one either learned Italian or did not), but somewhat more abstract because the causal factor is an event, state, or history rather than a physical object (see Meehl, 1992, for further discussion of this issue). Nevertheless, in both cases, the manifest behaviors are due to a common source that is shared by all members of the group.

An important implication of this idea is that *there will be negligible covariation between indicators within the taxon group because the manifestations are the result of a discrete source of influence.* Because there is no variability in the latent source (all members of the group share the entity, state, or history), variability in the indicators cannot be accounted for by variability in the latent source. As an example, consider the case of meningitis from organic medicine, discussed by Meehl (1995; see also Waller, Putnam, & Carlson, 1996). Individuals with meningitis often present with elevated temperature and report severe pain upon bending the neck. These symptoms *co-occur* for individuals with meningitis because they result from a single source (presence of bacteria or viruses in the meninges). However, they do not *covary* for members of the group because there is no variability *in the latent entity* giving rise to the manifestations.[5] Thus, within the taxon group, there is no systematic correlation between temperature and neck stiffness.

Importantly, in a mixed sample of individuals with and without meningitis, temperature and neck stiffness would be moderately correlated. In this case, indicator covariation reflects variability in the latent entity—that is, some individuals have meningitis whereas others do not. The latent source exerts a common "main effect" for the taxon group, resulting in higher mean levels on the indicators relative to nontaxon members. Thus, the positive association results, in part, from mixing two latent groups that differ in their mean levels on each indicator.

We illustrate the logic of this example in Figure 4.2. Notice in this scatterplot that the total sample correlation between x and y is quite strong ($r = .47$). This correlation results from mixing two groups that differ in their mean levels on each indicator. Within each group, however, the correlation between x and y is close to zero.

The situation depicted in the scatterplot can be succinctly expressed by an important theorem known as the General Covariance Mixture Theorem (Meehl, 1973). In words, this theorem states that the covariance between two indicators of a taxonic construct results from the weighted within-group covariances and the weighted indicator mean differences. Algebraically, the General Covariance Mixture Theorem can be expressed as follows:

$$\text{cov}_{xy} = p(\text{cov}_t) + q(\text{cov}_c) + pq(\bar{x}_t - \bar{x}_c)(\bar{y}_t - \bar{y}_c) \tag{1}$$

where: cov_{xy} denotes the observed covariance between indicators x and y in the mixed sample; p is the base rate of the taxon group (t); q is the base rate of the complement (nontaxon) group (c); and $pq(\bar{x}_t - \bar{x}_c)(\bar{y}_t - \bar{y}_c)$ is the weighted product of the indicator mean separations in the two groups (i.e., the product of the indicator validities). When the within-group indicator covariances (i.e., cov_t and cov_c) are negligible, the General Covariance Mixture Theorem can be expressed more compactly:

$$\text{cov}_{xy} \approx pq(\bar{x}_t - \bar{x}_c)(\bar{y}_t - \bar{y}_c) \tag{2}$$

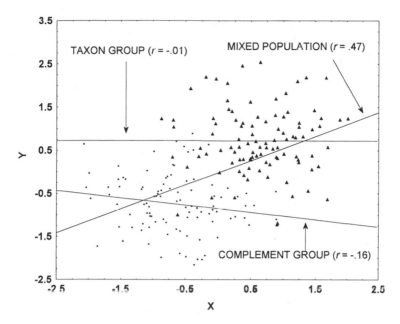

FIGURE 4.2. The correlation in this sample is due to mixing two latent groups with different mean levels on each indicator ($p = q = .5$). Within each group, the indicator correlations are close to zero. That is, for group members, the indicators *co-occur* but do not *covary*.

Thus, for a taxonic construct, the indicator covariances are a function of the mean differences between groups and the amount of taxon mixture in the sample (i.e., pq). This result provides a convenient way to test taxonic conjectures. For instance, let us return to our meningitis example. Suppose we have a sample of infected individuals. The covariance between temperature and neck stiffness in this sample will be essentially zero. Now, suppose that we add some healthy individuals to our sample. What happens to the covariation between temperature and neck stiffness? Importantly, as implied by Equation 2, the covariance between these indicators increases until the proportion of infected individuals in our sample reaches one-half. This occurs because the product term, pq, is greatest when $p = q = .5$. This important result provides the mathematical foundation for the two taxometric procedures described in the next section.

"Mean above Minus below a Cut" (MAMBAC) Procedure

MAMBAC ("mean above minus below a cut"; Meehl & Yonce, 1994) can be used whenever we have two continuously measured indicators—say, x and y—of a conjectured taxonic construct. To implement the procedure, cases on one indicator, for instance, x, are ordered from low to high. If x is a valid indicator of a taxonic construct, then low scores on x will tend to be produced by nontaxon members, whereas high scores will tend to be produced by taxon members. After sorting x we partition the scores into two groups by applying a *cut* score, or threshold point, toward the lower end of the x distribution. We then calculate the mean of y for individuals with x scores falling below the cut score and for individuals with x scores above the cut. That is, we calculate the average y value for the two partitioned groups. The difference between these means is calculated and recorded for later use (hence the name, mean above minus below a cut). Having completed this step, we slide the cut-point on x to a slightly higher position and repeat the aforementioned calculations. This process of gradually increasing the sliding cut-point on one indicator and comparing the group means on a second indicator is repeated until we have traversed the entire x-score range.

The goal of MAMBAC is to identify that point on x that results in the greatest mean differences on y. As discussed shortly, this point is identified by plotting the cut-score threshold points against the y group mean differences. When the latent situation is taxonic, a plot of the threshold points versus the group mean differences—that is, the MAMBAC function—will resemble a hill or convex parabola. The peak of this hill represents the point on x where the two groups formed by partitioning y contain relatively homogeneous samples of nontaxon and taxon members, respectively (for further details, see Meehl & Yonce, 1994; or Waller et al., 1996).

Importantly, the MAMBAC function takes on a different form if the latent situation is dimensional. Specifically, with dimensional constructs the MAMBAC function resembles a bowl, or concave parabola. Because there are no underlying groups, the differences between the partitioned group means will be minimized when the sample is cut at the mean of the score distribution. For instance, consider a hypothetical normal distribution. If we divide this distribution at the mean, the two groups represented by the lower and upper half of the distribution will have equivalent absolute means, and thus the difference between the group means will equal 0.00. Splitting the total sample at any other point along the distribution results in a positive value for the group mean differences.

MAMBAC functions for taxonic and dimensional constructs are presented in Figure 4.3. Panel A represents data that were generated from a latent taxonic model in which the correlation between the indicators is .5. This correlation arises because the group means on each indicator differ by two within-group standard deviations. Notice that, for reasons described earlier, the MAMBAC function resembles a hill. Now consider the plot depicted in the second panel of the figure. The data for this plot were sampled from a dimensional construct, and as predicted by the General Covariance Mixture Theorem (see Equations 1 and 2 above), the resulting MAMBAC plot has a clear dish-like appearance.

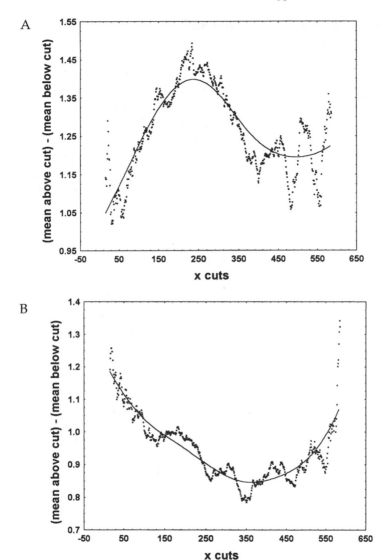

FIGURE 4.3. Panel A represents the MAMBAC function for the taxonic data presented in Figure 4.1. Panel B represents the MAMBAC function for the dimensional data in Figure 4.1. The MAMBAC functions reveal that the two data sets have different latent distributions.

The data used in these MAMBAC plots were presented earlier in Figure 4.1. Recall that a careful inspection of the distributions in Figure 4.1 revealed no clear signs of taxonicity in either the taxonic or dimensional cases. With MAMBAC, however, the structures of the latent distributions are easily distinguished. This illustrates that MAMBAC is a *structure uncovering* approach that allows investigators to test taxonic conjectures.

"Maximum Covariance-Hitmax" (MAXCOV) Procedure

In the maximum covariance-hitmax procedure (MAXCOV; Meehl, 1973; Meehl & Yonce, 1996) one indicator is designated as an "input variable" and two indicators are designated as "output variables." Suppose the indicators are labeled x, y, and z. With MAXCOV we study the covariances between the output variables (y and z) for cases falling in contiguous regions of the input variable (x). That is, we study the *conditional covariances* between the output variables. A plot of these covariances is called a MAXCOV plot. In less formal terms, imagine calculating the covariance between y and z separately for each interval on a histogram of x. The MAXCOV plot is simply a plot of the covariances against the x intervals.

Recall from our earlier discussion that when a latent taxonic variable generates indicator covariation in a mixed sample, indicator covariances within the taxon and nontaxon groups will be minimal. Hence, if an investigator examines the covariance between two indicators (y and z) of a taxonic construct in an interval on x, the size of the covariance is a simple function of the relative proportion of taxon and nontaxon members in the interval (as expressed by Equation 2). In intervals that contain primarily nontaxon members, the indicator covariances are smallish and tend toward zero. In these intervals, the proportion of nontaxon members, q, is substantially larger than p, the proportion of taxon members, and, thus, the product pq is small. For similar reasons, pq—and consequently, the indicator covariance—is small in subsamples that contain primarily taxon members (however, in this case, p is substantially larger than q). As implied by the General Covariance Mixture Theorem, the conditional covariance will often be greatest in the subsample that contains an equal number of taxon and nontaxon members (where $p = q = .5$).

The MAXCOV plot shown in Panel A of Figure 4.4 illustrates that the conditional covariances for the output indicators resembles a peak or a mountain when the latent variable is taxonic and the taxon base rate is close to .5. In samples where the base rate is less than .5, the peak is shifted to the right, whereas in samples where the base rate is larger than .5, the peak is shifted to the left (see Meehl & Yonce, 1996).

When working with quantitatively distributed constructs, the MAXCOV conditional covariances deviate randomly around a horizontal line (see Panel B of Figure 4.4). This occurs because there is no latent taxon and thus, in terms of the General Covariance Mixture Theorem, either p or q will equal 1.00.[6]

With multiple variables, MAXCOV (and also MAMBAC) can be repeatedly applied by interchanging the input variables. For example, the covariance of x and y can be observed along z, z and y along x, and x and z along y. Similarly, in MAMBAC, mean differences between partitionings on x can be observed along sliding cuts of y and vice versa.

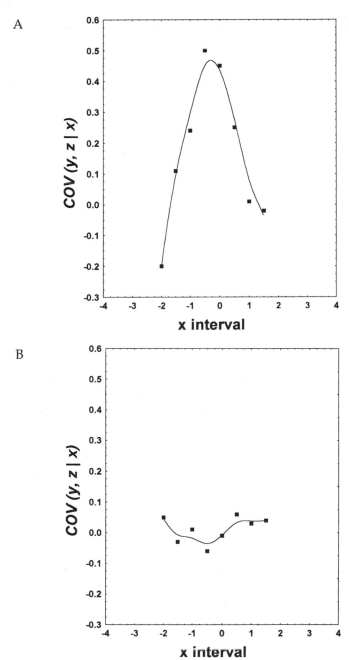

FIGURE 4.4. Panel A represents the MAXCOV function for taxonic data presented in Figure 4.2. As can be seen, the indicator covariances are essentially zero in low and high regions of the sorting variable. However, the covariances are higher in regions on the sorting variable where there is a mixture of taxon and nontaxon members. Panel B illustrates a typical MAXCOV curve that would be expected for dimensional data.

WHY IS A TAXOMETRIC ANALYSIS OF ATTACHMENT SECURITY WARRANTED?

As discussed at the beginning of this chapter, proponents of attachment theory have argued that, with respect to attachment security, individuals differ in kind rather than in degree. According to this view, insecure individuals possess qualitatively different working models than secure individuals. There are several theoretical reasons why this view may be correct. First, in many respects, the hypothesized dynamics of working models are functionally similar to the dynamics of recursive systems (see Hofstadter, 1979, for a clever description of the behavior of recursive systems). A dynamic system is recursive when the system output is also a system input variable. Recursive systems have the potential to exhibit *qualitatively* different behaviors because the state of the system at time *t* is a function of the state at *t*-1 and whatever other functional rules regulate the system.

Importantly, in recursive systems, qualitatively different states can result from different initial states. For example, when a microphone is held at some distance from its output amplifier, the system may be said to be a "very well-behaved communications device"; it amplifies input and does not cause any problems. However, when the microphone is located too close to its output amplifier, the output from the amplifier is fed back into the system (via the microphone). This process rapidly results in a loud, high-frequency screeching sound (sometimes called "feedback"). Individuals who temporarily lose their hearing because of such feedback may be inclined to say that audio systems come in two types: those that work and those that hurt.

In many respects, the dynamics of working models are similar to those of recursive systems. For example, working models of attachment are theoretically shaped by the responsiveness of the early caregiving environment (Ainsworth et al., 1978), but later come to shape the caregiving environment itself (see Bowlby's [1969/1982] concept of a goal-corrected partnership). Thus, the presence of a rejecting attachment figure may lead a child to develop an expectation that others are not available. This expectation may lead the child to avoid others when distressed, thereby reinforcing his or her negative expectations of others. Such a process could conceivably create a feedback loop and lead to a consolidation of beliefs that differ qualitatively from those of an individual who initially had a sensitive and responsive environment. Thus, depending on the sensitivity and responsiveness of the early caregiving environment, at least two kinds of working models could develop. Although no one has tested this model by fitting to data a simple recursive function ($\text{security}_{\text{time}(n)} = \text{security}_{\text{time}(n-1)} + \text{maternal responsiveness}_{\text{time}(n-1)} + \text{error}$), many findings in the literature support the idea (see Bartholomew & Horowitz, 1991; Hazan & Shaver, 1994).

It is interesting to note that such processes are an implicit assumption in many developmental theories. As Meehl (1992) has noted:

It is easy to understand how the environment molds the attitudes and beliefs into an ideological syndrome that is statistically tighter, and often more resistant to change, than many diseases recognized as taxa in internal medicine.... An environmental mold taxon emerges because persons subjected to certain (formal or informal) learning experiences—precepts, models, and reinforcement schedules—acquire motives, cathexes, cognitions, and act dispositions that the social group "teachers" tend to transmit together, at least stochastically.... If you major in subject S, or join political party P, or convert to religion R, or cultivate hobby H, you will learn to *want, value, perceive, believe, say,* and *do* such and such things with a higher probability than those not so educated. (p. 149)

A second reason for suspecting that attachment security may be *qualitatively* distributed is that many investigators of attachment phenomena note that certain indicators co-occur within the attachment types (Ainsworth et al., 1978; Bartholomew & Horowitz, 1991). For instance, Ainsworth et al. (1978) reported that the particular attachment behaviors they had observed tended to be patterned or clustered together. Thus, they sought "to examine the developmental histories of the individuals in question for common antecedent experiences that may be hypothesized to have an influence in the development of similar patterns in one group of individuals that distinguish them from other groups of individuals who have other patterns" (p. 57).

Moreover, Bartholomew's adult attachment typology implies that certain psychological features cluster for some individuals and not for others (Bartholomew & Horowitz, 1991). For instance, secure individuals are theoretically characterized "by a valuing of intimate friendships, the capacity to maintain close relationships without losing personal autonomy, and a coherence and thoughtfulness in discussing relationships and related issues" (p. 228). If these indicators co-occur for some individuals and not for others, then there are strong reasons to suspect that the latent source is qualitatively distributed.

There are also several reasons for suspecting that attachment security is a *dimensional* construct. First, within the identified attachment groups, there is a substantial degree of systematic variance that meaningfully correlates with nontest criteria. For example, Griffin and Bartholomew (1994a) found that dimensional measures of attachment security were reasonably correlated with various outcome measures *within* each of Bartholomew's attachment categories. For instance, the correlations between self model and interpersonal anxiety within each category ranged from −.48 to −.26 (average correlation = −.34); the correlations between other model and problems with warmth ranged from .25 to .40 (average correlation = .33). If the attachment categories were carving nature at its joints, we would expect these within-group covariances to be smaller.

A second reason why attachment security may be a dimensional construct is that the sources influencing the development of working models are likely to be diffuse and quantitatively distributed at the manifest level. Variability in attachment security likely results from several factors, such as variability in temperament, the sensitive responsiveness of primary caregivers, the trustworthiness of romantic partners, and previous experiences with loss and rejection. Although it is feasible that the conjunction of these factors determines whether working models are organized in a secure or an insecure manner (a threshold effect leading to qualitative differences; see Gangestad & Snyder, 1985), it is also feasible that these factors contribute quantitative variability to the ways in which working models are organized (particularly if models are continuously modified and updated by one's relationship experiences).

A third indication that attachment security may be a quantitative variable stems from what we call the "subgroup problem." Within each attachment group in the standard Ainsworth typology there are a number of subgroups which further delineate the different behavioral patterns exhibited by infants. For example, within Group B (secure) four subgroups of infants have been specified (B_1, B_2, B_3, and B_4 infants). Moreover, with the recent introduction of the D category (Main & Solomon, 1986, 1990), the Ainsworth classification scheme has grown to total of 11 subgroups. Attachment researchers working with adult romantic relationships have also felt the need to increase the number of attachment categories (Bartholomew, 1990; Latty-Mann & Davis, 1996; Sperling, Berman, & Fagen, 1992).

The increasing expansion and refinement of the original tripartite categorical system suggests that the typological approach overlooks important variation resulting from latent quantitative variability. Moreover, a sizable proportion of infants are not easily classified in the Ainsworth system—a result that would be expected if attachment security is quantitatively distributed. Main and Weston (1981) report that 14% of their subjects were unclassifiable with the standard Ainsworth categories. In the adult domain, Hazan and Shaver (1987, Study 1) report that 8% of their subjects either did not pick an attachment classification or picked more than one style as being descriptive of themselves. (Because subjects were instructed to pick only one style, this number may underestimate the proportion of individuals who were truly uncertain about which category best described them.) For psychometric reasons alone, if attachment security is continuously distributed, individuals who fall near the imposed psychometric cut scores will be difficult to classify.

DETERMINING THE LATENT DISTRIBUTION OF ATTACHMENT SECURITY

As we have emphasized throughout this chapter, attachment researchers have overwhelmingly conceptualized attachment security as a typological variable. This can be illustrated by examining the statistical models that attachment researchers use. For instance, in three popular outlets for attachment research—the *Journal of Personality and Social Psychology, Personality and Social Psychology Bulletin,* and *Personal Relationships*—73% of 22 published studies (see Table 4.1) used statistical techniques that are designed for categorical variables (e.g., ANOVA). Interestingly, 18% of the published studies used typological *and* dimensional techniques. These data indicate that, despite the popularity of the typological approach, there is a lack of consensus in the field concerning the taxonic status of attachment security. In the next section, we report the results of several taxometic analyses that suggest that a typological model of adult attachment is not consistent with our data.

Taxometric Analysis: Method

To assess the verisimilitude of the typological model, we applied two taxometric procedures (MAMBAC and MAXCOV) to attachment data from a large sample (n = 639) of undergraduates at the University of California, Davis. In this study, attachment security was measured by Griffin and Bartholomew's (1994a) 30-item Relationship Styles Questionnaire (RSQ). This questionnaire contains items from the attachment-style descriptions of Bartholomew (Bartholomew & Horowitz, 1991) and Hazan and Shaver (1987, as revised by Collins & Read, 1990). Each RSQ item is rated on a 7-point scale that ranges from 1, "absolutely disagree," to 7, "absolutely agree."

The RSQ can be scored in two ways. According to the *prototype* approach advocated by Griffin and Bartholomew (1994a), prototype scores are created by averaging the items corresponding to each of the four attachment style descriptions. These scores putatively reflect the degree to which a subject fits each attachment prototype. Theoretically, the secure and fearful prototypes are opposites of one another, as are the dismissing and preoccupied prototypes (Griffin & Bartholomew, 1994a, p. 25). Thus, prototype scores for security can be reverse-keyed as a second indicator of fearful-avoidance. Similarly, dismissing scores can be reverse-keyed to create a second indicator of anxiety or preoccupation.

According to the *dimensional* approach advocated by Griffin and Bartholomew (1994b), individuals are scored on the two dimensions of Anxiety and Avoidance thought to underlie the attachment categories. These dimensional scores can be obtained by combining the prototype scores in a manner described by Griffin and Bartholomew (1994b). They can also be obtained by factor analyzing the RSQ.

In the taxometric analyses reported in the next section, we used scores derived from the prototype *and* the dimensional approaches. Because the prototype approach yields two indicators for each attach-

TABLE 4.1. A Survey of Adult Attachment Distributional Assumptions from the *Journal of Personality and Social Psychology, Personal Relationships,* and *Personality and Social Psychology Bulletin* between 1987 and 1994

Authors	Typological assumption	Dimensional assumption
Hazan & Shaver (1987)	Y	
Collins & Read (1990)	Y	Y
Feeney & Noller (1990)	Y	
Hazan & Shaver (1990)	Y	
Mikulincer, Florian, & Tolmacz (1990)	Y	
Simpson (1990)		Y
Bartholomew & Horowitz (1991)	Y	Y
Kobak & Hazan (1991)		Y
Mikulincer & Nachshon (1991)	Y	
Shaver & Brennan (1992)	Y	Y
Simpson, Rholes, & Nelligan (1992)		Y
Baldwin, Fehr, Keedian, Seidel, & Thomson (1993)	Y	
Mikulincer, Florian, & Weller (1993)	Y	
Carnelley, Pietromonaco, & Jaffee (1994)		Y
Doherty, Hatfield, Thompson, & Choo (1994)	Y	
Feeney (1994)	Y	Y
Griffin & Bartholomew (1994b)		
Kirkpatrick & Davis (1994)	Y	
Kirkpatrick & Hazan (1994)	Y	
Pietromonaco & Carnelley (1994)	Y	
Scharfe & Bartholomew (1994)		Y
Sprecher et al. (1994)	Y	

Note. Methods classified as dimensional used correlational techniques such as Pearson correlations, regression, and path modeling. Methods classified as typological used categorical methods such as ANOVA and chi-square.

ment style, we used MAMBAC to test the taxonicity of the attachment prototypes. Because multiple items can be used to assess the dimensions, we used MAXCOV to test the taxonicity of the RSQ anxiety and avoidance subscales. All analyses were implemented in S-Plus (StatSci, 1995).

Taxometric Analysis: Results

MAMBAC Analysis of the Theoretical Prototypes

In our first set of analyses we examined the attachment prototypes (Griffin & Bartholomew, 1994a). As noted earlier, when variables measure a taxonic construct, the MAMBAC curve will resemble a hill. However, when the variables tap a dimensional construct, the MAMBAC curve will resemble a bowl.

Figure 4.5 presents the MAMBAC plots for the adult attachment data. As can be seen in this figure, the prototype scores provide no evidence for the taxonic hypothesis. On the contrary, the MAMBAC curves have an unambiguous bowl-like appearance—a shape that is consistent with the dimensional hypothesis.

MAXCOV Analysis of Avoidance and Anxiety

In our second set of analyses we used MAXCOV (Meehl & Yonce, 1996) to determine whether the set of factors (Avoidance and Anxiety) generally obtained in factor-analytic studies of attachment (see Feeney & Noller, 1996; Griffin & Bartholomew, 1994a, 1994b; Hazan & Shaver, 1994) reflect dimensions or types. Because latent dimensions and types can produce equivalent covariance matrices, factor analysis cannot be used to answer the types versus dimensions question (although see Waller & Meehl, in press, Chap. 5). The latent "factors" identified in factor analysis can represent quantitatively or qualitatively distributed variables. Fortunately, factor analysis *can* be used to identify items that covary in a mixed population or sample. In turn, the statistical behavior of these items can be investigated with appropriate taxometric procedures to determine whether a latent taxon or dimension is responsible for the pattern of covariances.

In the present study, we used principal-axis factoring to examine the data.[7] Two factors were extracted that clearly resembled the Avoidance and Anxiety dimensions in Bartholomew's model (Griffin & Bartholomew, 1994b). We conducted MAXCOV analyses with the items loading highest on each factor. The five highest loadings on the Avoidance factor ranged from .63 to .68; the five highest loadings on the Anxiety factor ranged from .51 to .58. These items and their intercorrelations are presented in Table 4.2.

With five indicators, we were able to conduct 30 nonredundant MAXCOV analyses for each latent variable. The averaged MAXCOV curves for the Anxiety and Avoidance items are presented in Figure 4.6. As can be seen in this figure, the MAXCOV plots provide no support for the taxonic hypothesis for either latent variable. On the contrary, the conditional covariances in both panels randomly vary around a flat line. These results are entirely consistent with those from the MAMBAC analyses reported above. In other words, our data suggest that adult attachment is best represented by a dimensional model.[8]

GENERAL DISCUSSION

Although adult attachment styles have primarily been conceptualized as representing different types of individuals, our analyses revealed no evidence of taxonicity. In contrast, our results suggest that individual differences in adult attachment organization are quantitatively distributed

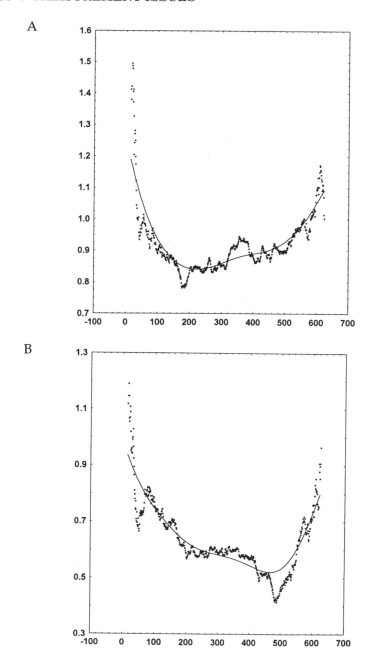

FIGURE 4.5. Results from the MAMBAC analysis of the attachment prototypes. Panel A represents the MAMBAC function for Fearful-Avoidance (or Security, reverse-keyed). Panel B represents the MAMBAC function for Preoccupation (or Dismissing, reverse-keyed). Both MAMBAC plots have an unambiguous bowl-like shape, indicating that these latent variables are dimensional.

TABLE 4.2. Intercorrelations of Attachment Items Used in the
MAXCOV Analyses

	Avoidance					Anxiety				
Items	a1	a2	a3	a4	a5	b1	b2	b3	b4	b5
a1 I find it difficult to trust others completely.	1.00									
a2 I am nervous when anyone gets too close to me.	.40	1.00								
a3 I am uncomfortable being close to others.	.36	.52	1.00							
a4 I am not sure that I can always depend on others to be there when I need them.	.51	.36	.36	1.00						
a5 I find it difficult to depend on other people.	.51	.38	.42	.50	1.00					
b1 I want to be completely emotionally intimate with others.	–.11	–.23	–.21	–.12	–.17	1.00				
b2 I want emotionally close relationships.	–.11	–.23	–.30	–.12	–.19	.55	1.00			
b3 I worry about being abandoned.	.35	.27	.24	.24	.12	.17	.14	1.00		
b4 I worry about being alone.	.18	.13	.04	.13	.01	.21	.26	.50	1.00	
b5 I want to merge completely with another person.	–.04	–.17	–.17	–.10	–.10	.59	.44	.12	.18	1.00

at both the manifest and latent levels. This conclusion holds for both the attachment prototypes (Griffin & Bartholomew, 1994a) and attachment factor scales (Griffin & Bartholomew, 1994b). We believe that our findings have important implications for both the conceptualization and measurement of adult attachment security. In the remainder of this chapter, we discuss three areas where our results are especially relevant.

Implications for the Etiology and Composition of Attachment Styles

Why are the latent variables associated with adult attachment styles continuously distributed? One possibility is that *numerous* variables contribute to variability in attachment organization. These variables are likely to include early caregiving experiences (e.g., sensitive responsiveness), as well as later attachment experiences (e.g., in previous or current romantic relationships). One goal for attachment research should be to identify the multiple factors that affect the development of working models and to measure the degree to which they do so. It would be interesting and

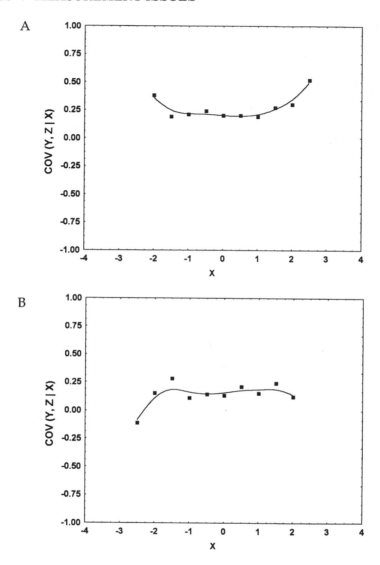

FIGURE 4.6. Results from the MAXCOV analysis of the attachment factor scales. Panel A represents the MAXCOV function for Avoidance. Panel B represents the MAXCOV function for Anxiety. Both MAXCOV plots indicate that latent dimensions, rather than latent types, are producing the observed covariances.

theoretically important to know whether adult attachment styles are better reflections of early parental representations, current parental representations, or current representations of romantic partners. Unfortunately, with the existing emphasis placed on the importance of early attachment relationships, it is unlikely that researchers will focus on other factors that may affect the organization of working models.

Although attachment researchers have never claimed that adult attachment organization is a function solely of early caregiving environments, it has been our experience that students often think that this *is* a claim of the theory. Even professional scholars have often misunderstood the theory as implying a strong continuity between early experiences and adult romantic relationship styles (Hendrick & Hendrick, 1994). We think that the typological approach to conceptualizing adult attachment styles may help promote the widespread belief that there is a single etiology. After all, the natural question to ask when a class of individuals is identified or proposed is, "What is it that all of these individuals have in common?" And rightly so. Such a question is appropriate in the taxonic case because, at one level of analysis, there is a single qualitative variable (a state, history, or entity) responsible for the behavioral patternings. When the qualitative assumption is warranted (e.g., when taxometic analyses of the data suggest that there is a taxonic source variable present), investigation into etiology is greatly facilitated because the investigator knows something about the distribution, prevalence, and structure of the possible cause. Consider a situation in which food poisoning at a local restaurant is the true, but unknown, source of illness for a group of individuals. It will be easier for investigators to determine the true source of illness if they know that whatever they are looking for is categorically distributed and that 20% of their patients belong to a taxon group. Such an investigation would proceed much differently than one in which the latent source of the illness was thought to be the result of numerous quantitatively distributed factors. The point here is that *the way a variable is conceptualized has a profound impact upon the kinds of questions that are asked about that variable.* By focusing on a typological conceptualization of adult attachment patterns we may be restricting the kinds of research questions that are addressed. Moreover, we may be inadvertently promoting misconceptions about the etiology and composition of adult attachment patterns. Thus, resolving the types versus dimensions issue is critical for the advancement of the adult attachment field; it is not just a simple matter of psychometric pedantic preference.

Implications for Reliability and Validity of Attachment Styles

A second implication of our findings is that the observed instability in attachment style classifications results from partitioning a quantitatively distributed variable. Baldwin and Fehr (1995) recently reviewed data on the stability of attachment "types" from a number of data sets. These authors report that, on average, 30% of participants changed their attachment classification over periods of time ranging from 1 week to 52 weeks. This degree of instability poses serious problems for researchers who are attempting to assess a relatively enduring aspect of an individual's psychological organization. However, Baldwin and Fehr propose that the observed instability is not a serious problem if attachment styles are not an enduring aspect of the person. If this is true, as these authors argue, then the instability in measurement reflects the nature of the construct rather than the nature of the measurement instruments themselves.

We would like to suggest an alternative explanation for these findings. Specifically, we propose that a large portion of the aforementioned instability can be accounted for by the crude measurement that inevitably results when a dimensional construct is assessed categorically. To understand why this may be the case, consider what happens when a continuous variable is dichotomized at its mean. The correlation between a dichotomized variable and its continuous "parent" is .80, on average (Cohen, 1983). Thus, by categorizing a continuous variable, about 36% of the variance $(1 - .80^2)$ in the original scores is tossed away (see Cohen, 1983, for a mathematical justification of this point). The problem gets worse when one is using less-than-perfect measures. When two continuous variables that correlate .80 are dichotomized at their means, the kappa for the dichotomized variables will only equal .59.[9] This indicates that, after accounting for the proportion of correct classifications that would be expected by chance, only 59% of the cases were classified the same on both measures. According to the data presented by Baldwin and Fehr (1995), the average kappa for the three-category attachment measures is about .51. Interestingly, this value is similar to that which would be expected if stable and normally distributed dimensions were dichotomized at their means.[10]

Because continuity and change in attachment patterns is a central issue in attachment research, we believe that it is critical to emphasize the deleterious consequences of categorizing continuous variables. *When a taxonic model is inappropriate, categorization will substantially underestimate true continuity.* Thus, if attachment security is a fairly stable construct, investigators using categorical measurements will inevitably draw incorrect conclusions. We think that categorization will become more problematic as more researchers begin to assess the continuity of attachment from early childhood to adulthood. Because there are so many factors that could contribute to the way working models are shaped throughout adolescence (as discussed earlier), the continuity of attachment patterns across time should be fairly modest. However, with the measurement noise introduced by categorical scales, the observed continuity may be remarkably small.

To illustrate this point more clearly, consider the data presented in Table 4.3. These data come from a longitudinal study on ego resiliency and ego control (Block, 1993, p. 33). The left-hand column presents correlations between ego resiliency (a construct similar to security) at age 3 and ages 7, 11, 14, 18, and 23 for a small group of males. As can be seen, the test–retest correlations decrease in a negative logarithmic manner over time, asymptoting between .22 and .31. These values indicate that there is a reasonable degree of continuity in ego resiliency over a 20-year period.

How would our conclusion about the continuity of ego resiliency differ if we were to categorize our scores? In the right-hand column of Table 4.3 we present the correlations that would result if the scores on ego resiliency at each time period had been dichotomized. As can be seen, the degree of continuity appears substantially lower. The new correlation between resiliency at age 3 and age 23 is only .14—a value that would probably lead some investigators to mistakenly dismiss the hypothesis of continuity completely.

These data indicate that the use of categorical measures of attachment may, in the long run, lead to the conclusion that attachment security is not stable over the life course—even if security is fairly stable. On the basis of Block's data, we predict that the correlation between categorical scores of attachment security in infancy and adulthood will randomly fluctuate around the value of .14. In other words, we predict that some investigators will see stability whereas others will see instability.

Implications for Statistical Power

The decrease in reliability resulting from categorization can result in high levels of measurement fuzziness and lead researchers to observe patterns that do not exist or to overlook natural patterns that do exist. These problems are much more severe than the classic Type I and Type II statistical errors because they directly concern the validity of the measurement model itself and cannot be solved by simply adjusting n, α, or β.

Nevertheless, classical statistical errors are also problematic when categorical models are used inappropriately. Type II errors (failures to detect true effects) should be a major source of concern for attachment researchers because the relative proportion of individuals who fall into the insecure categories (on forced-choice self-report and interview measures) is quite small. For example, about 20% of individuals are classified as dismissing–avoidant or preoccupied in samples using Bartholomew's model of individual differences (Feeney & Noller, 1996). To run a study that has at least an 80% probability of detecting a medium-sized effect ($d = .5$ or $r = .23$) between an insecure group (e.g., dismissing–avoidant) and any other group of equal size will require a minimum of 64 dismissing individuals (see Cohen, 1988, p. 37). To obtain a sample with 64 dismissing individuals one would need to test more than 320 people. To detect an equivalent effect with the same degree of power using a dimensional measure would require testing only 150 people.

The use of categorical measurement models introduces major problems concerning statistical power that can only be avoided by testing very large samples. We note, however, that issues of power are only relevant in the context of classic Neyman–Pearson statistical significance testing. In the last 30 years there has been a growing disenchantment with null-hypothesis

TABLE 4.3. Test–Retest Correlations between Age 3 Measures of Ego Resiliency and Retests at Different Ages

	Correlations between age 3 and retest age	
Retest age	Correlation for continuous variables	Phi correlation for dichotomized variables
4 years	.65	.41
7 years	.34	.22
11 years	.35	.22
14 years	.23	.15
18 years	.31	.20
23 years	.22	.14

Note. Correlations in the left-hand column are from Block (1993, p. 33).

testing (Cohen, 1994; Lykken, 1968; Meehl, 1978; Oakes, 1986/1990; Schmidt, 1996). One of our goals should be to accurately estimate the parameters of interest—a goal that has become obscured by the popular focus on dichotomous decision rules and tabular asterisks. Measurement accuracy can be improved by using large sample sizes (which serves to reduce the standard error of measurement), reliable measures, and models that map as closely as possible onto the constructs of interest.

ISSUES RAISED BY THE DIMENSIONAL APPROACH

Throughout this discussion we have argued that individual differences in the organization of the attachment system are quantitatively distributed. If we are correct, then dimensional models of adult attachment styles should be adopted by attachment researchers to maximize measurement precision and validity. Although we think the field will benefit enormously by making the move from categorical to dimensional models, there are some secondary questions that need to be addressed. First, will a dimensional conceptualization of the distribution of attachment security undermine the attachment field? Second, should individuals be scaled according to the two dimensions of Anxiety and Avoidance or according to the attachment prototypes?

Will Dimensional Conceptualizations Undermine the Field?

Several authors have claimed that typological models have contributed to the rapid development of attachment as a popular area of psychological inquiry. For instance, Brennan and Shaver (1995) state that

Ainsworth's three attachment styles [have been] viewed as coherent dynamic systems with biological and psychological functions—wholes

that are greater than the sum of their locations on a handful of dimensions. The field of attachment research has benefited enormously from
the dynamic-system conception, and it almost certainly would not have
advanced as rapidly in the past 20 years if it had been proposed in terms
of a matrix defined by several dimensions. (p. 280)

We agree that the dynamic conception of attachment has played a
role in attachment theory's popularity over the years. However, we
believe that the strength and appeal of the theory lies in its ethological
roots, its psychodynamic flavor, and its concept of dynamic–behavioral
systems—not in the typology itself. *Dynamic concepts neither assume nor
require typological models of individual differences.* For instance, the dynamic
systems that regulate body temperature can be organized in ways that
lead some individuals to be too cold most of the time and others to be too
warm. Nonetheless, it does not follow that there exist two types of people
in the world as far as body temperature is concerned (e.g., "warm-
blooded people" and "cold-blooded people"). Internal thresholds and
other latent factors that determine the operation of the systems can be
quantitatively distributed across individuals. Thus, the dynamic components that set attachment theory apart from other theories of social
behavior and personality (e.g., nondynamic interpretations of trait theory)
do not require that individuals be distributed into categories rather than
along dimensions. It is unnecessary to assume that variability in the
organization of dynamic systems needs to be categorically distributed.
    Nevertheless, even if the types themselves were responsible for
advancing the field in the beginning, they have the potential to cripple
the field in the long run. We have demonstrated that the use of categorical
measurement models in assessing continuously distributed constructs
seriously undermines reliability, validity, and statistical power. One long-
term consequence of using unreliable, invalid, and unpowerful measures
is an accumulation of seemingly contradictory or unreliable findings in
the research literature—a situation which may serve to undermine the
integrity of the field as a whole (Schmidt, 1996). Furthermore, young
researchers using unreliable categorical measures may become disen-
chanted with attachment theory, rather than attachment measures, when
they do not obtain the effects predicted by the theory. Such outcomes are
not desirable for the long-term development of a cumulative science.

Prototypes and Dimensions

Griffin and Bartholomew (1994a) have recently argued in favor of a
"four-category model of adult attachment that explicitly uses a prototype
approach" (p. 24). According to this approach the attachment types are
thought to have "fuzzy" rather than discrete boundaries. Furthermore,
according to Griffin and Bartholomew, the prototypes "are not simply

reducible to the two attachment dimensions" (p. 32) because they add predictive power over and above that afforded by the dimensions alone.

Although we agree with Griffin and Bartholomew that the typological approach to attachment is wanting, we do not think that the prototype approach is preferable to the dimensional approach for several reasons. First, their claim that the prototype approach adds predictive power above that afforded by the dimensions is questionable. To support their argument, Griffin and Bartholomew (1994a, pp. 38–39) presented the results of a two-step hierarchical regression analysis in which the four attachment prototype scores were entered following the two attachment dimensions. They found for men, but not for women, that the dimensions explained 2% of the variance in relationship satisfaction, whereas the prototype scores explained an additional 28% of the variance. However it is noteworthy that the dimensions were *created* from a combination of the prototypes (see Griffin & Bartholomew, 1994a, p. 38). Mathematically, each of the four prototype scores cannot account for additional variance in the dependent variable because of the redundancy between the dimensions and the prototype scores from which they were derived. In fact, when we tried a similar analysis in one of our data sets, we found that the prototype scores contributed less than 1% of the variance to relationship satisfaction over and above the dimensions, and that two of the four prototypes were excluded from the analysis due to tolerance or colinearity problems (the prototype scores of security and preoccupation were completely accounted for by fearful and dismissing prototype scores and the Anxiety and Avoidance dimensions). Therefore, we believe that the claim for the superior predictive power of the prototypes is unjustified. Because the attachment prototypes represent linear combinations of the two dimensions of Avoidance and Anxiety, they are, ipso facto, reducible to the two attachment dimensions.

The prototype approach is also problematic because it implies that there are four distinct "types," and that people vary in the degree to which they fit those typological patterns. The explicit focus on the four patterns has the potential, we believe, to obscure the psychological relations among the various regions in the two-dimensional space. If the two-dimensional model is correct, then the psychological mechanisms and behavior patterns that characterize highly Anxious people will be the "opposite" of those that characterize less Anxious people. Similarly, the psychology that characterizes theoretically dismissing people (high Avoidance, low Anxiety) (see Fraley, Davis, & Shaver, Chapter 10, this volume) will be the reverse of that of theoretically preoccupied people (low Avoidance, high Anxiety). In other words, the various regions of the space are not characterized by psychologically independent patterns and mechanisms, each with its own specific dynamics. In fact, the intercorrelations of prototype scores suggest that security (low Avoidance, low Anxiety) and fearful-avoidance (high Avoidance, high Anxiety) are psychological opposites, and that preoccupation and dismissing-avoidance are psychological opposites. Thus, it would be inappropriate to enter the prototype scores into a simultaneous regression equation where each prototype is considered to be orthogonal to the others.

Another reason why we favor the dimensional approach is because it makes it easier, we believe, to think about underlying mechanisms. Most factor analytic studies indicate that the two latent dimensions of Avoidance and Anxiety are important in explaining variation in peoples' thoughts, behaviors, and feelings in close relationships. Thus, the next major theoretical step is to investigate the nature of these dimensions, to find out exactly what they represent and how they operate. Unfortunately, the prototype approach does not promote this kind of investigation because it focuses on manifest, and according to our analyses, arbitrary types. An explicit focus on the latent dimensions, however, may facilitate inquiry into the underlying operation of the attachment system. Avoidance and Anxiety may influence emotion and behavior at different temporal stages of information processing and behavioral regulation. It is also possible that the dimension of Anxiety captures variation in physiological and emotional parameters rather than cognitive knowledge structures, whereas Avoidance captures variation in the organization of knowledge structures rather than emotional thresholds. Such hypotheses, of course, are best conceived within a theoretical model that explicitly focuses on latent dimensions, rather than conceptual prototypes.

Finally, we believe that the prototype approach leaves the ontological status of the attachment patterns unclear. Are the prototypes advocated by Griffin and Bartholomew supposed to represent "fuzzy" groups that exist in nature or "fuzzy" groups that exist in the minds of perceivers of nature? Cognitive research on prototypes has been concerned with the ways in which the real-world correlational structure is reflected in the cognitive systems of perceivers rather than the real-world correlational structure itself (e.g., Rosch, 1978). Thus, research on prototypes tells us more about the way perceivers perceive than the subject matter they are perceiving. When it comes to assessing individual differences in attachment security, our primary concern should be in identifying the real-world correlational structure rather than the degree to which individuals fit our theoretical ideals. As Loevinger noted in her classic 1957 article, there is a crucial distinction to be made between psychological traits and constructs: "Traits exist in people; constructs (here usually about traits) exist in the minds and magazines of psychologists" (p. 642). It seems to us that measurements focused on prototypes will better reflect how the attachment system is perceived by psychologists than the way in which it is organized in people.

SUMMARY

Our goal in this chapter has been to make a key contribution to the types versus dimensions debate by testing the latent structure of adult attachment organization with appropriate taxometric methods. Although we claimed at the beginning of the chapter that our goal was *to resolve* the debate, we recognize that a debate cannot be resolved by a single study. We are limited by our measures, sample, and methods. Therefore, we encourage other researchers to contribute to the resolution of this debate by testing the latent structure of their attachment data. We have attempted to present two taxometric techniques, MAMBAC and MAXCOV, in a clear, accessible way to facilitate the investigation of this issue.

As we noted at the outset of this chapter, attachment theory has the potential to organize a diverse set of findings in the fields of personality and close relationships. In order for this potential to be fulfilled, the measurement models used by attachment researchers must correspond to the phenomena being measured. Our data indicate that the typological model traditionally favored by attachment researchers does not capture the natural structure of attachment security. Rather, they indicate that adult attachment organization is a quantitatively distributed variable—a variable on which people differ in degree rather than in kind.

ACKNOWLEDGMENTS

We would like to thank Jim Cassandro, Paul Meehl, Steve Rholes, Phil Shaver, and Jeff Simpson for reading and making comments on previous drafts of this chapter.

NOTES

1. It is important to point out that Ainsworth et al. (1978) are somewhat ambiguous regarding the ontological status of the classificatory groups. At one point the groups are viewed as useful empirical tools: "We view [the classificatory system] as a first step toward grasping the organization of complex behavioral data. . . . the categories are tools, not 'absolutes' " (p. 56). However, at other points, Ainsworth et al. (1978) argue that the behaviors they observed were patterned in unique ways: "The behavior in the reunion episodes contributed the most convincing evidence of clustering behaviors, in contrast to a continuous distribution along one or even two major dimensions" (p. 59). Thus, it appears that Ainsworth and her colleagues did not want to argue in favor of a true typological status for the groups even though they (1) sought to maximize the clustering of behaviors via multiple empirical filters (see pp. 98–100) and (2) abandoned their continuous scales in favor of categorical scales.

2. This is an important point because, as we discuss later, attachment researchers have recently conceptualized attachment patterns as being "fuzzy" types or categories with imperfect boundaries (Griffin & Bartholomew, 1994a).

3. We neither require nor expect our imperfect measures to exhibit bimodality because of their high degree of measurement error. Moreover, even with highly reliable measures, bimodality will be observed only when the groups are separated by two or more within-group standard deviations (Murphy, 1964).

4. As an interesting exercise, we challenge readers to submit two continuous and uncorrelated variables to a cluster analysis. You will find that, if a four-group solution is selected, the group centroids will fall into separate quadrants in a two-dimensional space. This centroid arrangement does not provide evidence for four "distinct" groups because the "groups" were imposed on the data by the clustering algorithm. Clustering procedures are not appropriate for uncovering types because they discover 'types' in nontaxonic data.

5. Technically, there is variability in the latent entity because meningitis is a brain infection and the infection can vary in severity. However, this variation does not systematically affect the symptoms of the condition. The presence or absence of the infection is what gives rise to the covariation among symptoms, not the degree of infection.

6. In the dimensional case, the covariance between indicators does not vary as a function of the quantity of the latent trait present. Thus, in standard linear regression with quantitative indicators, a single slope is used to describe the amount of change in y with each change in x. It is assumed that the amount of change in y does not vary as a function of x.

7. It should be noted that we also examined several groups of items resulting from a cluster analysis of the data using Ward's method. This procedure generated clusters very similar to those generated by the factoring procedure. A MAXCOV analysis of these item clusters produced results consistent with those produced from factor analyses of the items. We have chosen not to present the MAXCOV analyses based on the clusters in order to preserve space.

8. It should be noted that we have conducted taxometric analyses on the items using several different item combinations, including the single-item prototype descriptions (Bartholomew & Horowitz's [1991] Relationship Questionnaire) and six-factor, as opposed to two-factor, solutions. In each case we obtained results consistent with the dimensional hypothesis. We have also replicated these results in a large community sample with Feeney et al.'s (1994) Attachment Style Questionnaire.

9. We arrived at this value through a series of simulations where the test–retest correlation between two continuous variables was varied. The results and details of this simulation are available from the authors.

10. We do not offer this example as a complete explanation of the observed instability in adult attachment classifications. We believe that there are several confounding factors (such as presentation order) which help determine the categories that individuals choose in forced-choice procedures. Because these factors have not been identified, we cannot model them in our example. Nevertheless, the example demonstrates an important point, namely, that apparent instability can arise when two highly stable dimensions are categorized.

REFERENCES

Ainsworth, M. D. (1967). *Infancy in Uganda*. Baltimore: John Hopkins Press.

Ainsworth, M. D. S., & Bell, S. M. (1970). Attachment, exploration, and separation: Illustrated by the behavior of one-year-olds in a strange situation. *Child Development, 41,* 49–67.

Ainsworth, M. D. S., Blehar, M. C., Waters, E., & Wall, S. (1978). *Patterns of attachment.* Hillsdale, NJ: Erlbaum.

Ainsworth, M. D. S., & Wittig, B. A. (1969). Attachment and exploratory behavior of one-year-olds in a Strange Situation. In B. M. Foss (Ed.), *Determinants of infant behavior* (Vol. 4, pp. 113–136). London: Methuen.

Baldwin, M. W., & Fehr, B. (1995). On the instability of attachment style ratings. *Personal Relationships, 2,* 247–261.

Baldwin, M. W., Fehr, B., Keedian, E., Seidel, M., & Thomson, D. W. (1993). An exploration of the relational schemata underlying attachment styles: Self-report and lexical decision approaches. *Personality and Social Psychology Bulletin, 19,* 746–754.

Bartholomew, K. (1990). Avoidance of intimacy: An attachment perspective. *Journal of Social and Personal Relationships, 7,* 147–178.

Bartholomew, K., & Horowitz, L. M. (1991). Attachment styles among young adults: A test of a four-category model. *Journal of Personality and Social Psychology, 61,* 226–244.

Blatz, W. E. (1966). *Human security: Some reflections.* Toronto: University of Toronto Press.

Block, J. (1993). Studying personality the long way. In D. C. Funder, R. D. Parke, C. Tomlinson-Keasy, & K. Widaman (Eds.), *Studying lives through time: Personality and development* (pp. 9–41). Washington, DC: American Psychological Association.

Bowlby, J. (1973). *Attachment and loss: Vol. 2. Separation: Anxiety and anger.* New York: Basic Books.

Bowlby, J. (1982). *Attachment and loss: Vol. 1. Attachment.* New York: Basic Books. (Original work published 1969)

Brennan, K. A., & Shaver, P. R. (1995). Dimensions of adult attachment, affect regulation, and romantic relationship functioning. *Personality and Social Psychology Bulletin, 21,* 267–283.

Brennan, K. A., Shaver, P. R., & Tobey, A. E. (1991). Attachment styles, gender and parental problem drinking. *Journal of Social and Personal Relationships, 8,* 451–466.

Carnelley, K. B., Pietromonaco, P. R., & Jaffe, K. (1994). Depression, working models of others, and relationship functioning. *Journal of Personality and Social Psychology, 66,* 127–140.

Cohen, J. (1983). The cost of dichotomization. *Applied Psychological Measurement, 7,* 249–253.

Cohen, J. (1988). *Statistical power analysis for the behavioral sciences* (2nd ed.). Hillsdale, NJ: Erlbaum.

Cohen, J. (1994). The earth is round ($p < .05$). *American Psychologist, 49,* 997–1003.

Colin, V. L. (1996). *Human attachment.* New York: McGraw-Hill.

Collins, N. L., & Read, S. J. (1990). Adult attachment, working models, and relationship quality in dating couples. *Journal of Personality and Social Psychology, 58,* 644–663.

Crittenden, P. M. (1988). Relationships at risk. In J. Belsky & T. Nezworski (Eds.), *Clinical implications of attachment* (pp. 136–174). Hillsdale, NJ: Erlbaum.

Cummings, E. M. (1990). Classification of attachment on a continuum of felt security: Illustrations from the study of children of depressed parents. In M. T. Greenberg, D. Cicchetti, & E. M. Cummings (Eds.), *Attachment in the preschool years: Theory, research, and intervention* (pp. 311–338). Chicago: University of Chicago Press.

Doherty, R. W., Hatfield, E., Thompson, K., & Choo, P. (1994). Cultural and ethnic influences on love and attachment. *Personal Relationships, 4,* 391–398.

Everitt, B. S. (1974). *Cluster analysis.* London: Heinemann.

Feeney, J. A. (1994). Attachment style, communication patterns, and satisfaction across the life cycle of marriage. *Personal Relationships, 4,* 333–348.

Feeney, B. C., & Kirkpatrick, L. A. (1996). Effects of adult attachment and presence of romantic partners on physiological responses to stress. *Journal of Personality and Social Psychology, 70,* 255–270.

Feeney, J. A., & Noller, P. (1990). Attachment styles as a predictor of adult romantic relationships. *Journal of Personality and Social Psychology, 58,* 281–291.

Fenney, J. A., & Noller, P. (1996). *Adult attachment.* Beverly Hills, CA: Sage.

Feeney, J. A., Noller, P., & Hanrahan, M. (1994). Assessing adult attachment: Developments in the conceptualization of Security and Insecurity. In M. B. Sperling & W. H. Berman (Eds.), *Attachment in adults: Clinical and developmental perspectives* (pp. 128–152). New York: Guilford Press.

Freud, S. (1953). The interpretation of dreams. In *Standard Edition* (Vols. 4 & 5). London: Hogarth Press. (Original work published 1900)

Gangestad, S., & Snyder, M. (1985). "To carve nature at its joints": On the existence of discrete classes in personality. *Psychological Review, 92,* 317–349.

George, C., Kaplan, N., & Main, M. (1985). *The Adult Attachment Interview.* Unpublished manuscript, Department of Psychology, University of California, Berkeley.

Grayson, D. A. (1987). Can categorical and dimensional views of psychiatric illness be distinguished? *British Journal of Psychiatry, 151,* 355–361.

Griffin, D. W., & Bartholomew, K. (1994a). The metaphysics of measurement: The case of adult attachment. In K. Bartholomew & D. Perlman (Eds.), *Advances in personal relationships: Vol. 5. Attachment processes in adulthood* (pp. 17–52). London: Jessica Kingsley.

Griffin, D. W., & Bartholomew, K. (1994b). Models of the self and other: Fundamental dimensions underlying measures of adult attachment. *Journal of Personality and Social Psychology, 67,* 430–445.

Hazan, C., & Shaver, P. R. (1987). Romantic love conceptualized as an attachment process. *Journal of Personality and Social Psychology, 59,* 511–524.

Hazan, C., & Shaver, P. R. (1990). Love and work: An attachment-theoretical perspective. *Journal of Personality and Social Psychology, 59,* 270–280.

Hazan, C., & Shaver, P. R. (1994). Attachment as an organizational framework for research on close relationships. *Psychological Inquiry, 5,* 1–22.

Hendrick, C., & Hendrick, S. S. (1994). Attachment theory and close relationships. *Psychological Inquiry, 5,* 38–41.

Hofstadter, D. (1979). *Gödel, Escher, and Bach: An eternal golden braid.* New York: Vintage.

Howes, C., & Hamilton, C. E. (1992). Children's relationships with caregivers: Mothers and child care teachers. *Child Development, 63,* 859–866.

Kirkpatrick, L. A., & Davis, K. E. (1994). Attachment style, gender, and relationship stability: A longitudinal analysis. *Journal of Personality and Social Psychology, 66,* 502–512.

Kirkpatrick, L. A., & Hazan, C. (1994). Attachment styles and close relationships: A four-year prospective study. *Personal Relationships, 1*, 123–142.

Kobak, R. R., & Hazan, C. (1991). Attachment in marriage: Effects of security and accuracy of working models. *Journal of Personality and Social Psychology, 60*, 861–869.

Latty-Mann, H., & Davis, K. E. (1996). Attachment theory and partner choice: Preference and actuality. *Journal of Social and Personal Relationships, 13*, 5–23.

Levy, M. B., & Davis, K. E. (1988). Lovestyles and attachment styles compared: Their relations to each other and to various relationship characteristics. *Journal of Social and Personal Relationships, 5*, 439–471.

Loevinger, J. (1957). Objective tests as instruments of psychological theory. *Psychological Reports, 3*, 635–694.

Lykken, D. (1968). Statistical significance in psychological research. *Psychological Bulletin, 70*, 151–159.

Main, M., & Solomon, J. (1986). Discovery of an insecure–disorganized/disoriented attachment pattern: Procedures, findings and implications for the classification of behavior. *Monographs of the Society for Research in Child Development, 50*, 66–104.

Main, M., & Solomon, J. (1990). Procedures for identifying infants as disorganized/disoriented during the Ainsworth Strange Situation. In M. Greenberg, D. Cicchetti, & M. Cummings (Eds.), *Attachment in the preschool years: Theory, research, and intervention* (pp. 121–160). Chicago: University of Chicago Press.

Main, M., & Weston, D. (1981). The quality of the toddler's relationship to mother and father: Related to conflict behavior and readiness to establish new relationships. *Child Development, 52*, 932–940.

Maxwell, S. E., & Delaney, H. D. (1993). Bivariate median splits and spurious statistical significance. *Psychological Bulletin, 113*, 181–190.

Meehl, P. E. (1973). MAXCOV-HITMAX: A taxonomic search method for loose genetic syndromes. *Psychodiagnosis: Selected papers* (pp. 200–224). Minneapolis: University of Minnesota Press.

Meehl, P. E. (1978). Theoretical risks and tabular asterisks: Sir Karl, Sir Ronald and the slow progress of soft psychology. *Journal of Consulting and Clinical Psychology, 46*, 806–834.

Meehl, P. E. (1992). Factors and taxa, traits and types, differences of degree and differences in kind. *Journal of Personality, 60*, 117–174.

Meehl, P. E. (1995). Bootstraps taxometrics: Solving the classification problem in psychopathology. *American Psychologist, 50*, 266–275.

Meehl, P. E., & Golden, R. (1982). Taxometric methods. In P. Kendall & J. Butcher (Eds.), *Handbook of research methods in clinical psychology* (pp. 127–181). New York: Wiley.

Meehl, P. E., & Yonce, L. J. (1994). Taxometric analysis: I. Detecting taxonicity with two quantitative indicators using means above and means below a sliding cut (MAMBAC procedure). *Psychological Reports, 74*, 1059–1274.

Meehl, P. E., & Yonce, L. J. (1996). Taxometric analysis: II. Detecting taxonicity using covariance of two quantitative indicators in successive intervals of a third indicator (MAXCOV procedure). *Psychological Reports, 78*, 1091–1227.

Mikulincer, M., Florian, V., & Tolmacz, R. (1990). Attachment styles and fear of personal death: A case study of affect regulation. *Journal of Personality and Social Psychology, 58*, 273–280.

Mikulincer, M., Florian, V., & Weller, A. (1993). Attachment styles, coping strategies, and posttraumatic psychological distress: The impact of the Gulf War in Israel. *Journal of Personality and Social Psychology, 64*, 817–826.

Mikulincer, M., & Nachshon, O. (1991). Attachment styles and patterns of self-disclosure. *Journal of Personality and Social Psychology, 61*, 321–331.

Mikulincer, M., & Orbach, I. (1995). Attachment styles and repressive defensiveness: The accessibility and architecture of affective memories. *Journal of Personality and Social Psychology, 68*, 917–925.

Murphy, E. A. (1964). One cause? Many causes?: The argument from the bimodal distribution. *Journal of Chronic Disease, 17*, 301–324.

Oakes, M. (1990). *Statistical inference*. Newton Lower Falls, MA: Epidemiology Resources. (Original work published 1986)

Pietromonaco, P. R., & Carnelley, K. B. (1994). Gender and working models of attachment: Consequences for perceptions of self and romantic relationships. *Personal Relationships, 1*, 63–82.

Richters, J. E., Waters, E., & Vaughn, B. E. (1988). Empirical classification of infant–mother relationships from interactive behavior and crying during reunion. *Child Development, 59*, 512–522.

Rosch, E. (1978). Principles of categorization. In E. Rosch & B. B. Lloyd (Eds.), *Cognition and categorization* (pp. 27–48). Hillsdale, NJ: Erlbaum.

Scharfe, E., & Bartholomew, K. (1994). Reliability and stability of adult attachment patterns. *Personal Relationships, 1*, 23–44.

Schmidt, F. L. (1996). Statistical significance testing and cumulative knowledge in psychology: Implications for training of researchers. *Psychological Methods, 1*, 115–129.

Shaver, P. R., & Brennan, K. A. (1992). Attachment styles and the "Big Five" personality traits: Their connections with each other and with romantic relationship outcomes. *Personality and Social Psychology Bulletin, 18*, 536–545.

Shaver, P. R., Hazan, C., & Bradshaw, D. (1988). Love as attachment: The integration of three behavioral systems. In R. J. Sternberg & M. L. Barnes (Eds.), *The psychology of love* (pp. 68–99). New Haven, CT: Yale University Press.

Shaver, P. R., Papalia, D., Clark, C. L., Koski, L. R., Tidwell, M. C., & Nalbone, D. (1996). Androgyny and attachment security: Two related models of optimal personality. *Personality and Social Psychology Bulletin, 22*, 582–597.

Simpson, J. (1990). The influence of attachment styles on romantic relationships. *Journal of Personality and Social Psychology, 59*, 971–980.

Simpson, J., Rholes, W. S., & Nelligan, J. S. (1992). Support-seeking and support-giving within couples members in an anxiety-provoking situation: The role of attachment styles. *Journal of Personality and Social Psychology, 62*, 434–446.

Sperling, M. B., & Berman, W. H. (1994). The structure and function of adult attachment. In M. B. Sperling & W. H. Berman (Eds.), *Attachment in adults: Clinical and developmental perspectives* (pp. 3–28). New York: Guilford Press.

Sperling, M. B., & Berman, W. H., & Fagen, G. (1992). Classification of adult attachment: An integrative taxonomy from attachment and psychoanalytic theories. *Journal of Personality Assessment, 59*(2), 239–247.

Sprecher, S., Aron, A., Hatfield, E., Cortese, A., Potapova, E., & Levitskaya, A. (1994). Love: American style, Russian style, and Japanese style. *Personal Relationships, 4*, 349–370.

Sroufe, L. A. (1990, Autumn). The role of training in attachment assessment. *Society for Research in Child Development Newsletter,* pp. 1–2.

Sroufe, L. A., & Waters, E. (1977). Attachment as an organizational construct. *Child Development, 48,* 1184–1199.

StatSci. (1995). *S-Plus for Windows user manual.* (Statistical Sciences, Inc., 1700 Westlake Ave. N., Suite 500, Seattle, WA 98109)

Tatsuoska, M. M. (1970). *Discriminant analysis: The study of group differences.* Champaign, IL: Institute for Personality Ability Testing.

Tellegen, A., & Lubinski, D. (1983). Some methodological comments on labels, traits, interaction, and types in the study of "Femininity" and "Masculinity": Reply to Spence. *Journal of Personality and Social Psychology, 44,* 447–455.

Van Dam, M., & van IJzendoorn, M. H. (1988). Measuring attachment security: Concurrent and predictive validity of the parental attachment Q-set. *Journal of Genetic Psychology, 149,* 447–457.

Waller, N. G., & Meehl, P. E. (in press). *Multivariate taxometric procedures: Distinguishing types from continua.* Newbury Park, CA: Sage.

Waller, N. G., Putnam, F. W., & Carlson, E. B. (1996). Types of dissociation and dissociative types: A taxometric analysis of dissociative experiences. *Psychological Methods, 1,* 300–321.

Waters, E., & Deane, K. E. (1985). Defining and assessing individual differences in attachment relationships: Q-methodology and the organization of behavior in infancy and early childhood. In I. Bretherton & E. Waters (Eds.), Growing points of attachment theory and research. *Monographs of the Society for Research in Child Development, 50*(1–2, Serial No. 209), 41–65.

5

Working Models of Attachment

A Theory-Based Prototype Approach

EVA C. KLOHNEN
OLIVER P. JOHN

What are working models of adult attachment, how should we measure them, and do they change across adulthood? According to attachment theory, early attachments form the prototype for later attachments via *internal working models of "self" and "other."* Internal working models include expectations about the individual's own worth vis-à-vis the attachment figure and about the availability and responsivity of that attachment figure. Because working models are thought to form the underlying basis of attachment styles, we need to better understand the content and structure of these models and find more comprehensive ways of measuring them.

In this chapter we first summarize Bowlby's (e.g., 1973, 1980) theorizing about working models, describe Bartholomew's (1990; Bartholomew & Horowitz, 1991) four-category model of adult attachment styles, and briefly review existing research on working models of attachment in adults. We then summarize our recent research on expert-based prototypes (Klohnen & John, 1996, 1997) which we developed to assess working models in adulthood. Finally, we report new evidence for the validity of these working model prototypes in a longitudinal study of adult development. In particular, we ask whether individual differences on these prototypes are stable over 25 years and whether individuals change over time, becoming more secure from early to middle adulthood, as suggested by a recent cross-sectional study of different age groups (Mickelson, Kessler, & Shaver, in press).

INTERNAL WORKING MODELS
OF SELF AND OTHER

Starting with Bowlby (1973), the concept of internal working models has been inextricably intertwined with attachment theory. Bowlby suggested that infants construct models of how their significant caregivers may be expected to behave, how the infant is expected to behave, and how the two interact with each other. As cognitive development increases and infant–environment transactions become more differentiated, these models become increasingly more elaborated, complex, and abstract. Although early working models are assumed to be a function of the primary infant–caregiver relationships, they become internalized over time, eventually characterizing the individual as much as the specific attachment relationship. Infants thus develop mental representations of self, attachment figures, and the social world out of the repeated interpersonal transactions they experience with caregivers and other important attachment figures.

The basic character and affective tone of the emerging working models reflect answers to two fundamental questions: (1) Am I a worthy and lovable person? and (2) Are others (the attachment figures) trustworthy and caring? According to Bowlby (1973), if caregivers consistently recognize and respond appropriately to the child's needs for comfort, security, and independent exploration, the child is likely to develop a model of self as valued and self-sufficient (i.e., positive), and a model of other as trustworthy and caring (i.e., positive). If, on the other hand, the caregiver routinely rejects the child's overtures for protection and comfort and also interferes with the infant's desire for independent exploration, the infant is likely to develop and internalize a model of self as worthless and incompetent (i.e., negative), and a model of other as unreliable and rejecting (i.e., negative). These two components of working models of attachment have come to be called *models of self* and *models of others* and are thought to vary in valence from emotionally negative to positive.

Two-Dimensional Model of Adult Attachment Styles

Bartholomew (1990; Bartholomew & Horowitz, 1991) incorporated Bowlby's ideas about positive and negative models of self and of other into a two-dimensional system which, she proposed, gives rise to four adult attachment patterns (see Figure 5.1). As Bowlby had suggested,

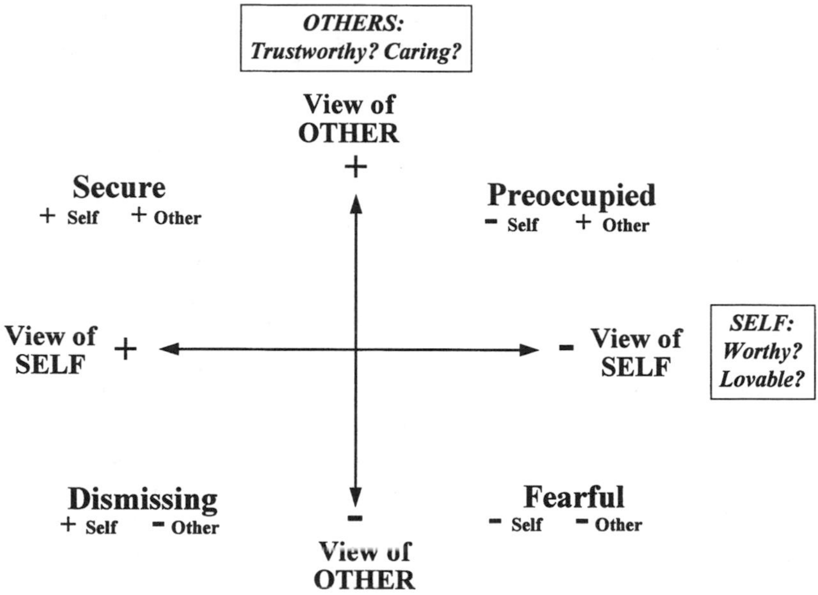

FIGURE 5.1. Fourfold attachment classification system.

models of self and other are often complementary—both models are positive or both are negative in valence. Thus, the majority of individuals fall either in the *secure* quadrant (positive self and positive other) or the *fearful* quadrant (negative self and negative other). The other two cells are more complex, combining both positive and negative models. According to the theory summarized in Figure 5.1, *preoccupied* individuals desire close relationships (positive other) but feel insecure or even worthless (negative self); conversely, *dismissing* individuals feel competent and self-sufficient (positive self) but view others as undependable or even rejecting (negative other).

Thus, Bartholomew's model distinguishes three different insecure attachment styles—preoccupied, fearful, and dismissing. All three are assumed to arise out of negative, or at least not consistently positive, experiences with attachment figures. How, then, is it possible that two of the insecure styles—preoccupied and dismissing—maintain evaluatively inconsistent models of self and other? The argument is that each of the four attachment styles represents a different way of coping adaptively with the caregiving and attachment experiences the individual has encountered. Note that the underlying self and other models are defined at the level of consciously maintained beliefs about self and other. However, it is possible that the two "mixed" insecure styles have split off negative components of their working models so that these components have become less consciously accessible. Indeed, as Bartholomew noted (cited in Scharfe et al., 1996):

> At some unconscious level prototypical dismissing individuals do feel negatively about themselves, and their adoption of a detached stance toward others is a way of defending a fragile sense of self from potential hurt by others. Similarly, the positive model of the preoccupied masks a less conscious negative model of others, with the tendency to idealize others acting as a defense against acknowledging that significant others are, at least at times, uncaring and unavailable. (p. 5)

More generally, it is possible to understand the disparate working models of preoccupied and dismissing individuals in terms of Bowlby's ideas about the formation and coexistence of multiple working models. Bowlby (1973, 1980) proposed that individuals may hold two or more models of themselves, as well as multiple, potentially inconsistent working models of attachment figures (Main, 1991). He suggested that when multiple models exist, they are likely to differ with respect to their origin, their dominance, and the extent to which they are in conscious awareness (Bowlby, 1973). Defensive processes serve to keep potentially painful experiences out of awareness and to reconcile contradictory interpretations of the same experiences, thus blocking from consciousness some object representations or at least the affect associated with them (Bowlby, 1980).

In line with Bowlby's theorizing, working models have been characterized as a network of interconnected models that vary in their levels of generality, complexity, and conscious accessibility. Collins and Read (1994), for example, have proposed that working models include four interrelated components: (1) memories of attachment-related experience; (2) beliefs, attitudes, and expectations about self and others in relation to attachment; (3) attachment-related goals and needs; and (4) strategies and plans associated with achieving attachment goals. To date, most researchers have focused on those aspects of working models that are consciously accessible and relatively general in nature, that is, the second component in Collins and Read's taxonomy. In this chapter, we also are concerned with beliefs and attitudes that are consciously accessible and fairly general.

A Short Review of Previous Research on Internal Working Models

Research on the relations between attachment styles and working models in adults has often used measures of self-concept and personality to tap aspects of the self-model and other-model dimensions (see Shaver, Collins, & Clark, 1996; Shaver & Hazan, 1993, for reviews). Bartholomew and

Horowitz (1991; see also Griffin & Bartholomew, 1994b) focused on the four-category model of attachment and asked participants to complete a wide range of measures to tap models of self and models of other. They used measures of self-esteem, self-acceptance, and distress (i.e., anxiety, depression, and hostility) to capture aspects of the self-model dimension, and measures of sociability (vs. shyness) and interpersonal warmth to capture the other-model dimension. As predicted, secure and dismissing individuals scored higher on self-esteem and self-acceptance and lower on distress than preoccupied and fearful individuals. Regarding the other-model dimension, secure and preoccupied individuals indeed reported being more sociable than dismissing and fearful subjects.

A number of studies have focused on the earlier three-category model of attachment proposed by Hazan and Shaver (1987). Their model postulates similar categories for secure and preoccupied attachment, plus an avoidant category that includes the fearful and dismissing styles subsequently differentiated in Bartholomew's (1990) model. These studies have found similar differences in working models (e.g., Collins & Read, 1990; Feeney & Noller, 1990; Hazan & Shaver, 1987; Shaver & Brennan, 1992). Secures seem to have positive models of both self and others: They report high self-esteem and self-confidence, and they have high regard for others, as implied by their high scores on measures such as trust and altruism. Preoccupieds seem to have evaluatively mixed models. Their model of self appears to be negative—they have relatively low self-esteem—but their model of others seems to be positive, at least in the sense that they view closeness to others as highly desirable. However, they do not seem to hold uniformly positive views of others; like avoidant individuals, they are less likely to believe others have good intentions (Hazan & Shaver, 1987) and they endorse less favorable beliefs about human nature (Collins & Read, 1990). Findings for avoidant adults have been less conclusive, at least with regard to the self-model dimension. Whereas avoidant individuals showed the expected lack of trust in others, their scores on self-esteem measures, for example, tended to fall between those obtained by secure and preoccupied individuals. This finding makes sense in terms of the two-dimensional model described in Figure 5.1: The avoidant category subsumes both dismissing–avoidant and fearful–avoidant individuals; both have negative other models, but they differ in the valence of their self models.

As we have seen, most research on adult working models has used existing instruments that assess various aspects of self-concept and personality to test predictions about working models. Given the central role of working models in attachment theory, an important next step is to work toward a more detailed understanding of the models that characterize each attachment style. In an effort in that direction, Klohnen and Bera (in press) selected self-descriptive adjectives from a larger set of items that had been administered to the participants in the Mills Longitudinal Study of women (Helson & Wink, 1992). To differentiate the working models of avoidant and secure individuals, Klohnen and Bera (in press) defined five domains of working models: (1) interpersonal closeness (e.g., affectionate, sympathetic), (2) emotional distance (e.g., unemotional, aloof), (3) self-reliance (e.g., independent, not dependent), (4) distrust (e.g., distrustful, wary), and (5) social confidence (e.g., outgoing, sociable). Attachment style classifications at age 52 were based on Hazan and Shaver's (1987) three-category measure. As hypothesized, the avoidant women described themselves as relatively less interpersonally close, more emotionally detached, more self-reliant, more distrustful, and less socially confident than the secures.

The self-descriptive adjectives used by Klohnen and Bera (in press) help elaborate the content of avoidant and secure working models, thus beginning to map the features of these working models in greater detail. Nonetheless, this research focused on only two of the four major attachment styles, and had to rely on items from a preexisting item pool that had been administered to the Mills Longitudinal sample. The research summarized in the remainder of this chapter aims to overcome the limitations of this initial work.

Our goal was to develop a broad-based measure that would enable us to explicate the content and structure of all four adult attachment styles in the Bartholomew and Horowitz (1991) model. We began with a comprehensive set of descriptors that were chosen on the basis of their theoretical relevance to attachment. To translate theoretical notions about the content of working models into explicit constructs that can be operationalized and measured, we used experts to define theoretical prototypes of the working models for each attachment style. We first summarize the steps we took to develop these expert-based prototypes (see Klohnen & John, 1997, for more detail), then consider evidence for their reliability, structural fidelity, and validity, and finally report a new study examining their consistency and change over 25 years of adulthood.

DEVELOPMENT OF EXPERT DEFINITIONS OF PROTOTYPICAL WORKING MODELS

Derivation of Working Model Prototypes

We developed our prototype measure of working models in several steps, which are summarized in Figure 5.2. In the first step, our aim was to assemble a comprehensive set of items that would allow us to capture as many aspects of working models as possible. For this purpose, we reviewed widely used self-concept and personality measures and culled from them all the adjectival descriptors and short phrases that seemed potentially or even vaguely related to attachment (see Figure 5.2). After

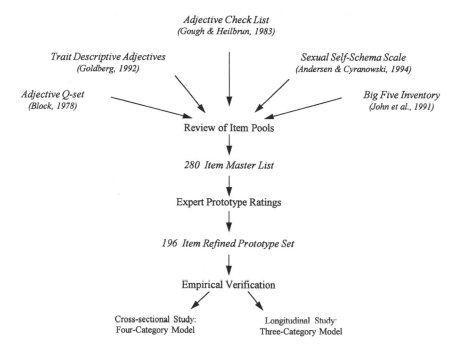

Adjective Check List
(Gough & Heilbrun, 1983)

Trait Descriptive Adjectives
(Goldberg, 1992)

Sexual Self-Schema Scale
(Andersen & Cyranowski, 1994)

Adjective Q-set
(Block, 1978)

Big Five Inventory
(John et al., 1991)

Review of Item Pools

280 Item Master List

Expert Prototype Ratings

196 Item Refined Prototype Set

Empirical Verification

Cross-sectional Study:
Four-Category Model

Longitudinal Study:
Three-Category Model

FIGURE 5.2. Steps in developing prototypes of working models of attachment.

eliminating redundancy in item content (e.g., trusting and trustful) and adding theoretically relevant descriptors not yet sufficiently represented (e.g., values autonomy, romantic, needy, detached), we arrived at a master list of 280 descriptors. Obviously, this master list was overinclusive—at this step, we retained items whose theoretical relevance to attachment was only tenuous. An examination of this list showed that it contained many items relevant to the Big Five dimensions Extraversion, Agreeableness, and Neuroticism but relatively few items relevant to Openness to experience (or intellect) and Conscientiousness (John, 1990)—a finding consistent with research showing that among the Big Five dimensions Openness and Conscientiousness are least closely related to adult attachment (Griffin & Bartholomew, 1994a; Shaver & Brennan, 1992).

In the second step, we used this master list to obtain expert ratings. Seven individuals familiar with the adult attachment literature provided prototypicality ratings of each item for four working models, one for each of the four attachment styles.[1] That is, the experts rated the degree to which prototypical preoccupied, fearful, dismissing, or secure individuals would view each item as characteristic (or uncharacteristic) of themselves. In our instructions to the experts, we emphasized that they should consider how the members of each attachment style would see *themselves* on these descriptors, not how others might perceive them. This is a difficult task that requires both expertise in attachment theory and psychological insight into people's conscious self-perceptions of their working models: The experts had to step into the "character" of each attachment style (as they conceptualize it theoretically) and rate how individuals who are preoccupied, fearful, dismissing, or secure would see and describe themselves. These prototypicality ratings were made on a 5-point rating scale that ranged from "definitely uncharacteristic" (–2) to "definitely characteristic" (+2), with a middle response option (0) to indicate that an item was "unrelated or irrelevant" to that attachment style. Thus, each judge provided four ratings (i.e., one for each attachment style) for all 280 items.

Shared Theoretical Conceptions: Did the Experts Agree on the Four Working Model Prototypes?

Our first question was whether the experts agreed. Obviously, we had hoped agreement would be substantial, but we realized it might be limited because the experts differed somewhat in their theoretical orientation and background on adult attachment. As described in Klohnen and John (1997), the experts achieved considerable interrater agreement. Interrater alphas for the composite of the seven judges were .94 for the secure prototype, .91 for preoccupied, .85 for fearful, and .87 for dismissing. Note that agreement was substantial even for the fearful and dismissing styles (Bartholomew, 1990) which represent two variants of the earlier avoidant style (Hazan & Shaver, 1987). In light of the substantial agreement among the judges, we derived composite working model prototype descriptions for each attachment style by averaging the ratings for each descriptor across all seven raters.

Content of the Working Models: What Are the Characteristic Attributes of the Four Prototypes?

The consensual prototype descriptions represent the experts' shared theoretical conceptions of the working models associated with each attachment style. What were the most characteristic and uncharacteristic attributes of the four working model prototypes? Examples of characteristic attributes of the secure prototype included confident, good-natured, dependable, and understanding; uncharacteristic attributes were insecure, unstable, cold, and suspicious. For the preoccupied prototype, characteristic attributes were expressive, dependent, needs approval, and self-revealing, whereas unemotional, aloof, self-reliant, and calm were among the most uncharacteristic attributes. The most characteristic attributes of the fearful prototype included vulnerable, doubting, timid, and distrustful, as contrasted with secure, optimistic, adaptable, and outgoing. Finally, the dismissing prototype was characterized by such features as independent, competent, rational, and sarcastic; uncharacteristic features were clingy, affectionate, jealous, and vulnerable. These attributes make good conceptual sense and seem to correspond closely to recent theoretical accounts of working models (e.g., Bartholomew & Horowitz, 1991; Collins & Read, 1994; Shaver, Collins, & Clark, 1996). Because attachment researchers might be interested in using the prototypes or the individual items in their research, Appendix 5.1 includes the 196 most relevant items and the experts' mean prototype ratings for all four attachment styles.

Structure of the Working Models: How Were the Prototypes Related?

The theory that underlies Bartholomew's (1990) conceptualization of attachment specifies that the four attachment styles fall into quadrants as shown in Figure 5.1. It follows from this conceptualization that diagonally opposite attachment styles—and their underlying working models—should be highly negatively correlated, whereas adjacent attachment styles should be correlated only moderately. Indeed, we found that the intercorrelations among the four expert prototypes conformed to these theoretical expectations (see Klohnen & John, 1997). The secure prototype was strongly negatively correlated with the fearful prototype, as were the preoccupied and dismissing prototypes. Moreover, as expected, the intercorrelations among theoretically adjacent prototypes were smaller in magnitude than those obtained for diagonally opposite styles; all four correlations were moderate in size, and none reached .40. The adjacent correlations differed from each other in potentially interesting ways. The secure and dismissing prototypes, and the preoccupied and fearful prototypes, were somewhat more similar to each other than were the secure and preoccupied prototypes and the dismissing and fearful prototypes. This pattern of correlations suggests that the prototypes for attachment styles assumed to be similar on the self-model dimension were more alike than the prototypes for styles assumed to be similar on the other-model dimension.

In evaluating these structural relations, it is important to keep in mind that they reflect the conceptual relations among the working model prototypes across the 280 items *as rated by the experts*, rather than their observed co-occurrence in a sample of individuals. Thus, the correlational findings might reflect the current understanding of working models in the attachment literature: Researchers might find it easier to conceptualize the self-model dimension than the other-model dimension. For example, Griffin and Bartholomew (1994a) have noted that the other-model dimension is more complex and more difficult to capture than the self-model dimension.

Regardless of the particular interpretation of the specific findings, however, the overall pattern of intercorrelations among the four working model prototypes indicates that the prototypes lined up as theory predicted: The diagonally opposite prototypes were most dissimilar, whereas adjacent styles showed only modest intercorrelations.

Reduction of the Master List: Were There Theoretically Irrelevant Items?

To ensure the representation of a broad range of item content, we had designed our master list of 280 items to be overinclusive. It contained a fair number of items that turned out to be conceptually unrelated to any of the four working models. Indeed, an examination of the expert ratings showed that some items received ratings of zero (irrelevant or unrelated) from all seven judges across all four prototypes, including intelligent, neat, innovative, and conventional. These items seemed unlikely to contribute much to the measurement of the working model prototypes and were therefore discarded.

More generally, we limited our item set to those items that differentiated reliably and substantially between at least two of the four attachment styles. To determine these items, we used a pairwise discrimination index expressed as an effect size in standard (z) score metric. In particular, we created pairwise comparisons by subtracting the composite rating (averaged across all seven judges) of each descriptor for one prototype from that for another prototype and divided the resulting difference score by the standard deviation (SD) of the seven expert ratings for that descriptor (i.e., the average of the SDs on the two prototypes being compared). This index takes the standard form of an effect size measure and reflects the difference between the two mean ratings in standard deviation units. We retained only those items that obtained values of at least plus or minus 2.0 on this index (i.e., a difference of at least two SDs); this cut-off ensured that the prototype ratings differed by at least two SDs (a sizable effect size) in at least one of the six possible pairwise comparisons between prototypes (e.g., secure vs. dismissing). Expressed in terms of a pairwise t-test, this cutoff corresponds to a $p < .004$ significance level. In this way we were able to reduce the number of items needed to score the working model prototypes to 196 items.

How Valid Are These Theory-Based Conceptualizations of Working Models?

So far, our findings suggested that we were able to capture a shared theoretical definition of the content of the four working models and that these definitions are in line with attachment theory: Agreement among the experts defining the prototypes was substantial, and the correlations among the conceptually derived prototypes approximated the theoretical structure postulated by Bartholomew (e.g., 1990; Bartholomew & Horowitz, 1991). However, reliability and structural fidelity do not address the crucial question of external validity: Do the theory-based working model prototypes capture how individuals with different attachment styles actually perceive and describe themselves? To evaluate how the four attachment groups would score on the working model prototypes, we needed to obtain prototype scores for a sample of individuals. It was thus necessary to collect self-ratings on the 196 items that define the refined working model prototypes. Prototype scores could then be computed for each participant, indicating the similarity of each participant's self-ratings to each of the four prototypes—that is, the correlation between the self-ratings and each prototype across all 196 items.

Initial evidence for the validity of the prototypes came from a large sample of undergraduates collected by Brennan, Clark, and Shaver (Chapter 3, this volume).[2] On the basis of their responses to a large number of attachment questionnaire items, participants were classified into one of the four attachment groups and also completed our 196-item prototype measure. As described in Klohnen and John (1996, 1997), each of the four attachment groups scored highest on their own working model prototype and lowest on the diagonally opposite one. Thus, secure individuals scored highest on the secure and lowest on the fearful prototype, preoccupied individuals highest on the preoccupied and lowest on the dismissing prototype, fearful individuals highest on the fearful and lowest on the secure prototype, and dismissing individuals highest on the dismissing and lowest on the preoccupied prototype. Again, these findings were consistent with Bartholomew's (e.g., Bartholomew & Horowitz, 1991) prediction that diagonally opposite styles should show the greatest dissimilarity. In short, our expert-based, theory-driven operationalization of working models showed promising construct validity; the empirical results suggested that they indeed capture differences in the ways individuals with different attachment styles perceive and describe themselves.

VALIDITY, STABILITY, AND CHANGE OF WORKING MODEL PROTOTYPES: FINDINGS FROM A 25-YEAR LONGITUDINAL STUDY

The validity of the working model prototypes in this cross-sectional study were encouraging. However, a more stringent test is possible if we can compare how individuals with different attachment styles score on the working model prototypes across time. If it is true that individual differences in attachment are maintained over time by internal working models (e.g., Main, Kaplan, & Cassidy, 1985; Rothbard & Shaver, 1994), then the working models themselves should be stable over time, and they should differ across attachment styles not only concurrently but also over time. To test these crucial assumptions, we used data from the Mills Longitudinal Study (Helson, 1967; Helson, Mitchell, & Moane, 1984; Helson & Wink, 1992). Helson and her colleagues have followed a sample of women who graduated from Mills College in the late 1950s over three decades of their adult lives. In the present study we made use of data collected at the age 27, 43, and 52 assessments.

Mills Longitudinal Data

Attachment style classifications were based on Hazan and Shaver's (1987) three-category measure when the women were 52 years old. The women were asked to choose the one paragraph description that best described their feelings about relationships. The following frequencies were obtained: 70% (n = 65) secure, 25% (n = 23) avoidant, and 5% (n = 4) preoccupied. This distribution of attachment styles for midlife women closely mirrors the distribution obtained for the age group of 45–54 year-old men and women in a recent study of a nationally representative sample (Mickelson et al., in press). As was the case in our sample, that study found very few preoccupied adults in this age group: 64% secure, 23% avoidant, and 8% preoccupied (with 5% unclassified). Note that this distribution of attachment styles in middle-aged samples differs from that usually found in college and young-adult samples, which tend to include more preoccupied individuals (about 20%) and fewer secure individuals (about 50%). The longitudinal design of the present study will allow us to examine whether these differences in attachment style frequencies are due to generational cohort differences or may be attributed to developmental *changes* in attachment style within the same individual over time.

To derive a measure of our working model prototypes, we used self-reports on the Adjective Check List (ACL; Gough & Heilbrun, 1983), a 300-item instrument containing a broad range of adjectives administered in checklist format (i.e., participants check only those adjectives that are self-descriptive). Self-reports on the ACL have been obtained at three Mills follow-up assessments spanning 25 years of adult development—at ages 27, 43, and 52.

Because the ACL was one of the instruments from which we had selected items for our initial master list, there was considerable item overlap between the 300 ACL items and our 196-item prototype measure. Specifically, 70% of the working model items also appear on the ACL. Using these 138 overlapping items (i.e., a slightly abbreviated set), we were able to compute working model prototype scores for each participant. In particular, we computed the similarity of each participant's self-description to each of the expert-based prototypes; that is, we computed the correlations between the self-descriptions and the prototypes across the 138 overlapping items.

Note that in the age 52 Mills follow-up assessment, conducted in 1989, only the original three attachment styles (Hazan & Shaver, 1987) could be measured. Thus, to map our four working model prototypes onto these three styles, we needed to derive an overall "avoidant" prototype. Because both the fearful and dismissing styles are considered variants of the broader avoidant style, we averaged the expert ratings of the fearful and dismissing prototypes. The descriptors most characteristic (or most uncharacteristic) of the resulting composite should thus be those descriptors that the experts rated very characteristic (or very uncharacteristic) of both the fearful and the dismissing styles; attributes considered characteristic of one but not the other style would end up "in the middle" as relatively unimportant (or irrelevant) attributes. According to theory (e.g., Bartholomew, 1990), the most characteristic attributes should be those that describe the negative other model that the two avoidant styles are thought to share. In line with this expectation, examples of the most characteristic adjectives on the ACL-based avoidant prototype were distrustful and reserved, as opposed to trusting and affectionate, which were least characteristic. Thus, using the ACL-based secure, preoccupied, and avoidant prototypes, we obtained three prototype-similarity scores for each individual at three ages (27, 43, and 52 years old). Higher scores indicate greater similarity, whereas lower scores (e.g., negative correlation coefficients) indicate relative dissimilarity.

Temporal Stability from Age 27 to 52

The longitudinal design of this research allowed us to ask several questions regarding the consistency of internal working models across adulthood. First, are individual differences in working models maintained over time? We addressed this question by examining the rank-order stability correlations for each of the working model prototypes across the three ages. Table 5.1 provides the temporal consistencies for each prototype score. The correlations were quite substantial, with an overall mean of .62. Most of the correlations were in the .50s and .60s. As expected, the

TABLE 5.1. Rank-Order Stability Correlations for Working Model Prototype Scores across 25 Years of Adult Development

Age period	Prototype scores			
	Secure	Preoccupied	Avoidant	Mean
27–43 years old	.52	.64	.57	.58
27–52 years old	.58	.58	.49	.55
43–52 years old	.75	.69	.70	.71
Mean	.63	.64	.60	.62

Note. Correlations are based on those subjects who had participated at all age periods and had attachment style ratings ($n = 70$).

rank-order stabilities were somewhat lower for the longest time period from age 27 to 52 (mean r = .55) than across the 9-year period from age 43 to 52 (mean r = .71). The column means in Table 5.1 show that overall the temporal stability coefficients for the three working model prototypes were quite similar to each other, with mean correlations ranging only from .60 for the avoidant to .64 for the preoccupied prototype scores. Finally, it is worth noting that these temporal stability correlations are similar to those obtained for personality scales on the ACL over the same time periods (e.g., Helson & Moane, 1987; Helson & Wink, 1992). Although the working model prototypes are unlike personality trait scales in that they represent broad patterns of diverse attributes, they nevertheless showed very similar levels of stability over time.

Differences between Attachment Styles over Time

Next we examined how the Mills Longitudinal Study women differed on the three working model prototypes and whether their scores changed over time. More specifically, how did secure, preoccupied, and avoidant women score on each of the three working model prototypes at age 52, when their attachment styles were assessed? And how did the women score when they were 27 years old and 43 years old, many years prior to the age 52 attachment classifications? Did their working model scores change—either decrease or increase—over time? Our longitudinal data speak to the cross-sectional findings reviewed earlier that fewer preoccupied and more secure individuals are found in later adulthood than in young adulthood. If these cross-sectional findings reflect developmental trends, then we should find that overall the Mills women became less preoccupied and more secure over time. In other words, they should decrease on the preoccupied working model prototype, increase on the secure working model prototype, and not change systematically on the avoidant prototype. We examined these questions using an ANOVA design, with time as a repeated-measures factor and attachment group as a between-subjects factor.

The three panels in Figure 5.3 show how secure, preoccupied, and avoidant women scored on each of the three working model prototypes at the three times of testing. Panel a shows the secure prototype scores, Panel b the preoccupied prototype scores, and Panel c the avoidant prototype scores. To facilitate interpretation and make effect sizes directly comparable across the three working model prototype scores in the three panels and across the three times of testing, the values in Figure 5.3 are given in standard score metric, with the z-scores computed across all three times of testing in order to preserve changes in mean levels over time.

Panel a in Figure 5.3 shows the respective mean scores on the secure prototype at ages 27, 43, and 52 for the women classified as either secure, preoccupied, or avoidant at age 52. Looking only at the concurrent data

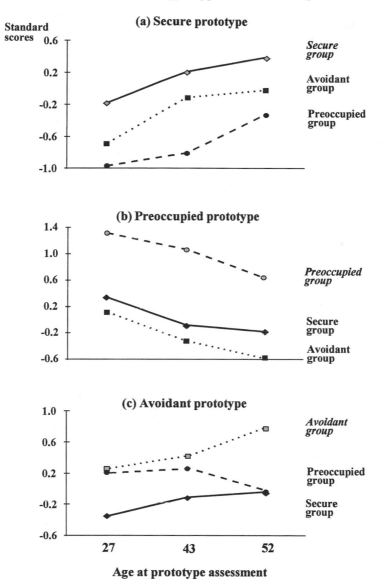

FIGURE 5.3. Mean level changes in working models across 25 years of adulthood by attachment classifications at age 52: secure prototype scores (Panel a), preoccupied prototype scores (Panel b), and avoidant prototype scores (Panel c).

(i.e., attachment and working model at age 52), the figure demonstrates that the secure women scored higher on the secure prototype than the women who were either preoccupied or avoidant. The results for the two earlier times of testing show that this difference in working models was already in place 9 years earlier, at age 43, and even 25 years earlier, at age 27. Across all three assessment periods, secure women scored about four-fifths of a standard deviation higher on the secure working model than preoccupied and avoidant women.

A second notable observation in Panel a was a general temporal trend: Scores on the secure prototype increased over time for all three groups. In ANOVA terms, these two observations—the maintenance of differences in working model prototype scores across time and mean level changes in prototype scores over time—suggest a main effect of attachment group, a main effect of time, and no interaction between attachment and time.

To test these effects more formally, we conducted a 3×3 ANOVA for each working model prototype, with attachment group (secure, preoccupied, avoidant) as a between-subjects factor, and time (age 27, 43, 52) as a repeated-measures factor. As expected, the ANOVA for the secure prototype showed a main effect of attachment group, $F(2, 67) = 2.8$, $p < .07$, and a main effect of time, $F(2,67) = 5.7$, $p < .01$, but no interaction.

Panels b and c in Figure 5.3 show the findings for the other two working model prototypes. For the preoccupied prototype, the ANOVA results showed a main effect of attachment group, $F(2, 67) = 3.2$, $p < .05$, a main effect of time, $F(2,67) = 6.3$, $p < .01$, and again no interaction. As expected, the preoccupied group scored highest at all three times, and the difference from the secure group was substantial, with an effect size of about one standard deviation. Moreover, as shown in Panel b, the main effect of time indicated a general drop in preoccupied prototype scores, and this effect held for all three attachment groups.

Finally, the ANOVA for the avoidant prototype also showed the expected main effect of attachment group, $F(2, 67) = 3.9$, $p < .05$, but no main effect of time and no interaction. Thus, although the Mills women changed significantly on the secure and preoccupied prototypes, we found no evidence of systematic change on the avoidant prototype. With respect to the differences among the three attachment groups, the findings for the avoidant prototype were weaker than for the other two prototypes. Although the avoidant group scored substantially higher than the secure group at all three times, with an effect size of about one-half of a standard deviation, it did not differ substantially from the other insecure group (the preoccupieds) at ages 27 and 43. In summary, the consistent main effects for attachment group and the lack of interactions between attachment group and time provide evidence for the validity of the working model prototypes across a 25-year period.

Implications of the Longitudinal Findings

These longitudinal findings are encouraging. Despite having to rely on abbreviated ACL-based working model prototypes, we found further support for the validity and usefulness of these prototypes. Because of the large number of items included on the expert prototypes, it was feasible to score sufficiently reliable and valid prototype scores from the ACL. Our concurrent analyses at age 52 suggest that the three groups indeed differed in their working models at the time when the attachment classifications were obtained; each of the attachment groups scored highest on its corresponding working model prototype. In addition to these systematic differences at midlife, our analyses suggest that most of these differences were already in place up to 25 years earlier. The substantial temporal stabilities—at .60 or above—for all three prototypes also suggest that individuals tend to maintain their relative standing on the prototypes. These are important findings: If working models of attachment are indeed part of the mechanism that fosters continuity in attachment organization across time, a minimum requirement is that these working models be fairly consistent over time. Our findings suggest they are.

In addition to the main effects of attachment style and the robust rank-order stabilities over time, we also obtained two intriguing main effects of time. Over 25 years of adulthood, the sample decreased on the preoccupied prototype (by about one-half a standard deviation) and increased on the secure prototype (by about one-half a standard deviation) but did not change on the avoidant prototype. These are provocative results because they complement the cross-sectional finding that the percentages of preoccupied and secure individuals differ from young to middle adulthood (Mickelson et al., in press): Whereas the percentage of avoidants stays roughly the same, the percentage of preoccupieds tends to be smaller at midlife and the percentage of secures tends to be greater. The present longitudinal findings of change in the *same individuals over time* suggest that these effects may be developmental, rather than generational. Thus, the combined cross-sectional and longitudinal findings suggest that over the course of young and middle adulthood, individuals might indeed become less preoccupied and increasingly more secure.

Why and how do these changes come about? At this point, we can only speculate about the underlying causes and mechanisms. One possibility is that young adults who show a preoccupied attachment style during early adulthood subsequently encounter life events and circumstances that foster security. For example, initially preoccupied individuals may find stable and loving relationship partners, and these positive relationship experiences may generalize to their underlying working models. Or, they might seek out forms of therapy that are conducive to positive changes in their working models. In contrast, avoidant individuals might forgo such experiences because they avoid getting emotionally close and involved with others, be it with a long-term relationship partner or with a therapist. This explanation may have some merit, as Klohnen and Bera (in press) have shown that by age 52 the avoidant women in the Mills sample were less likely to have had a long-term relationship, suggesting that they did not get exposed to relationship experiences sufficiently positive to disconfirm and alter their underlying working models.

Whereas these accounts highlight situational and experiential effects on internal representations of attachment relationships, general maturational changes may provide another explanation. One possibility is that preoccupation with romantic relationships becomes less important as people become older and more mature. This interpretation would be consistent with Helson and colleagues' (Helson & Moane, 1987; Helson & Wink, 1992) findings regarding personality change from early to middle adulthood: The Mills women increased in independence and decreased in traditional aspects of femininity, implying that in terms of their interests and identities they became less dependent on their partners. More generally, we suspect that both experiential and maturational factors will prove important, as researchers begin to document changes in adult attachment styles and unravel the underlying mechanisms and determinants.

CONCLUSIONS AND IMPLICATIONS

What Have We Learned?

In this chapter we have reviewed and summarized research on internal working models, focusing on their content, structure, and development in adulthood. Like much research in this area, our own work has examined those aspects of working models that are consciously accessible and relatively general in nature—that is, generalized beliefs and attitudes relevant to the self and relationships. In our research on expert prototypes (Klohnen & John, 1996, 1997), we began by culling potentially relevant items from commonly used inventories to create a large and comprehensive set of items that would allow us to capture as many aspects of working models as possible. In an effort to explicate existing theory, we asked experts to rate the relevance of each item to the particular working model assumed to underlie each of Bartholomew's (1990) four adult attachment styles.

The psychometric characteristics of the resulting expert-based working model prototypes were promising: We found considerable agreement among the expert ratings, and the prototypical attributes of each working model made conceptual sense. Moreover, the pattern of intercorrelations among the working model prototypes conformed to the theoretically expected structure. Across two studies, one using the three-category and the other the four-category attachment classification, we found that each attachment group indeed scored highest on its corresponding working model prototype, thus providing some support for construct validity. When we examined differences in working model prototype scores among secure, preoccupied, and avoidant women over a 25-year period, we found that the three attachment groups had fairly distinct working models that were maintained over time. Finally, we found that the sample as a whole decreased in their scores on the preoccupied prototype and increased on the secure prototype; these results, considered in conjunction with earlier cross-sectional findings, suggest developmental changes, rather than differences among generational cohorts. Tracing and understanding these developmental changes is one of the challenging tasks for the next wave of research on adult attachment. Focused longitudinal studies of adult development are needed to test experiential and maturational explanations for these changes.

Limitations

The available evidence for the validity of our working model prototypes, based on a cross-sectional and a longitudinal sample, appears quite promising. Nonetheless, this work has a number of limitations.

First, although we tried to be as inclusive as possible in our initial item selection, there might nevertheless be some attributes of working models that we have overlooked. However, now that we have available an explicit set of attributes to characterize the working model associated with each attachment style, it is possible to study how well we can predict each style from working model data; systematic differences in our ability to predict the four styles might suggest areas in which more theory and instrument development are needed. For example, a comparison of the fearful and dismissing prototypes might identify item content particularly suited to help differentiate these two kinds of avoidant groups.

A second limitation involves the number of expert judges. Ideally, every attachment researcher in the field would have served as an expert judge, and we had initially worried that seven judges might be too small a number to derive reliable and valid prototypes. However, the substantial levels of interjudge agreement provide some reassurance on that matter, indicating that adding more judges would not fundamentally change the prototype definitions obtained by Klohnen and John (1996, 1997) and presented here in Appendix 5.1.

Third, the development of our prototypes is tied to Bartholomew's (1990) four-category system. Although this system is currently the most influential account of adult attachment in the personality/social literature, there are other approaches. For example, we did not obtain a prototype for Hazan and Shaver's (1987) original avoidant style, nor does Bartholomew's (1990) four-category system map directly onto the categories defined and measured by the Adult Attachment Interview developed by Main and her colleagues (George, Kaplan, & Main, 1985; Main & Goldwyn, in press). Future research should examine how the four working model prototypes developed here relate to these other classificatory systems.

Fourth, more extensive evidence is needed to evaluate construct validity. Future research should extend the present findings to other data sources, such as peer reports of attachment styles.

Fifth, although the longitudinal findings presented here are intriguing, our sample was not large and included only women with college degrees. These findings need to be replicated in larger, more heterogeneous samples. Moreover, the prototype scores in this longitudinal study were based on the smaller and less comprehensive set of items included on the ACL. These prototype scores are likely to have somewhat lower reliabilities and validities, therefore leading to lower-bound effect sizes. Finally, the avoidant prototype had to be measured as the average of the dismissive and fearful prototypes, a theoretically justified but certainly suboptimal procedure. Indeed, the somewhat weaker findings for this prototype might be due, in part, to this limitation.

Future Directions

We now consider the present research in the context of the four-category model of attachment summarized in Figure 5.1. Which parts of that model are measured by our four working model prototypes? Note that our prototypes do not directly measure the positivity of a person's model of self or the positivity of a person's model of others. Rather, the prototypes measure the four particular *combinations* of self and other models that define the four attachment patterns in Figure 5.1. Consider the working model prototype we developed for the secure style. For example, the experts rated "optimistic" and "cooperative" as highly characteristic of this working model because these attributes imply both a positive view of self *and* a positive view of others. Similarly, "clingy" and "jealous," attributes rated as highly characteristic of the preoccupied working model, imply both negative views of self and positive views of others.

An alternative strategy to understanding and measuring working models would be to focus more directly on the content of the self and the other models. Consider the attribute "competent," which suggests a positive view of self but is neutral with respect to the other model; not surprisingly, the experts rated this attribute as highly characteristic of both the secure and the dismissive working models, which share a positive model of self. Similarly, "loving" was highly characteristic of both the secure and the preoccupied prototypes, which share a positive view of others. These examples show that one can identify attributes that uniquely define the self-model dimension and the other-model dimension.

Ultimately, the two approaches, one focusing on the four attachment patterns and the other on self and other models, need to be combined, as suggested by Figure 5.1 (see Klohnen & John, 1996, 1997). We can then think of the attributes associated with the four attachment patterns as particular combinations of the self- and other-model dimensions. For example, the combination of "competent" (positive self) and "loving" (positive other) yields attributes such as "optimistic" and "cooperative," which the experts rated as highly characteristic of the working model associated with the secure attachment style. Similarly, the combination of "affectionate" (positive other) and "anxious" (negative self) yields "clingy" and "jealous," attributes that the experts rated as characteristic of the working model associated with the preoccupied attachment style.

These examples show that it is possible to develop separate working model measures—one set focused directly on the content of the four attachment patterns (i.e., secure, preoccupied, fearful, and dismissing) and another set focused on the two poles defining the self-model dimension and the other-model dimension (i.e., positive self, negative self, positive other, and negative other). This measurement approach results in eight working model scales that should theoretically conform to the circumplex structure implied by Figure 5.1. As we have recently shown (Klohnen & John, 1996, 1997), there is considerable evidence for this circumplex structure.

A second broad issue in research on working models involves the conceptual justification for the method used to assess the self- and other-model dimensions. The self model is conceptualized and measured quite straightforwardly via the individual's judgments about his or her subjectively experienced self-worth. The other model, however, is more complex. Studies of the four-category system have used self-reports of interpersonal orientations to assess the other-model dimension. In other words, rather than asking direct questions about specific or generalized others (e.g., "Do you think others are trustworthy?"), the other-model dimension has mostly been inferred from questions about the interpersonal characteristics of the self (e.g., "Do you trust others?"). In the research summarized here, we also have taken the latter approach, asking individuals to rate how trusting, outgoing, or jealous they are.

Note, however, that two earlier studies of the three-category system used measures of the other-model dimension that were less explicitly focused on judgments about the self, namely, questions about individuals' beliefs about others, human nature, and the larger world (Collins & Read, 1990; Hazan & Shaver, 1987). Future research on the four-category system should examine how individuals with different attachment styles perceive and describe others, both the "hypothetical others" invoked by attachment theorists (e.g., Bartholomew & Horowitz, 1991) and the "real" individuals that are important in people's lives. One approach to measure the "hypothetical other" is to ask individuals to rate how frequent they think particular attributes are among people in general. Whereas this approach focuses on a rather abstract notion of other, a second approach would focus on specific others, such as romantic partners, friends, and family members. At this point, little is known about the connections between attachment and the expectations individuals hold about people in general as contrasted with those they hold about specific individuals. For example, it remains to be seen whether dismissing individuals expect people in general to be untrustworthy and whether they describe their best friends and lovers in more negative terms than do securely attached individuals.

In conclusion, we hope that this research on conceptualizing and measuring components of working models will prove helpful for understanding the ways in which working models are acquired, how they change over time, and how they mediate the effects of the attachment system on behavioral and life outcomes in adulthood. The longitudinal analyses presented in this chapter provide an initial step in this direction. With new and more flexible measurement instruments at our disposal, the next decade of research on adult attachment promises to be an exciting time.

Appendix 5.1

MEAN EXPERT RATINGS OF THE PROTOTYPES FOR SECURE, PREOCCUPIED, FEARFUL, AND DISMISSING WORKING MODELS FOR 196 DESCRIPTORS

Item	Sec	Preoc	Fear	Dism	Item	Sec	Preoc	Fear	Dism
Acts without thinking	−.57	1.29	−.57	−.71	Complaining	−1.00	1.14	.71	−.71
					Complex	.29	.43	.57	−.29
Adaptable	1.71	−.43	−1.29	.86	Confident	2.00	−1.43	−1.57	1.71
Adventurous	1.00	.14	−1.43	.71	Confused	−1.14	1.29	1.14	−1.29
Affectionate	1.71	1.57	−.86	−1.29	Considerate	1.57	1.29	.43	.00
Aggressive	−.43	−.14	−.71	.57	Contented	1.57	−1.57	−1.14	1.14
Agreeable	1.43	.86	−.29	−.29	Cool	−.57	−1.29	−.14	1.00
Aloof	−1.29	−1.86	.29	.71	Cooperative	1.57	1.14	.29	.00
Ambitious	.57	.29	.00	1.57	Creative	.57	.29	−.43	−.14
Ambivalent	−1.43	.43	1.00	−1.00	Critical	−.43	.57	.57	.86
Anxious	−1.14	1.43	1.43	−1.71	Cynical	−1.00	−.57	.71	1.00
Appreciative	1.14	1.00	.14	−.14	Daring	.57	.29	−1.00	.86
Assertive	1.43	−.14	−1.43	1.43	Deep	.00	.86	.14	−.29
Attractive	.86	.00	−.71	.86	Defensive	−.86	.71	.57	−1.43
Autonomous	1.57	−1.43	−.86	2.00	Deliberate	.29	−1.00	−.14	.71
Avoidant	−1.29	−1.29	1.43	1.00	Demanding	−.57	.00	.29	−.29
Bashful	−.71	−.29	1.14	−1.00	Dependable	2.00	.57	.29	.29
Bold	.86	.29	−1.00	1.00	Dependent	−.14	2.00	.29	−1.86
Calm	1.71	−1.57	−1.00	.86	Depressed, blue	−1.43	1.29	1.43	−1.14
Can be counted on	2.00	.71	−.29	.43	Detached	−1.43	−1.43	.57	1.14
Capable	1.86	−.43	−.86	1.71	Dismissive	−1.29	−1.71	.00	1.29
Cautious	−.14	−.71	1.43	.29	Dissatisfied	−1.43	1.43	1.29	−.71
Changeable	.43	.71	−.14	−.57	Distant	−1.43	−1.86	.86	1.29
Charming	.71	1.00	−.57	.43	Distractible	−.57	1.14	−.14	−.29
Cheerful	1.57	.29	−1.14	.14	Distressed	−1.43	1.71	1.43	−1.43
Clingy	−1.00	1.57	−.57	−2.00	Distrustful	−1.43	.86	1.57	.57
Cold	−1.57	−1.57	.29	.29	Doesn't show feelings	−1.14	−1.86	.43	1.43
Competent	1.71	−.71	−1.14	1.71					
Competitive	.57	.29	−.29	1.43	Dominant	.71	−.57	−1.29	1.00

Item	Sec	Preoc	Fear	Dism	Item	Sec	Preoc	Fear	Dism
Doubting	-.57	1.00	1.57	-.57	Not easily satisfied	-.43	.43	.71	.43
Easily upset	-1.00	2.00	1.00	-1.71	Obliging	.14	.71	.29	-.71
Easy-going	1.43	-.71	-.86	.86	Optimistic	1.71	.43	-1.43	.29
Emotional	.43	2.00	.14	-1.57	Outgoing	1.43	1.00	-1.29	.00
Energetic	1.00	.57	-.57	.43	Outspoken	.29	.29	-.86	.14
Enthusiastic	1.43	1.00	-.71	.14	Passionate	1.14	1.57	-.29	-1.00
Envious	-.71	1.57	.86	-1.00	Patient	.86	-.57	-.29	-.29
Evasive	-.71	-.71	.43	.43	Pessimistic	-1.43	.29	1.57	.00
Excitable	.29	1.43	-.14	-.71	Playful	1.29	.71	-.57	.14
Expressive	1.43	2.00	-.29	-1.14	Pleasure-seeking	.86	.86	-.43	.43
Extraverted	1.29	.86	-.86	.29	Practical	.43	-.71	.14	.86
Fearful	-.86	.71	1.86	-1.29	Preoccupied	-1.00	1.00	.71	-1.00
Feminine	.00	.86	.43	-1.00	Proud	.43	-.43	-.43	.57
Flirtatious	.14	1.14	-.57	.14	Prudent	.71	-.71	.00	.57
Forceful	.57	-.29	-1.00	1.00	Prudish	-.43	-1.14	.57	-.14
Forgiving	1.43	.14	-.43	-.71	Quiet	-.29	-.86	1.14	.00
Fretful	-.86	.71	1.14	-.86	Rational	.57	-1.43	.00	1.43
Friendly	1.71	1.14	-.57	.14	Realistic	.71	-.57	.43	1.00
Frustrated	-1.29	1.43	1.14	-.57	Reflective	.71	.86	.71	-.86
Generous	1.14	.86	.00	.00	Relaxed	1.43	-1.14	-1.00	.71
Gentle	1.14	.86	.57	-.43	Reliable	1.29	.29	.29	.29
Giving	1.14	1.29	.00	.00	Resentful	-1.29	1.00	1.14	.29
Gloomy	-.71	.57	1.00	.43	Reserved	-.71	-1.29	1.57	.86
Good-natured	2.00	1.14	.71	.71	Responsive to others	1.86	1.57	-.14	-.29
Hard-headed	-.14	-.43	.14	.86	Restless, fidgety	-.29	1.00	.00	-.57
Harsh	-.71	-.71	-.29	.43	Rigid	-1.00	-.71	.57	.00
Headstrong	.00	.29	-.43	1.14	Robust	.71	-.86	-1.14	.71
High-strung	-1.00	1.57	.57	-1.43	Romantic	1.14	2.00	-.14	-.71
Honest	.86	.00	.14	.43	Ruminative	-.71	1.57	1.43	-1.14
Hostile	-1.43	.14	-.14	.14	Sarcastic	-.86	.00	.71	1.29
Idealistic	.71	1.14	-.86	-.57	Secure	1.86	-1.57	-1.71	.57
Immature	-.71	.29	-.14	-.57	Seeks reassurance	-.14	1.86	1.14	-2.00
Impatient	-.71	1.00	.29	.71	Self-centered	-1.14	1.00	.00	-.14
Impulsive	-.43	1.29	.14	-.86	Self-conscious	-.71	.29	1.43	-1.00
Inconsistent	-.43	1.00	.00	-1.00	Self-controlled	.43	-1.29	.29	1.00
Independent	1.29	-1.43	.00	2.00	Self-denying	-.57	-1.00	.29	.57
Indifferent	-1.00	-1.14	-.29	1.14	Self-pitying	-1.29	1.00	1.00	-1.29
Individualistic	.00	-.86	-.14	1.14	Self-protective	-.43	.43	1.29	.71
Inhibited	-1.29	-1.14	1.29	-.29	Self-reliant	1.29	-1.57	.57	1.86
Insecure	-1.57	1.86	1.71	-.43	Self-revealing	.86	1.86	-.43	-1.00
Introspective	.43	.71	.57	-.57	Selfish	-.57	-.14	-.14	.14
Introverted	-.86	.14	1.29	-.43	Sensible	1.00	-.86	-.29	1.14
Irritable	-.86	.43	.29	.43	Sensitive	.86	1.57	.71	-.86
Jealous	-.43	2.00	.71	-1.86	Sentimental	.29	1.43	.14	-1.43
Kind	1.43	1.00	.29	-.14	Sexy	.57	.71	-.57	.57
Likes to be center of attention	.00	1.00	-1.43	.29	Show-off	.00	1.43	-1.43	-.57
					Shy	-1.14	-.43	1.86	-.14
Likes to be with others	1.86	2.00	.00	-.57	Sociable	1.57	1.14	-.86	-.29
Logical	.14	-.14	.00	.86	Soft-hearted	.86	1.14	.43	-1.29
Loving	1.71	1.57	.00	-.43	Spontaneous	1.00	1.43	-.57	-.29
Masculine	.29	-1.00	-.29	1.00	Stable	1.57	-1.14	-.71	1.29
Modest	.14	-.29	.57	.00	Stern	-.29	-.57	-.14	.29
Moody	-1.00	1.43	.71	-1.00	Strong	1.00	-.86	-1.14	1.29
Nagging	-.71	.86	-.29	-.43	Stubborn	-.57	.29	.43	.57
Natural	.57	.29	-.29	.00	Submissive	-1.29	-.43	1.29	-1.71
Needs approval	-.29	1.86	1.43	-1.86	Suggestible	-.43	.86	.14	-1.14
Needy	-1.00	1.86	1.14	-1.86					
Nervous	-1.29	1.29	1.29	-1.43					

Item	Sec	Preoc	Fear	Dism	Item	Sec	Preoc	Fear	Dism
Sulky	−.43	.86	.43	−.71	Understanding	1.86	.71	.29	.14
Superstitious	−.29	.57	.14	−.71	Unemotional	−.86	−2.00	−.71	1.29
Suspicious	−1.43	1.00	1.29	.00	Uninhibited	.43	1.29	−1.43	−.71
Sympathetic	1.43	1.00	−.14	−.29	Unrestrained	.14	1.14	−.86	−.86
Takes initiative	.71	.43	−.86	.86	Unstable	−1.57	1.57	1.00	−.71
Talkative	.57	1.29	−.86	−.14	Values	1.14	−.86	.43	1.86
Temperamental	−.71	1.57	.71	−1.00	autonomy				
Tense	−1.57	1.14	.86	−.57	Versatile	1.29	−.29	−.43	.86
Timid	−1.14	−.14	1.71	−1.00	Vulnerable	−.86	1.43	1.86	−1.71
Tolerant	1.29	1.00	.00	−.14	Warm	1.86	1.57	−.14	.43
Touchy	−1.14	1.00	.57	−.86	Wary	−.71	.71	1.43	.14
Tough	.00	−.86	−.86	1.43	Weak	−.71	1.00	.57	−1.86
Trusting	1.57	−.14	−1.86	−1.00	Withdrawn	−1.29	−1.00	1.57	−.43
Unassuming	.29	−.29	1.00	.29	Worrying	−1.29	1.86	1.57	−1.29

Note. Sec, Secure; Preoc, Preoccupied; Fear, Fearful; Dism, Dismissing. Mean ratings are based on seven expert judges; experts made prototypicality ratings on a 5-point rating scale that ranged from "definitely uncharacteristic" (−2) to "definitely characteristic" (+2), with a middle response option (0) to indicate that an item was "unrelated or irrelevant" to that attachment style.

ACKNOWLEDGMENTS

The preparation of this chapter was supported by Grant Nos. MH43948 and MH49255 from the National Institute of Health. We are indebted to Kelly A. Brennan for including our prototype measure in her large-scale attachment measurement study, and to Ravenna Helson for giving us access to the Mills Longitudinal study and for her tangible and intangible support of our research. We also thank Kim Bartholomew, Ravenna Helson, Jennifer L. Pals, W. Steven Rholes, and Jeffry A. Simpson for their comments on an earlier version of this chapter.

NOTES

1. The prototype raters were Kelly Brennan, Kevin Carlson, Per Gjerde, Debbie Jacobvitz, Oliver John, Eva Klohnen, and Phillip Shaver, who completed the ratings in consultation with Catherine Clark and Chris Fraley. We are indebted to them for donating their time to complete the prototype ratings on which this work is based.

2. We are particularly grateful to Kelly A. Brennan, who collected these ratings as part of her larger project and made them available to us.

REFERENCES

Andersen, B. L., & Cyranowski, J. M. (1994). Women's sexual self-schema. *Journal of Personality and Social Psychology, 67,* 1079–1100.

Bartholomew, K. (1990). Avoidance of intimacy: An attachment perspective. *Journal of Social and Personal Relationships, 7,* 147–178.

Bartholomew, K., & Horowitz, L. M. (1991). Attachment styles among young adults: A test of a four-category model. *Journal of Personality and Social Psychology, 61,* 226–244.

Bowlby, J. (1973). *Attachment and loss: Vol. 2. Separation: Anxiety and anger.* New York: Basic Books.

Bowlby, J. (1980). *Attachment and loss: Vol. 3. Loss: Sadness and depression.* New York: Basic Books.

Collins, N. L., & Read, S. J. (1990). Adult attachment, working models, and relationship quality in dating couples. *Journal of Personality and Social Psychology, 58,* 644–663.

Collins, N. L., & Read, S. J. (1994). Cognitive representations of attachment: The structure and function of working models. In K. Bartholomew & D. Perlman (Eds.), *Attachment processes in adulthood: Advances in personal relationships* (pp. 53–90). London: Jessica Kingsley.

Feeney, J. A., & Noller, P. (1990). Attachment style as a predictor of adult romantic relationships. *Journal of Personality and Social Psychology, 58,* 281–291.

George, C., Kaplan, N., & Main, M. (1985). *Adult Attachment Interview.* Unpublished manuscript, University of California, Berkeley.

Goldberg, L. R. (1992). The development of markers for the Big Five factor structure. *Psychological Assessment, 4,* 26–42.

Gough, H. G., & Heilbrun, A. B., Jr. (1983). *The Adjective Check List manual.* Palo Alto, CA: Consulting Psychologists Press.

Griffin, D. W., & Bartholomew, K. (1994a). The metaphysics of measurement: The case of adult attachment. In K. Bartholomew & D. Perlman (Eds.), *Attachment processes in adulthood: Advances in personal relationships* (pp. 17–51). London: Jessica Kingsley.

Griffin, D. W., & Bartholomew, K. (1994b). Models of the self and other: Fundamental dimensions underlying measures of adult attachment. *Journal of Personality and Social Psychology, 67,* 430–445.

Hazan, C., & Shaver, P. (1987). Romantic love conceptualized as an attachment process. *Journal of Personality and Social Psychology, 52,* 511–524.

Helson, R. (1967). Personality characteristics and developmental history of creative college women. *Genetic Psychology Monographs, 76,* 205–256.

Helson, R., Mitchell, V., & Moane, G. (1984). Personality and patterns of adherence and non-adherence to the social clock. *Journal of Personality and Social Psychology, 46,* 1079–1096.

Helson, R., & Moane, G. (1987). Personality change in women from college to midlife. *Journal of Personality and Social Psychology, 53,* 176–186.

Helson, R., & Wink, P. (1992). Personality change in women from the early 40s to early 50s. *Psychology and Aging, 7,* 45–55.

John, O. P. (1990). The "Big Five" factor taxonomy: Dimensions of personality in the natural language and in questionnaires. In L. A. Pervin (Ed.), *Handbook of personality: Theory and research* (pp. 66–100). New York: Guilford Press.

John, O. P., Donahue, E. M., & Kentle, R. L. (1991). *The Big Five Inventory: Versions 4a and 54* (Technical report). University of California, Berkeley: Institute of Personality and Social Research.

Klohnen, E. C., & Bera, S. (in press). Behavioral and experiential patterns of avoidantly and securely attached women across adulthood: A 30-year longitudinal perspective. *Journal of Personality and Social Psychology.*

Klohnen, E. C., & John, O. P. (1996, August). *Attachment styles and a circumplex measure of internal working models.* Poster presented at the biannual conference of the International Society for the Study of Personal Relationships, Banff, Canada.

Klohnen, E. C., & John, O. P. (1997). *A circumplex conception of internal working models of attachment.* Manuscript submitted for publication.

Main, M. (1991). Metacognitive knowledge, metacognitive monitoring, and singular (coherent) vs. multiple (incoherent) model of attachment: Findings and directions for future research. In C. M. Parkes, J. Stevenson-Hinde, & P. Marris (Eds.), *Attachment across the life cycle* (pp. 127–159). London: Tavistock/Routledge.

Main, M., & Goldwyn, R. (in press). Interview-based adult attachment classifications: Related to infant–mother and infant–father attachment. *Developmental Psychology.*

Main, M., Kaplan, N., & Cassidy, J. (1985). Security in infancy, childhood, and adulthood: A move to the level of representation. *Monographs of the Society for Research in Child Development, 50,* 66–104.

Mickelson, K. D., Kessler, R. C., & Shaver, P. R. (in press). Adult attachment in a nationally representative sample. *Journal of Personality and Social Psychology.*

Rothbard, J. C., & Shaver, P. R. (1994). Continuity of attachment across the life span. In M. B. Sperling & W. H. Berman (Eds.), *Attachment in adults: Clinical and developmental perspectives* (pp. 31–71). New York: Guilford Press.

Scharfe, E., Bartholomew, K., Henderson, A., Trinke, S., Cobb, R., Poole, J., Callander, L., & Servello, S. (1996, August). *Four-category model of adult attachment: Measurement issues, prototype descriptions, and other tidbits.* Workshop given at the biannual conference of the International Society for the Study of Personal Relationships, Banff, Canada.

Shaver, P. R., & Brennan, K. A. (1992). Attachment styles and the "Big Five" personality traits: Their connections with each other and with romantic relationship outcomes. *Personality and Social Psychology Bulletin, 18,* 536–545.

Shaver, P. R., Collins, N., & Clark, C. L. (1996). Attachment styles and internal working models of self and relationship partners. In G. J. O. Fletcher & J. Fitness (Eds.), *Knowledge structures in close relationships: A social psychological approach* (pp. 25–62). Mahwah, NJ: Erlbaum.

Shaver, P., & Hazan, C. (1993). Adult romantic attachment: Theory and evidence. In D. Perlman & W. Jones (Eds.), *Advances in personal relationships* (pp. 29–70). London: Jessica Kingsley.

PART III

Affect Regulation

6

The Relationship between Adult Attachment Styles and Emotional and Cognitive Reactions to Stressful Events

MARIO MIKULINCER
VICTOR FLORIAN

Toward the end of the 20th century, the issue of coping and adaptation to stress has become one of the hot areas of psychological theory, research, and practice. Although numerous studies have been published on this issue, there is still a lively debate on the personal and contextual factors that may influence the ability to cope with stressful experiences. One of the major theoretical trends in psychological literature emphasizes the central role that individual differences may play in the process of coping and adaptation (e.g., Kobasa, 1982; Lazarus & Folkman, 1984). In this context, the present chapter focuses on Bowlby's (1973, 1988) idea that attachment working models may function as inner structures upon which people organize experience and handle distress. Our basic premise is that secure attachment is an inner resource that may help a person to positively appraise stressful experiences, to constructively cope with these events, and to improve his or her well-being and adjustment. In contrast, insecure attachment, either avoidant or anxious–ambivalent, can be viewed as a potential risk factor, leading to poor coping and to maladjustment.

Although Bowlby's theory mainly deals with developmental and interpersonal issues, the association between the attachment system and reactions to life stress is one of the basic pillars of this theoretical framework. First of all, attachment theory was originally formulated in order to understand animal and human reactions to two major life stressors, loss and separation. Second, Bowlby (1969, 1973) proposed that attachment processes in the early relationship between child and caretaker function as protective mechanisms in encounters with danger and threat. In his view, the attachment system is activated when infants experience distress, and the goal of attachment responses is to maintain proximity to a nurturing adult, who is expected to help the infant to manage the distress and to promote a sense of well-being and security. Third, the original empirical test of attachment theory—the Strange Situation paradigm (Ainsworth, Blehar, Waters, & Wall, 1978)—was conducted under the assumption that attachment working models may determine one's reactions to two basic stressors—maternal separation and the presence of a stranger. Fourth, the sorting of insecurely attached persons into avoidant and anxious–ambivalent groups reflects the idea that attachment working models include defensive strategies that guide people in coping with stress (Bowlby, 1988).

In analyzing Bowlby's theory, it is clear that the basic concept of security in attachment can be viewed as an "inner resource" that may help the individual to cope successfully with life adversities. Security in attachment develops from the early relationship with a nurturing adult who is responsive and sensitive to one's signals of distress and who is available in times of need. These positive experiences help to create basic trust in the world and the self, to build a sense of a "secure base" (Bowlby, 1973), and to develop expectations that stressful experiences, although painful and requiring effort, can be manageable (Bowlby, 1988; Shaver & Hazan, 1993). Furthermore, security in attachment may evolve into optimistic expectations, a strong sense of control and self-efficacy, and self-confidence in seeking outside help in times of need (e.g., Bartholomew & Horowitz, 1991; Collins & Read, 1990; Shaver & Hazan, 1993). When achieved, this sense of security may become a stable personality aspect and a main source of continuity throughout the entire life span. In our view, all these components of secure attachment can be viewed as resilience factors, which may foster a constructive attitude toward life and buffer the psychological distress resulting from the encounters adversity.

Bowlby's theory also implies that insecure attachment can be viewed as a risk factor that may detract from the individual's resilience in times of stress. The early attachment experience of insecure persons (both anxious–ambivalent and avoidant) is characterized by unstable and inadequate regulation of distress by the caretaker and a sense of personal inefficacy in relieving discomfort (Bowlby, 1973; Shaver & Hazan, 1993). These experiences may obstruct the development of the inner resources necessary for successful coping with, and adaptation to, life stressors.

With regard to anxious–ambivalent persons, these experiences may foster a generalized working model that exaggerates the appraisal of adversities as threatening, irreversible, and uncontrollable. When facing such situations, these persons may react with strong emotional distress, continuing even after the actual threat has terminated. It is possible that their sense of smallness and helplessness and the lack of a sense of permanence and support provided by secure attachment bonds may impair their ability to put the distress behind them. In the case of avoidant persons, such early experiences may lead to working models that emphasize the threatening and untrustworthy nature of significant others, the need to rely exclusively on oneself, and the importance of maintaining distance from attachment figures and relationships, which may cause distress. Although these avoidant strategies may reduce overt expressions of distress, they may unable in the long run to mitigate internalized sources of attachment insecurity and pain.

Support for this reasoning can be found in recent studies that have examined the association between attachment style and cognitive and emotional aspects of maladjustment. Avoidant and anxious–ambivalent people seem to be more anxious and more hostile than secure people (Kobak & Sceery, 1988), and to have more negative and mistrusting views of the social world and of human nature in general (Collins & Read, 1990). Anxious–ambivalent people were found to have more negative self-views than secure people (Bartholomew & Horowitz, 1991; Collins & Read, 1990; Mikulincer, 1995), and to show signs of distress related to disagreement and conflict with attachment figures (see Feeney, Chapter 8, this volume). Avoidant people were not likely to use partners as sources of reassurance in anxiety-arousing conditions (Simpson, Rholes, & Nelligan, 1992), and tended to show signs of distress in situations that might decrease the psychological distance from attachment figures (see Rholes, Simpson, & Grich Stevens, Chapter 7, this volume). In addition, as compared to secure persons, both types of insecure attachment have been found to be related to loneliness (Hazan & Shaver, 1987), physical symptoms (Hazan & Shaver, 1990), negative affect (Simpson, 1990), alcohol consumption, eating disorders (Brennan, Shaver, & Tobey, 1991), and shame, anger, fear of negative evaluation and pathological narcissism (Wagner & Tangney, 1991). It seems that "insecure attachment at adulthood, as in infancy, places individuals at risk for a variety of problems with which they are poorly equipped to cope" (Shaver & Hazan, 1993).

Another implication of Bowlby's theory involves the role that attachment working models may play in determining the selection of particular coping strategies for dealing with stress. In our terms, these working models are cognitive schemata that provide people with guidelines about the ways to cope with life adversities. Even in the early Ainsworth (e.g., Ainsworth et al., 1978) studies, we can observe the infant's adoption of different strategies for coping with the stress of maternal separation.

While anxious–ambivalent infants tend to adopt a clinging and hypervigilant attitude toward the source of stress, avoidant infants adopt a strategy of detachment from this source. Moreover, it is obvious that one basic difference between secure and insecure infants is the use of the caretaker as a resource for managing distress. While secure infants tend to seek the caretaker's proximity during stressful episodes and to rely on him or her as a source of security, insecure infants may be more reluctant to seek the help of the caretaker. These early differences in the coping process also may be manifested in adulthood, every time individuals are confronted with stressful events.

The attachment literature describes secure persons as dealing with distress by acknowledging it, enacting instrumental constructive actions, and turning to others for emotional and instrumental support (Bowlby, 1988; Kobak & Sceery, 1988; Shaver & Hazan, 1993). Securely attached persons are hypothesized to be more tolerant of stressful events and to allow accessibility of unpleasant emotions, without being overwhelmed by the resulting distress. In Lazarus and Folkman's (1984) terms, it seems that secure persons deal with distress by relying mainly on problem-focused and support-seeking strategies.

People characterized by the anxious–ambivalent pattern of attachment are hypothesized to deal with stressful events by directing attention toward distress in a hypervigilant manner and by mentally ruminating on negative thoughts, memories, and affect (Kobak & Sceery, 1988; Mikulincer & Orbach, 1995; Shaver & Hazan, 1993). In Main, Kaplan, and Cassidy's (1985) terms, anxious–ambivalent people have free access to confused and negative affect and memories, which produce high levels of distress. These persons seem to be unable to repress negative emotions, to suppress negative thoughts, and to detach from inner pain, and thereby cannot limit the autonomous spreading of distress to other life areas (Mikulincer & Orbach, 1995). In Lazarus and Folkman's (1984) terms, anxious–ambivalent persons might deal with distress by relying mainly on passive, ruminative, emotion-focused strategies.

Avoidant people may deal with stressful events by restricting the acknowledgment of distress and by adopting what Bowlby (1973) labels "compulsive self-reliance" (Shaver & Hazan, 1993). Such a strategy is manifested in emphasis on autonomy and self-reliance, dismissal of the importance of the source of stress, and inhibition of display of negative emotions (Bowlby, 1973; Kobak & Sceery, 1988; Main et al., 1985). Mikulincer and Orbach (1995) argued that avoidant persons inhibit accessibility to unpleasant affect and thoughts, erect barriers against external or internal sources of distress, and escape from any direct or symbolic confrontation with life adversities. This defensive armor seems to be accompanied by underlying anxiety, which reflects the failure to achieve a "secure base" with attachment figures. In Lazarus and Folkman's (1984) terms, avoidant persons might deal with distress by relying on distancing withdrawal strategies.

In the following sections we review empirical evidence examining the idea that adult attachment styles may play an important role in determining the level of psychological distress that people experience during specific stressful circumstances. We also review the strategies they may use for coping with these events. In other words, we ask whether secure attachment serves as an inner resource in times of stress and whether insecure attachment may be a risk factor that increases vulnerability and distress. Specifically, we present data on the ways adult attachment styles seem to affect one's coping and emotional reactions to (1) the terror of personal death, (2) military and war-related stressors, (3) interpersonal losses, (4) personal failure, (5) parenthood-related stressors, and (6) chronic pain.

THE TERROR OF PERSONAL DEATH

Among the wide variety of stressors to which we are exposed during the life span, the threat of one's own death may be the most prominent one. Death has generally been seen as a source of fear and anxiety (e.g., Wass & Neimeyer, 1995). However, although the fear of death seems to be a universal phenomenon, there is wide agreement that basic individual differences exist in the way people react to and cope with the terror of their own mortality. In our view, attachment style, which seems to guide people in coping with stress, may be an important factor in explaining these individual differences.

In two separate studies in our laboratory (Florian & Mikulincer, in press; Mikulincer, Florian, & Tolmacz, 1990), we examined whether and how adult attachment style is related to the various expressions of the fear of personal death as well as to the psychological devices used for dealing with this fear. The basic theoretical assumption of these studies is that the encounter with death activates attachment-related working models and strategies of affect regulation. From our perspective, death not only entails a loss of oneself, but also involves an irreversible separation from loved persons. Fear of death may symbolically represent the infant's fear of separation from his or her primary attachment figures (e.g., Kalish, 1985).

In the first study (Mikulincer et al., 1990), we assessed differences among attachment styles in the overt meanings that people attribute to their fear of death and in below-level-of-awareness expressions of this fear (responses to projective Thematic Apperception Test [TAT] cards; Florian, Kravetz, & Frankel, 1984). This multilevel approach seems to be highly relevant, since the threat of death should activate defense mechanisms, such as denial, that reveal attachment-related styles of affect regulation. Eighty Israeli university students completed the Adult Attachment Style Scale (Hazan & Shaver, 1987) and the Fear of Personal Death Scale (FPDS), and wrote stories in response to four TAT death-relevant cards. The FPDS, a well-validated measure (Florian & Kravetz, 1983), taps three psychological meanings of fear of death: intrapersonal, interpersonal, and transpersonal consequences of death. Fear of death may involve fear of the expected impact on mind and body, social identity, or loved ones, or it may arise from beliefs about the transcendental nature of the self and punishment in the hereafter.

In the second study (Florian & Mikulincer, in press), we employed the theoretical framework of symbolic immortality introduced by Lifton (1979) in order to examine whether adult attachment style explains individual differences in the way people cope with the terror of their own death. The construct of symbolic immortality refers to the cognitive and behavioral attempts to preserve and develop a personal sense of continuity and lastingness, which can help people to transcend the fear of their own finitude (Lifton, 1979). Lifton hypothesizes that this anticipatory coping response to the terror of death can be attained through generational continuity, creative contributions to culture and society, the feeling of being a part of a universe that is beyond oneself, spiritual and religious attainments, and the capacity to lose oneself in ecstatic peak experiences. Two-hundred and seventy Israeli students filled out the adult attachment style scale (Hazan & Shaver, 1987), the FPDS, and the symbolic immortality scale (Mathews & Kling, 1988).

The two preceding studies provided a consistent pattern of findings. In general, secure persons reported less fear of death than insecure persons. Specifically, anxious–ambivalent persons exhibited higher fear of death at both conscious and below-conscious levels of awareness, whereas avoidant persons evidenced higher fear of death only at a lower level of awareness. Moreover, anxious–ambivalent persons were more likely to attribute their fear of death to the loss of social identity, whereas avoidant persons were more likely to overtly fear the unknown nature of death. Findings of the second study revealed that attachment styles differ in the sense of symbolic immortality as well as in its association with fear of death. Secure and anxious–ambivalent persons reported higher symbolic immortality than avoidant persons. However, while secure persons evidenced an inverse association between symbolic immortality and fear of death, anxious–ambivalent and avoidant persons showed a positive association between the two constructs.

In integrating the results of the two studies, one can conclude that securely attached persons, who have experienced warm attachment relationships in the past and developed a sense of secure base, are able to develop a corresponding sense of symbolic immortality, which, in turn, seems to protect them against the terror of their own mortality. It may be that the secure persons' positive attitude toward life helps them in developing a sense of personal continuity and in transcending the terror of death. In fact, Lifton (1973) proposed that a positive and secure attachment to the world is a basic prerequisite for the development of a sense of symbolic immortality.

Avoidant persons revealed an interesting pattern of symbolic immortality and fear of death. These persons, who have experienced insecure attachment relationships in the past and do not hold a positive connection to the world, fail to attain a sense of symbolic immortality. However, this lack of a sense of personal continuity is only reflected in the transpersonal meaning of fear of death as well as in below-awareness expressions of this fear. This pattern of fear of death may suggest that avoidant persons deal with death in the same way that they habitually regulate negative affect. They might reduce the expression of the components of fear of death related to social rejection, but might be overwhelmed by the unknown components of their own demise as well as by below-awareness expressions of this fear. In addition, they may try to suppress their fear of death and thereby make irrelevant the need to develop a sense of personal continuity.

In the case of anxious–ambivalent persons, the fact that they reveal a high sense of symbolic immortality together with high level of fear of death may result from their inability to distance themselves from negative emotions and ruminative worries about their social identity and value. In facing the terror of death, their hypersensitivity to social rejection leads them to perceive their personal demise egocentrically, as yet another separation episode in which they might be rejected by significant others, thereby losing their social identity. Moreover, they may also feel unable to suppress or deny this fear and may constantly search for other coping mechanisms, like a sense of symbolic immortality, that might provide some kind of release from their worries. However, even though anxious–ambivalent persons try to develop a sense of symbolic immortality, this cognitive shield may be inefficient in reducing their terror of death.

The findings of the two studies reviewed here support our view that adult attachment style shapes the way people cope with the terror of their own mortality. It seems that security or insecurity in one's connection to the world has a strong impact not only on how people cope with life adversities but also on how they manage the terror of their own death.

COPING WITH MILITARY AND WAR-RELATED STRESS

In contrast to civilian life, military activities in general and wartime experiences in particular expose the individual to more intense and dangerous kinds of stressful events. Although many studies have examined the short-term and long-term emotional effects of such stressors, relatively few studies have related personality constructs to the process of coping and adjustment in these kinds of dangerous life circumstances (e.g., Solomon, Mikulincer, & Avitzur, 1988). In some cases, emotional balance and well-being is restored with the end of the stressful period; in others, profound and prolonged mental health sequelae may ensue in the form of various psychopathological disturbances, such as posttraumatic stress disorder (e.g., Solomon, Weisenberg, Schwarzwald, & Mikulincer, 1987). Our review of the literature identifies only a handful of studies that have investigated the role of attachment style in explaining cognitive and emotional reactions to military and war-related stressful events.

The first systematic study that attempted to examine the role of adult attachment style was conducted on the reactions of young adults to the Iraqi Scud missile attacks on Israeli cities during the Gulf War (Mikulincer, Florian, & Weller, 1993). One hundred and forty university students who lived in places that either did or did not receive Iraqi Scud missile attacks were approached 2 weeks after the end of the Gulf War and asked to complete a series of measures on attachment style, coping with the missile attacks, and posttraumatic stress emotional reactions.

The findings supported the hypothesis that attachment style is a useful construct for explaining individual differences in coping and ad-justment with war-related stress. Specifically, secure subjects tended to seek more support during the missile attacks and to show lower levels of posttraumatic stress than insecure subjects. Anxious–ambivalent persons were found to show heightened reliance on maladaptive emotion-focused coping and reported higher levels of posttraumatic emotional distress in response to the missile attacks. Finally, avoidant persons were found to rely more on distancing coping for dealing with the missile attacks and suppressing anxiety and depression from their emotional responses, while expressing distress indirectly through higher somatization and hostility after the war.

Unexpectedly, the three attachment groups did not differ in the use of problem-focused coping. While secure persons were expected to use more of this strategy, Mikulincer et al. (1993) believed that the particular characteristics of the missile attacks in Israel may have nullified this difference. They argued that both before and during the Gulf War, the Israeli public was exposed to mass media instructions on what to do in the event of a missile attack. This exposure may have guided everyone in Israel, regardless of individual differences, to deal with a missile attack in a similar, problem-focused way.

Findings also indicated that people with different attachment styles differed in their emotional reactions, particularly under conditions of high stress (living in places that actually received missile attacks). While one could suggest that psychological distress is a definitional component of insecure attachment, this finding shows that distress reflects a maladap-tive response to particular aspects of the stressful situation. That is, insecure attachment seems to be a risk factor to maladjustment, which becomes evident in highly stressful situations.

Following these findings, Mikulincer and Florian (1995) attempted to refine and expand the association between attachment style and coping with military and war-related stressors by exploring the reactions of young Israeli recruits undergoing a demanding 4-month combat training period. Even in the initial period of military training, recruits are exposed to a wide variety of stressful demands inherent to the military setting. Soldiers are routinely stripped of some aspects of their personal identities. They have to wear uniforms, cut their hair, don the signs and symbols of the new establishment, obey orders, and perform duties even when these conflict with their personal inclinations. These demands are exacerbated for soldiers who undergo combat training. These soldiers are exposed to many physical and psychological demands, such as long periods of physical exercise and short periods of sleep.

Ninety-two young Israeli recruits reported their attachment style at the beginning of their combat training, and then filled out Folkman and Lazarus' (1985) appraisal and coping measures regarding their current experiences 4 months later (1 week before ending this training). In general, the findings about coping strategies replicated Mikulincer et al.'s (1993) findings. While the three attachment groups did not differ in reliance on problem-focused coping during the training, anxious–ambivalent persons reported more emotion-focused strategies, avoidant persons reported more distancing coping, and secure persons reported seeking more support. However, contrary to Mikulincer et al.'s study, anxious–ambivalent persons, like secure persons, showed a tendency to seek support during the training.

Mikulincer and Florian (1995) explained the inconsistency between the two studies regarding support seeking in two possible ways. First, while coping in the Gulf War study was assessed retrospectively, Mikulincer and Florian (1995) assessed the ongoing use of coping strategies during the period of combat training. It is possible that ambivalent persons seek support when exposed to stressful events, but after these events end they may dismiss their reliance on others so that their memories could fit to their views of the world as nonsupportive. Second, the inconsistency may be related to the sources of support available during the stressful period. While people experienced the stress of the Gulf War isolated in their homes, the stress in Mikulincer and Florian's study was experienced while soldiers were in intensive interactions with their peers. It is possible that anxious–ambivalent persons seek support mainly when they find themselves in the company of others who experience the same stress. This explanation is consistent with Simpson et al.'s (1992) findings.

The results also expand the usefulness of attachment theory for understanding the cognitive appraisal component of the process of coping with stress. The working model of secure persons was reflected in a benign appraisal of the combat training and a sense of inner strength to cope with it. In contrast, anxious–ambivalent persons were found to be characterized by an exaggerated appraisal of threat and a sense of personal inadequacy and helplessness in dealing with the combat training.

Interestingly, the appraisal of avoidant persons reveals two basic conflicting facets of their working models. On the one hand, their strong need for autonomy and control was manifested in avoidant persons' appraisal of themselves as capable of managing the demands of the training. On the other hand, their basic insecurity was expressed in their appraisal of the training as a threatening period.

In a recent study, Solomon, Ginzburg, Mikulincer, Neria, and Ohry (in press) examined the impact of attachment style on retrospective accounts of the experience of captivity and long-term psychological adjustment of prisoners of war (POWs). One-hundred and sixty-four Israeli ex-POWs of the Yom Kippur War and 184 matched controls were interviewed 18 years after the war. Findings on long-term adjustment replicated Mikulincer et al.'s (1993) results, showing that attachment style explained individual differences in mental health, particularly under high stress conditions. While among control veterans attachment style had no significant effect on their current mental health status, among ex-POWs, both avoidant and anxious–ambivalent veterans reported more severe psychiatric symptomatology, more posttraumatic stress symptoms, and more problems in functioning than secure ex-POWs. Quite interestingly, even 18 years after the end of the traumatic experience, insecure ex-POWs still had a poorer mental health status than matched controls. Only among secure persons did the long-term detrimental impact of captivity on mental health vanish, emphasizing their ability to cope successfully with this extreme traumatic condition.

These adjustment patterns were associated with the observed differences among attachment groups in the retrospective accounts of the experience of captivity. Compared to insecure subjects, the secure ex-POWs' experience was less negative. They reported lower levels of suffering and less helplessness, felt less abandoned and less hostile toward the army, and relied on more active coping strategies. It may be that secure ex-POWs dealt effectively with the helpless nature of captivity by recruiting their inner resources in the form of positive memories or imaginary encounters with significant others, which, in turn, may have evoked a sense of security and warmth, served as positive coping models, and enhanced the sense of meaningfulness in the empty reality. The subjective experience of insecure ex-POWs reflected their inner working models and habitual ways of dealing with stress. The helplessness and suffering of anxious–ambivalent subjects was mainly characterized by feelings of abandonment and loss of control, which may reflect their habitual oversensitivity and preoccupation with rejection. The negative experience of avoidant persons was colored by hostile feelings and reactions toward the army, which can be viewed as a manifestation of their mistrust toward nonsupportive others.

In general, the three studies reviewed in this section present a consistent pattern of findings. All of them clearly found the hypothesized patterns of coping and adjustment of the three attachment groups in dealing with man-made stressful situations.

REACTIONS TO INTERPERSONAL LOSS

According to Bowlby (1973, 1980), reactions to loss should depend on the attachment experiences one had with the lost person. There is evidence that dependent feelings toward a person lead to negative emotional reactions and adjustment difficulties after the loss of this person (Maddison & Viola, 1968; Parkes & Weiss, 1983). A similar pattern of findings was reported by Scharlach (1991), who found that the more clinging the relationship of adult daughters with their parents, the more intense their negative reactions were 1–5 years after the parents' death. In addition, Parkes and Weiss (1983) reported that persons who felt more ambivalence toward their spouses reported more anxiety and depression after the spouse's death. Weiss (1993) suggests that ambivalence toward an attachment figure can impede emotional acceptance of the loss because there will be confusion regarding the nature of feelings, and because remorse may compound the pain of loss.

The quality of early experiences with attachment figures also has been found to shape a person's responses to loss in adulthood. For example, Douglas (1990) reported that, even many years after the death of parents, adults who recollected negative childhood memories about their interactions with parents reported more pathological grief reactions. Brown (1982) found that early loss experiences were apt to lead to anxious attachment and to increase the risk of adult women's depression after the loss of a spouse. In a recent research, Stoll (1993) also found that widows who reported negative relationships with attachment figures during childhood, and who experienced more separation episodes and more threats of loss of primary caretakers, reported higher levels of depression and psychosomatic symptoms between 6 and 24 months after the death of their husbands. Similar findings were reported by Goidel (1993) in another sample of widows and widowers, and by Sable (1989) in a study of aged widows.

In a recent study by our team (Birnbaum, Orr, Mikulincer, & Florian, 1997), we focused on the three attachment styles and assessed the ways in which these styles affect coping and adaptation to divorce. A sample of 123 subjects who were involved in a long process of divorce were classified according to their attachment style, using Hazan and Shaver's (1987) attachment style prototypes, and compared to a matched group of married subjects using a measure of mental health. In addition, they also reported on how they appraised and coped with the stressful experience of the divorce.

The results corroborated the basic assumption that adult attachment style is related to the ways people cope with and adjust to the divorce process. As expected, secure persons appraised themselves as more capable of coping with the divorce, appraised this crisis in less threatening terms, relied on more adaptive coping strategies (e.g., seeking support, problem-focused coping), and experienced less distress than avoidant and anxious–ambivalent persons. Secure persons, who constructively handle interpersonal separations and learn that separation is a resolvable episode, react to the reconstruction of this experience as it reappears in divorce with less distress. In our view, secure persons may suffer much distress after the loss of a loved person, but, at the same time, may also have sufficient inner resources to cope effectively with the loss and to buffer inner pain.

These findings also support the hypothesis that insecure attachment is related to more distress after the loss of a significant person. For anxious–ambivalent persons, the divorce process may further increase the level of distress they habitually experience. The observed reactions of avoidant persons may indicate that their habitual working models (detachment, self-reliance) prove to be ineffective in dealing with a major loss. During the divorce process, the pseudo-safe world of avoidant persons is shattered, and they may find themselves helpless in the face of the loss. Divorce may reactivate early unresolved separations from attachment figures and lead to a flood of negative feelings, which avoidant persons find difficult to repress.

REACTIONS TO PERSONAL FAILURE

Extensive research has demonstrated that personal failures have deleterious effects on functioning and well-being (see Mikulincer, 1994, for a review). Specifically, the experience of failure may reduce the expenditure of effort toward pursuing the lost goal, impair subsequent performance on related tasks, raise anxiety and other stress-related emotions, damage a person's sense of self-worth and esteem, and divert attention away from problem solving or instrumental thoughts (Mikulincer, 1994). In this section, we present an illustration of the possible effects of the individual's attachment style on his or her cognitive and behavioral reactions to personal failure.

Ninety undergraduate students, previously classified according to their attachment style (30 subjects per style), were asked to perform four concept learning tasks in which they received either failure feedback or no feedback. They then completed a new task (a visual memory scanning task), and their performance was assessed. Finally, they answered questions about the frequency of off-task thoughts experienced during the experiment. The findings indicated that attachment style indeed moderated the effects of personal failure on task performance and cognitive interference (see Table 6.1). Specifically, the experience of failure led to

TABLE 6.1. Means and Standard Deviations of Performance, Negative Emotions, and Interfering Thoughts According to Attachment Style and Personal Failure

	Secure		Avoidant		Ambivalent	
	M	*SD*	*M*	*SD*	*M*	*SD*
Performance measure						
Control group	4.84$_a$	0.66	4.73$_a$	1.14	5.16$_a$	0.79
Failure group	4.38$_a$	0.56	3.38$_b$	0.55	3.33$_b$	0.52
Interfering thoughts						
Control group	2.19$_a$	0.70	2.20$_a$	0.48	2.49$_a$	0.74
Failure group	2.55$_a$	0.66	2.44$_a$	0.41	3.83$_b$	0.64

Note. Higher scores reflect better performance and more interfering thoughts. Means with different subscripts are significantly different ($p < .05$).

worse performance on the second task than no feedback only for avoidant and anxious–ambivalent subjects, but not for secure subjects. In addition, failure produced more interfering thoughts than no feedback only for anxious–ambivalent subjects, but not for secure and avoidant subjects.

Overall, the findings again indicate the adaptive advantage of security in attachment. It seems that secure persons are more resistant to the detrimental effects of personal failure. Interestingly, avoidant persons who, like secure persons, showed no cognitive reaction to failure still exhibited problems in functioning after failure, as did anxious–ambivalent persons. This finding might reflect the behavioral cost that avoidant persons pay for repressing interfering thoughts during stressful episodes.

COPING WITH PARENTHOOD TASKS

In the psychological literature, it is well recognized that normative developmental changes may involve a certain amount of stress. One of these expected developmental processes is the task of becoming a parent. This process usually starts with pregnancy, continues with the growing of the offspring throughout the life span, and sometimes involves taking care of children with special needs. In this section, we review findings from a series of four new studies conducted in our laboratory, each dealing with the possible impact of mother's attachment style on several aspects of parenthood.

In the first study, we assessed the association between attachment style and women's anxieties during pregnancy. Pregnancy is viewed as a normative developmental change that demands readjustment of women's roles and identity and temporarily taxes their coping resources. Pregnancy is a time of emotional upheaval, which may produce profound biological and neuroendocrinological changes. It generates strong negative emotional reactions, such as fear and anxiety related to one's own and the newborn's physical health (Gaffney, 1986). The main question we asked was whether attachment style may contribute to the arousal of anxiety during pregnancy.

The adult attachment-style scale (Hazan & Shaver, 1987) and six items tapping fear and anxiety about one's physical health and the health of one's baby (Gaffney, 1986) were completed by 255 first-time pregnant, young, healthy women. Forty-seven women completed the scales during the first trimester of their pregnancy, 91 during the second trimester, and 118 women during the third trimester. As expected, findings revealed significant positive correlations between women's anxiety and both the avoidant and anxious–ambivalent attachment styles (rs = .34 and .36, respectively) and a significant inverse correlation with the secure attachment style (r = −.24). One should note that these correlations were significant only when women were interviewed during the first and second trimesters of pregnancy, but not when the scales were completed during the third trimester. It is possible that, at the third trimester, the adaptation process reaches an asymptote, thereby attenuating existing individual differences. Overall, the findings support the hypothesized positive role that security in attachment plays during the first and second trimesters of pregnancy.

One may wonder whether the contribution of attachment style to parental adaptation continues after delivery, when women become mothers. Traditionally, the transition to motherhood has been viewed as a major life change, demanding important short-term adjustments (Dyer, 1963; LeMasters, 1957). Several studies have documented the stressful aspects of this transition (e.g., Power & Parke, 1984; Terry, 1991; Tessier, Piche, Tarabulsy, & Muckle, 1992) and have identified the arrival of a child as a source of stress that may lead to psychological disorders (e.g., McLanahan & Sorensen, 1984). However, studies have also demonstrated that a large number of factors may mediate mother's adjustment after the birth of a child, such as the presence of coping resources, cognitive appraisals of the situation, and the strategies mothers use to deal with stressful aspects of young motherhood (e.g., Tessier et al., 1992). The mother's attachment working models may contribute to these factors, thereby moderating her reactions to the birth of a child.

To examine these ideas, we conducted a second study assessing the impact of mother's attachment style on coping with, and adjustment to, the birth of a first child. For this purpose, we approached 80 healthy young women who delivered their first child 2–3 months before the study, along with a matched group of 80 married women who did not yet have a child. All the subjects completed the attachment-style scale (Hazan & Shaver, 1987) and the Mental Health Inventory (Veit & Ware, 1983). In addition, only the new mothers completed Lazarus and Folkman's (1984) appraisal scale, tapping the way they appraised the task of being a parent, and the Ways of Coping checklist (Folkman & Lazarus, 1985), tapping the strategies they used to deal with parenthood.

Findings clearly revealed that attachment style moderated the impact of becoming a mother on mental health (see Table 6.2). New mothers reported higher levels of psychological distress than control women. However, this effect was significant only among anxious–ambivalent and avoidant women, but not among securely attached women. It appears that secure new mothers are more resilient to the situation and show better mental health than insecure mothers. Findings also revealed that secure women appraised the task of being a mother in less threatening terms than avoidant and anxious ambivalent women, and reported having used more problem-focused strategies in coping with the parenthood task. Again, findings point to the adaptive advantage of secure attachment.

The first two studies dealt with the impact of attachment style on the "normal" developmental task of becoming a parent. However, as sometimes can happen, the stressful nature of parenthood may be compounded

TABLE 6.2. Means and Standard Deviations of Mental Health and Coping Measures According to Attachment Style in Parenthood Studies

	Secure		Avoidant		Ambivalent	
	M	SD	M	SD	M	SD
New mothers						
Psychological distress						
Control group	2.28_a	0.53	2.49_a	0.74	2.55_a	0.55
Study group	2.33_a	0.58	3.15_b	0.72	3.11_b	0.63
Threat appraisal						
Study group	3.20_a	0.91	3.97_b	1.15	4.05_b	0.69
Problem-focused coping						
Study group	2.57_a	0.43	1.85_b	0.32	1.92_b	0.33
Mothers of children with mild retardation						
Psychological distress						
Control group	2.27_a	0.75	2.07_a	0.67	2.51_a	0.79
Study group	2.24_a	0.66	2.95_b	0.55	3.06_b	0.82
Support seeking						
Study group	3.80_a	1.11	2.77_b	0.42	2.97_b	0.92
Mothers of hospitalized adolescents						
Psychological distress						
Control group	2.12_a	0.67	1.94_a	0.61	2.27_a	0.79
Study group	2.11_a	0.51	2.70_b	0.34	2.95_b	0.54
Problem-focused coping						
Study group	3.25_a	0.41	2.65_b	0.79	2.63_b	1.01
Support seeking						
Study group	3.06_a	0.58	2.36_b	0.64	2.48_b	0.89

Note. Means with different subscripts are significantly different ($p < .05$).

by unexpected physical and mental health problems of the offspring. Sabbeth (1984) contended that the impact of these problems in a family can affect a wide variety of life domains, including financial, social, somatic, and behavioral (e.g., the accumulation of stressors related to medical concerns, increased financial and housing burdens, modification of family activities, and strained family relationships). In the long run, the demands of caring for a child with a chronic illness or disability require the mobilization of parents' internal and external resources as well as complex and flexible coping strategies. From our point of view, mothers' attachment style may be one important inner resource in dealing with these demands.

In order to examine the role of attachment style in the process of coping with children's handicapping conditions, we conducted two small-scale studies. In one study, we interviewed 44 mothers of 4–5 year-old children who had mild mental retardation. In the second study, we interviewed 39 mothers of adolescents who were hospitalized due to psychiatric disorders. In both studies, mothers answered the attachment-style scale (Hazan & Shaver, 1987), the Mental Health Inventory (Veit & Ware, 1983), and the Ways of Coping checklist (Folkman & Lazarus, 1985). Their scores on these measures were then compared to matched groups of mothers of healthy children.

In both studies, the findings revealed the importance of security in attachment for coping with being a mother of a handicapped child (see Table 6.2). In general, mothers in the study groups reported higher levels of psychological distress than mothers in the control groups. However, this difference was significant only for avoidant and anxious–ambivalent mothers, but not for secure mothers. Again, security in attachment seems to provide a shield against the detrimental effects of stressful experiences. Moreover, secure mothers in the study groups reported having relied on more constructive strategies (e.g., support seeking, problem solving) for dealing with their predicament than avoidant and anxious–ambivalent mothers.

Overall, these four studies reveal a consistent and clear pattern of findings. It seems that security in attachment serves as a reliable protective inner resource that helps mothers in the adjustment to their parental role and demands. Moreover, it appears that insecurity in attachment may hinder mothers' abilities to successfully cope with parenthood and, therefore, may serve as a valid diagnostic indicator of difficulties in fulfilling the maternal role.

COPING WITH CHRONIC PAIN

Chronic pain is defined as pain that persists beyond normally expected healing time (Bonica, 1985). Although persons who suffer from chronic pain may display a number of adjustment problems, many of these persons appear to function relatively well (Taylor & Curran, 1985). Several models of stress and coping have been developed to explain adjustment differences among chronic pain patients (e.g., Revenson & Felton, 1989; Turner, Clancy, & Vitaliano, 1987). These models view chronic pain as a source of stress. Cognitive appraisals of the pain as well as coping efforts to manage it are believed to play a central role in mediating patients' emotional reactions and in determining their overall sense of well-being. In general, studies tend to find positive associations between efficacy beliefs (e.g., appraisal of one's ability to control the pain) and the endorsement of active coping strategies, on the one hand, and indices of psychological and physical functioning, on the other (see Jensen, Turner, Romano, & Karoly, 1991, for a review). In this section, we discuss the possible repercussions of attachment working models on emotional and cognitive reactions to chronic pain.

A recent study by our team assessed the impact of attachment style on coping with, and adjustment to, chronic low back pain. We approached 85 men who were clinically diagnosed as suffering from chronic low back pain for more than 6 months, and compared them to a matched sample of 85 healthy men. Both samples completed the adult attachment-style scale (Hazan & Shaver, 1987) and the Mental Health Inventory (Veit & Ware, 1983). In addition, subjects with low back pain completed Lazarus and Folkman's (1984) appraisal scale, tapping the way they appraised their pain, and the Ways of Coping checklist (Folkman & Lazarus, 1985), tapping strategies they used to deal with pain.

Findings revealed that attachment style moderated the impact of chronic pain on mental health (see Table 6.3). Although the study group reported higher levels of psychological distress than the control group, this was true only for avoidant and anxious–ambivalent persons, not for

TABLE 6.3. Means and Standard Deviations of Mental Health and Coping Measures According to Attachment Style in the Chronic Pain Study

	Secure		Avoidant		Ambivalent	
	M	SD	M	SD	M	SD
Psychological distress						
Control group	2.42_a	0.66	2.22_a	0.85	2.61_a	0.84
Study group	2.31_a	0.70	2.78_b	0.83	3.34_b	1.41
Study group's coping measures						
Threat appraisal	4.07_a	1.24	4.93_b	1.06	5.02_b	0.83
Ability appraisal	3.70_a	1.11	2.66_b	0.82	2.72_b	1.42
Emotion-focused coping	1.90_a	0.51	2.40_b	0.48	2.57_b	0.75
Problem-focused coping	3.09_a	0.61	2.66_b	0.60	2.58_b	0.73

Note. Means with different subscripts are significantly different ($p < .05$).

secure persons. In fact, even when suffering from low back pain, secure persons showed better mental health than their insecure counterparts. In addition, attachment style seemed to contribute to the appraisal of, and coping with, physical pain. As expected, secure persons appraised their back pain in less threatening terms, appraised themselves as being more able to deal with the pain, and relied on more problem-focused strategies and less emotion-focused strategies in coping with pain than both avoidant and anxious–ambivalent persons.

CONCLUSIONS

An overall look at the studies reviewed indicates the importance of adult attachment style as a key factor in determining success or failure in adaptation to stress. Bowlby's theoretical formulation has clear implications for a wide range of life events, involving issues related to life and death, physical and emotional threats, normative and non-normative developmental tasks, and personal and interpersonal losses. In all of these life domains, attachment working models seem to shape the way people appraise and cope with stressors and to moderate their emotional reactions to these events.

One major conclusion is that secure attachment seems to be an inner resource that facilitates adjustment and improves well-being in times of stress. This adaptational role could derive from three major sources. The first source is the secure persons' cognitive appraisal of the world. The optimistic attitude secure persons have toward life and their basic trust of the world may serve as a shield against unexpected adversities. Moreover, secure persons tend to appraise stressful situations in benign terms, which seems to be necessary for the adoption of constructive coping and the management of distress.

The second source of resilience may be the way in which secure persons construct their self-views. Mikulincer (1995) found that secure persons describe themselves in positive terms yet admit negative self-attributes, exhibit a highly differentiated and integrated self-schema, and reveal relatively low discrepancies between domains of the self. The positive view secure persons have of themselves may allow them to confront life problems with a sense of mastery, whereas their ability to organize experiences into differentiated self-schemata may allow them to encapsulate distress and to prevent it from spreading to the entire self-structure. In addition, the coherence of their self-structure may prevent the experience of distress every time they fail in meeting their own personal standards.

The third possible source of resilience might be the attitude secure persons have toward information processing and cognitive activity. Mikulincer (1997) found that secure persons have a positive attitude toward information processing. Specifically, this attitude is manifested in secure persons' engagement in information search; their high tolerance for unpredictability, disorder, and ambiguity; their reluctance to endorse rigid beliefs; and their tendency to integrate new evidence within cognitive structures when making social judgments. The search for information and the integration of new data within one's schemata may facilitate the learning of more appropriate skills for dealing with life adversities. Moreover, the openness of secure persons to new information and their tendency to revise schemata in the face of new information may be a sign of cognitive flexibility, which allows them to adjust to environmental changes and to develop more realistic coping plans. This cognitive openness may also allow secure persons to avoid cognitive or motivational entrapments that may create distress.

An additional conclusion is that adult attachment style is a valid predictor of the way in which people cope with stressful events. In the vast majority of studies, the working models of secure people, in which significant others are available when needed to bring relief and comfort (e.g., Hazan & Shaver, 1987), are manifested in the tendency to seek support when coping with stressful experiences. The reviewed findings also fit with the theoretical description of avoidant individuals as inhibiting emotional display, denying negative affect and memories, and devaluing events that may cause painful feelings (Hazan & Shaver, 1987; Mikulincer et al., 1990). The hypothesized working models of anxious–ambivalent persons are seen in their high reliance on passive, contemplative, and emotion-focused coping.

Another interesting idea emanating from this literature review is the emergence of two alternative patterns of associations between avoidant attachment and mental health. In everyday circumstances, avoidant persons may have the required abilities to endure minor hassles and stressors and to display self-confidence, which prevent them from experiencing strong distress and allow them to maintain adequate functioning. In these circumstances, researchers may find it difficult to differentiate between avoidant and secure persons in terms of their overt behavior and mental health. However, when facing a serious stressful event or period, the facade may crumble, and the basic insecurity of avoidant persons may become overtly manifested by ineffective ways of coping and the experience of high levels of distress. In such cases, avoidant persons are likely to become distressed and to resemble anxious–ambivalent persons. Attachment theory is a rich source for further exploration of the process of coping and adaptation (see Rholes, Simpson, & Grich Stevens, Chapter 7, this volume). Future studies should attempt to expand the reviewed data to other kinds of stressors and to other populations, taking advantage of cross-cultural comparisons. In addition, the contribution of attachment style should be examined in the context of other possible inner resources and personality characteristics. Attachment style also should be studied in interaction with contextual factors that may moderate its impact on the process of coping and adaptation. Finally, more attention should be given to the implications of the data for diagnostic and therapeutic issues.

REFERENCES

Ainsworth, M. D. S., Blehar, M. C., Waters, E., & Wall, S. (1978). *Patterns of attachment: A psychological study of the Strange Situation.* Hillsdale, NJ: Erlbaum.

Bartholomew, K., & Horowitz, L. M. (1991). Attachment styles among young adults: A test of a four-category model. *Journal of Personality and Social Psychology, 61,* 226–244.

Birnbaum, G. E., Orr, I., Mikulincer, M., & Florian, V. (1997). When marriage breaks up—Does attachment style contribute to coping and mental health? *Journal of Social and Personal Relationships, 14,* 643–654.

Bonica, J. J. (1985). Importance of the problem. In G. A. Aronoff (Ed.), *Evaluation and treatment of chronic pain* (pp. xxxi–xliv). Baltimore: Urban & Schwarzenberg.

Bowlby, J. (1969). *Attachment and loss: Vol. 1. Attachment.* New York: Basic Books.

Bowlby, J. (1973). *Attachment and loss: Vol. 2. Separation: Anxiety and anger.* New York: Basic Books.

Bowlby, J. (1980). *Attachment and loss: Vol. 3. Loss: Sadness and depression.* New York: Basic Books.

Bowlby, J. (1988). *A secure base: Clinical applications of attachment theory.* London: Routledge.

Brennan, K. A., Shaver, P. R., & Tobey, A. E. (1991). Attachment styles, gender, and parental problem drinking. *Journal of Social and Personal Relationships, 8,* 451–466.

Brown, G. W. (1982). Early loss and depression. In C. W. Parkes & J. Stevenson-Hinde (Eds.), *The place of attachment in human social behavior* (pp. 161–183). New York: Basic Books.

Collins, N. L., & Read, S. J. (1990). Adult attachment, working models, and relationship quality in dating couples. *Journal of Personality and Social Psychology, 58,* 644–663.

Douglas, J. D. (1990). Patterns of change following parent death in midlife adults. *Omega, 22,* 123–137.

Dyer, E. D. (1963). Parenthood as crisis: A restudy. *Marriage and Family Living, 25,* 196–201.

Florian, V., & Kravetz, S. (1983). Fear of personal death: Attribution, structure, and relation to religious belief. *Journal of Personality and Social Psychology, 44,* 600–607.

Florian, V., Kravetz, S., & Frankel, J. (1984). Aspects of fear of personal death, levels of awareness, and religious commitment. *Journal of Research in Personality, 18,* 289–304.

Florian, V., & Mikulincer, M. (in press). Does symbolic immortality contribute to transcend the terror of death?: The moderating role of attachment style. *Journal of Personality and Social Psychology.*

Folkman, S., & Lazarus, R. S. (1985). If it changes it must be a process: Study of emotion and coping during three stages of a college examination. *Journal of Personality and Social Psychology, 48,* 150–170.

Gaffney, K. F. (1986). Maternal–fetal attachment in relation to self-concept and anxiety. *Maternal Child Nursing Journal, 15,* 91–101.

Goidel, J. (1993). Social, situational, and psychological factors in the adjustment of widows and widowers. In K. Pottharst (Ed.), *Research explorations in adult attachment* (pp. 257–268). New York: Lang.

Hazan, C., & Shaver, P. (1987). Romantic love conceptualized as an attachment process. *Journal of Personality and Social Psychology, 52,* 511–524.

Hazan, C., & Shaver, P. (1990). Love and work: An attachment-theoretical perspective. *Journal of Personality and Social Psychology, 59,* 270–280.

Jensen, M. P., Turner, J. A., Romano, J. M., & Karoly, P. (1991). Coping with chronic pain: A critical review of the literature. *Pain, 47,* 249–283.

Kalish, R. A. (1985). *Death, grief, and caring relationships.* New York: Cole.

Kobak, R. R., & Sceery, A. (1988). Attachment in late adolescence: Working models, affect regulation, and representations of self and others. *Child Development, 59,* 135–146.

Kobasa, S. C. (1982). Commitment and coping in stress resistance among lawyers. *Journal of Personality and Social Psychology, 42,* 707–717.

Lazarus, R. S., & Folkman, S. (1984). *Stress, appraisal, and coping.* New York: Springer.

LeMasters, E. E. (1957). Parenthood as a crisis. *Marriage and Family Living, 19,* 352–355.

Lifton, R. J. (1973). The sense of immortality: On death and the continuity of life. *American Journal of Psychoanalysis, 33,* 3–15.

Lifton, R. J. (1979). *The broken connection.* New York: Simon & Schuster.

Maddison, D., & Viola, A. (1968). The health of widows in the year after bereavement. *Journal of Psychoanalytic Research, 12,* 297–306.

Main, M., Kaplan, N., & Cassidy, J. (1985). Security in infancy, childhood, and adulthood: A move to the level of representation. *Monographs of the Society for Research in Child Development, 50,* 66–104.

Mathews, R. C., & Kling, K. J. (1988). Self-transcendence, time perspective, and prosocial behavior. *Journal of Voluntary Action Research, 17,* 4–24.

McLanahan, S. S., & Sorensen, A. B. (1984). Life events and psychological well-being: A reexamination of theoretical and methodological issues. *Social Science Research, 13,* 111–128.

Mikulincer, M. (1994). *Human learned helplessness: A coping perspective.* New York: Plenum Press.

Mikulincer, M. (1995). Attachment style and the mental representation of the self. *Journal of Personality and Social Psychology, 69,* 1203–1215.

Mikulincer, M. (1997). Adult attachment style and information processing: Individual differences in curiosity and cognitive closure. *Journal of Personality and Social Psychology, 72,* 1217–1230.

Mikulincer, M., & Florian, V. (1995). Appraisal and coping with a real-life stressful situation: The contribution of attachment styles. *Personality and Social Psychology Bulletin, 21,* 406–414.

Mikulincer, M., Florian, V., & Tolmacz, R. (1990). Attachment styles and fear of personal death: A case study of affect regulation. *Journal of Personality and Social Psychology, 58,* 273–280.

Mikulincer, M., Florian, V., & Weller, A. (1993). Attachment styles, coping strategies, and post-traumatic psychological distress: The impact of the Gulf War in Israel. *Journal of Personality and Social Psychology, 64,* 817–826.

Mikulincer, M., & Orbach, I. (1995). Attachment styles and repressive defensiveness: The accessibility and architecture of affective memories. *Journal of Personality and Social Psychology, 68,* 917–925.

Parkes, C. M., & Weiss, R. S. (1983). *Recovery from bereavement.* New York: Basic Books.

Power, T. G., & Parke, R. D. (1984). Social network factors and the transition to parenthood. *Sex Roles, 10,* 949–972.

Revenson, T. A., & Felton, B. J. (1989). Disability and coping as predictors of psychological adjustment to rheumatoid arthritis. *Journal of Consulting and Clinical Psychology, 57,* 344–348.

Sabbeth, B. (1984). Understanding the impact of chronic childhood illness on families. *Pediatric Clinics of North America, 31,* 47–57.

Sable, P. (1989). Attachment, anxiety, and loss of a husband. *American Journal of Orthopsychiatry, 59,* 550–556.

Scharlach, A. E. (1991). Factors associated with filial grief following the death of an elderly parent. *American Journal of Orthopsychiatry, 61,* 307–313.

Shaver, P. R., & Hazan, C. (1993). Adult romantic attachment: Theory and evidence. In D. Perlman & W. Jones (Eds.), *Advances in personal relationships* (Vol. 4, pp. 29–70). London: Kingsley

Simpson, J. A. (1990). The influence of attachment styles on romantic relationships. *Journal of Personality and Social Psychology, 59,* 273–280.

Simpson, J. A., Rholes, W. S., & Nelligan, J. S. (1992). Support seeking and support giving within couples in an anxiety-provoking situation: The role of attachment styles. *Journal of Personality and Social Psychology, 62,* 434–446.

Solomon, Z., Ginzburg, K., Mikulincer, M., Neria, Y., & Ohry, U. (in press). Attachment style and long-term adjustment to captivity in war. *European Journal of Personality.*

Solomon, Z., Mikulincer, M., & Avitzur, E. (1988). Coping, locus of control, social support, and combat-related posttraumatic stress disorder. *Journal of Personality and Social Psychology, 55,* 279–285.

Solomon, Z., Weisenberg, M., Schwarzwald, J., & Mikulincer, M. (1987). Post-traumatic stress disorder among front-line soldiers with combat stress reaction: The 1982 Israeli experience. *American Journal of Psychiatry, 144,* 448–454.

Stoll, M. (1993). Predictors of middle aged widows' psychological adjustment. In K. Pottharst (Ed.), *Research explorations in adult attachment* (pp. 219–255). New York: Lang.

Taylor, H., & Curran, N. M. (1985). *The Nuprin pain report* (Study No. 851017). New York: Louis Harris.

Terry, D. J. (1991). Stress, coping, and adaptation to new parenthood. *Journal of Social and Personal Relationships, 8,* 527–547.

Tessier, R., Piche, C., Tarabulsy, G. M., & Muckle, G. (1992). Mothers' experience of stress following the birth of a first child: Identification of stressors and coping resources. *Journal of Applied Social Psychology, 22,* 1319–1339.

Turner, J. A., Clancy, S., & Vitaliano, P. P. (1987). Relationships of stress, appraisal, and coping to chronic low back pain. *Behaviour Research and Therapy, 25,* 281–288.

Veit, C. T., & Ware, J. E. (1983). The structure of psychological stress and well-being in general populations. *Journal of Consulting and Clinical Psychology, 51,* 730–742.

Wagner, P. E., & Tangney, J. P. (1991). *Affective style, aspects of the self, and psychological symptoms.* Unpublished manuscript, Department of Psychology, George Mason University, Fairfax, VA.

Wass, H., & Neimeyer, R. A. (1995). *Dying—Facing the facts.* Washington, DC: Taylor & Francis.

Weiss, R. S. (1993). Loss and recovery. In M. S. Stroebe, W. Stroebe, & R. O. Hansson (Eds.), *Handbook of bereavement* (pp. 271–284). New York: Cambridge University Press.

7

Attachment Orientations, Social Support, and Conflict Resolution in Close Relationships

W. STEVEN RHOLES
JEFFRY A. SIMPSON
JAMI GRICH STEVENS

From the viewpoint of the position adopted, adult personality is seen as a product of an individual's interactions with key figures during all his years of immaturity, especially of his interactions with attachment figures. Thus an individual who has been fortunate in having grown up in an ordinary good home with ordinarily affectionate parents has always known people from whom he can seek support, comfort, and protection, and where they are to be found. So deeply established are his expectations and so repeatedly have they been confirmed that, as an adult, he finds it difficult to imagine any other kind of world.

Others, who have grown up in other circumstances, may have been much less fortunate. For some the very existence of caretaking and supportive figures is unknown; for others the whereabouts of such figures have been constantly uncertain. For many more the likelihood that a caretaking figure would respond in a supportive and protective way has been at best hazardous and at worst nil. When such people become adults, it is hardly surprising that they have no confidence that a caretaking figure will ever be truly available and dependable. Through their eyes the world is seen as comfortless and unpredictable; and they respond either by shrinking from it or by doing battle with it.

—BOWLBY (1973, pp. 208–209)

The C baby fears that he will not get enough of what he wants; the A baby fears what he wants.

—AINSWORTH, BLEHAR, WATERS, and WALL (1978, p. 130)

These quotations, taken from two of the landmark volumes on attachment theory, express themes that are of central importance to the theory—namely, that the influence of childhood relationships extends well into adulthood and that inadequate relationships early in life can lead to opposing, but equally dysfunctional, orientations toward the interpersonal world. As Bowlby and Ainsworth state, persons who experience impoverished relationships in childhood may either shrink from potential attachment figures in fear or struggle vigorously to receive their care and support. In this chapter, we describe two behavioral observation studies, both of which are based on the premise that these types of behavior are the joint product of attachment history and current involvement in interpersonal situations that serve to trigger or "release" affective and behavioral patterns formed through prior experience with attachment figures. Before describing these studies, however, we first review the theoretical context from which they derive.

ATTACHMENT THEORY: BOWLBY AND AINSWORTH

Early in his work on attachment, Bowlby noticed that infants of many species in addition to humans experience considerable anxiety when separated from their primary caretaker. Combining principles from several disciplines, most notably ethology and control theory, Bowlby concluded that the typical response to separation—anxiety and protest, despair, and finally detachment—is the product of an innate system designed to encourage proximity between vulnerable infants and their stronger, wiser caregivers. Maintenance of proximity, he argued, enhances reproductive fitness by increasing the probability that infants will survive to the reproductive years.

Although the desire for proximity is virtually universal in human infants, the way in which it is expressed depends on the infant's history of interactions with attachment figures. Using the Strange Situation test, Ainsworth, Blehar, Waters, and Wall (1978) identified three fundamental patterns of proximity (or attachment) behavior. Infants who have *secure* relationships with their caregivers use them as a source of comfort and support to control feelings of distress when they arise. For these infants, the caregiver's presence signals safety and is an unequivocal source of comfort. Infants who have *anxious–ambivalent* relationships with their caregivers make conflicted and often unsuccessful attempts to derive support from them. Their behavior seems to reflect uncertainty about the caregiver's ultimate availability and willingness to provide support. Finally, infants who develop *avoidant* relationships do not actively seek support from their caregivers when they are distressed. Instead, they cope internally without relying on social support, at least in any obvious way.

Their behavior suggests that they wish to remain independent of their caregivers.

Children who develop ambivalent or avoidant patterns of attachment usually have lost confidence that their caregivers are accessible and willing to offer support in times of need (Bowlby, 1973). Decreased confidence can be brought about by a variety of experiences, such as prolonged separations from attachment figures or habitual threats of separation (e.g., when threats to abandon are routinely used as a disciplinary tactic). Confidence also can be undermined when responses to bids for support are unpredictable, when caregivers refuse to respond, or when bids are met with sarcasm, irritation, scolding, or moralization. Other experiences capable of undermining confidence include intense childhood bereavement, role reversals in which the child assumes responsibility for the parent's emotional state, and the use of conditional love as a control tactic (Bowlby, 1973, 1980). Ambivalence frequently emerges in environments characterized by genuine love and sensitive care mixed with lengthy separations, periods of nonresponsiveness, role reversal, bereavement, or related factors, whereas avoidance usually stems from environments containing little genuine affection and cold or derisive responses to bids for comfort and support.

Consequences of Attachment Orientations

A cardinal feature of the ambivalent orientation, especially in adulthood, is the need for control in relationships. Fearing abandonment and obsessively questioning their attachment figure's availability and commitment, ambivalent persons often become clingy, suspicious, dependent, jealous, and controlling, sometimes to the point of being domineering (Hazan & Shaver, 1994). The hallmark of the avoidant orientation, in contrast, is a deep desire to avoid emotional dependence. This tendency isolates avoidant persons from an awareness of both their own emotional needs and those of others, thereby limiting their capacity for developing truly intimate relationships. Despite their differences, both ambivalent and avoidant adults find it difficult to obtain social support from significant others. They often fail to seek support because they believe none will be forthcoming or because they want to retain independence. They also may alienate potential helpers through possessive, dependent, or controlling behavior, or they may reject help because they erroneously perceive criticism, hostility, or malevolent intent on the part of potential helpers (Bowlby, 1973).

Both avoidant and ambivalent individuals often feel helpless and guilty about their inability to form close bonds (Bowlby, 1973). Beneath these feelings, however, lies anger and resentment toward childhood attachment figures that can quickly resurface in their close relationships in adulthood. Bowlby (1973, 1980) describes two types of anger: functional ("the anger of hope") and dysfunctional ("the anger of despair"). Functional anger is expressed in the service of maintaining attachment bonds. It usually is witnessed when a partner has been inattentive or neglectful, and its purpose is to discourage similar behavior in the future. Examples of this form of anger include the pouting child whom parents encounter upon returning home after a long trip and the spouse who angrily reproaches his or her partner for paying too little attention to the relationship. Functional anger becomes dysfunctional when it is so intense or persistent that the partner is alienated or when its principal goal is malice or revenge rather than deterrence. Dysfunctional anger in adulthood can have numerous sources. It can spring from the redirection of submerged anger from childhood toward current attachment figures, the projection of the rejecting, demanding, or hostile qualities of early attachment figures onto the current partner, or the modeling and reenactment of angry behavior exhibited by attachment figures during childhood (Bowlby, 1973).

Environmental Releasers

Like many behaviors with evolutionary origins, specific cues in the immediate environment play a significant role in eliciting attachment-related behaviors. A major releaser is simple unfamiliarity. According to Bowlby, environments that were unfamiliar should have been more dangerous to our ancestors throughout evolutionary history. Thus, anxiety that drew family members closer together in such situations should have been adaptive. Unfamiliarity, however, is merely one releasing factor. Bowlby (1969) describes two general categories of releasers in children. The first deals with the location or availability of attachment figures. If, for example, attachment figures are absent, out of sight (or seen departing), or observed caring for other children, infants and young children often make vigorous attempts to reestablish contact with them. The second category concerns events that generate anxiety, sadness, self-doubt, and related forms of negative affect. Unfamiliar environments, rebuffs from significant others, loss experiences, and alarming events—real or imagined—all fall into this second category, as do fatigue, hunger, ill-health, pain, and other conditions indicative of vulnerability or weakness.

Elaborating on Bowlby, Kobak and Duemmler (1994) discuss three types of situations that activate the attachment system in adults: fear-provoking situations, which motivate adults to seek out significant others as *safe havens*; challenging situations, which lead adults to make contact with those who provide a *secure base*; and conflictual interactions, which accentuate the importance of maintaining a *cooperative partnership*. Like

Bowlby, Kobak and Duemmler view releasers primarily from a normative (or "species-typical") perspective, and they focus on conditions that lead to the style of proximity-seeking behaviors most characteristic of secure adults. In the following review of our research, we adopt an individual difference, rather than normative, perspective; that is, we contend that prototypical avoidant and ambivalent behaviors are elicited in avoidant and ambivalent persons, respectively, by very different kinds of events.

At base, attachment orientations reflect different styles of affect regulation in interpersonal settings (cf. Sroufe & Waters, 1977). The major adult attachment orientations, therefore, should serve to maintain a comfortable level of proximity to attachment figures (cf. Main, 1981). Beset with fears of loss and abandonment, ambivalent persons seek to minimize distance between themselves and their attachment figures through clingy, possessive, and controlling behavior (see Feeney, Chapter 8, this volume). Thus, ambivalent attachment behavior should be triggered by events that make salient the underlying fear that attachment figures cannot be counted on for support. Metaphorically speaking, events that suggest actual or potential movement away from the ambivalent person should instigate behaviors designed to bring the partner back and keep him or her close. Such events might include actual separations or overt threats of separation, or events which suggest that loss or abandonment may be imminent, including long-standing conflict (especially if it is initiated by the partner), efforts by the partner to resist control, and circumstances that give the partner greater freedom to leave the relationship. All of these events should increase efforts by ambivalent persons to keep the partner close. Paradoxically, they also may lead ambivalent people to devalue the partner or relationship in order to lessen the impact of anticipated loss or abandonment.

Fearing intimacy and rejection and wishing to keep their partners at a safe emotional distance, avoidant persons should display prototypically avoidant, or distancing, behavior when their emotional zone of comfort is violated. Events that might trigger such behavior include situations involving support seeking reminiscent of that for which avoidant persons were rebuffed during childhood or the need to provide emotional support to a partner. Avoidant behaviors also might be elicited by events that heighten the potential for rejection or force avoidant persons to confront the poverty of their relationship history (Mikulincer & Florian, Chapter 6, this volume). To summarize, ambivalent behavior may be most readily observed when psychological "distance" from attachment figures increases, activating fears about abandonment or loss. Conversely, avoidant behavior may be most evident when psychological distance is decreased, undermining avoidant persons' strong desire to maintain independence and suppress the attachment system. In either case, the purpose of the activated behavior is to reestablish a comfortable interpersonal distance.

ADULT ATTACHMENT RESEARCH

Attachment theory proposes four general hypotheses about personality and behavior. First, it holds that attachment orientations form during childhood largely in response to interactions with primary attachment figures. Second, it maintains that attachment orientations remain relatively stable, at least from late childhood and early adolescence into adulthood. Third, it claims that early attachment experiences affect relationships in adulthood. Fourth, it predicts that parents' attachment orientations influence the nature of their children's attachment to them. Main and her colleagues have tested the second and fourth predictions using the Adult Attachment Interview (AAI) to assess adult orientations.

The AAI (George, Kaplan, & Main, 1996) classifies respondents into one of three attachment categories based on an hour-long interview that focuses on the respondent's relationship with his or her parents during childhood. The categories are: Dismissing (Ds), Secure–Autonomous (F), and Preoccupied (E).[1] The Ds category is the adult equivalent of Ainsworth's avoidant infant category, the F category is the adult equivalent of Ainsworth's secure infant category, and the E category is the adult equivalent of the ambivalent infant category. In support of Hypothesis 4, Main and others have shown that parents' AAI classifications correspond closely to their children's classifications in the Strange Situation. Parents in the F category typically have infants who are classified as secure, parents in the Ds category typically have infants classified as avoidant, and parents in the E category typically have infants classified as ambivalent (Main, Kaplan, & Cassidy, 1985; van IJzendoorn, 1995). Recent research also has provided initial support for the longitudinal stability hypothesis (Hypothesis 2). Both Hamilton (1995) and Waters, Merrick, Albersheim, and Treboux (1995) report that persons who were insecurely attached as infants (i.e., classified as A or C babies in the Strange Situation) tend to be classified as insecure (either Ds or E) by the AAI as adolescents (cited in George et al., 1996).

In addition to the AAI, one other interview measure (see Bartholomew & Horowitz, 1991) and several self-report measures of adult attachment orientations also have been developed (see Brennan, Clark, & Shaver, Chapter 3, this volume; Collins & Read, 1990; Feeney, Noller, & Callan, 1994; Hazan & Shaver, 1987; Simpson, Rholes, & Phillips, 1996). These measures differ from the AAI in that they assess orientations toward current romantic relationships rather than past nuclear family relationships (see Simpson & Rholes, Chapter 1, this volume). Classifications using these measures tend to be uncorrelated with AAI classifications (Main, personal communication; see Bartholomew & Shaver, Chapter 2, this volume.) Thus, they are not simply different markers of the construct assessed by the AAI. Both types of measures, however, relate to behavior in ways that are consistent with major tenets of attachment theory.

Many researchers who study adult attachment have examined questions about the nature and quality of romantic relationships among persons with secure, ambivalent, and avoidant orientations (Hypothesis 3). They have found that securely attached adults have positive working models of both themselves and significant others (Bartholomew & Horowitz, 1991). Secure people consider themselves as worthy of others' concern, care, and affection and perceive significant others as being accessible, reliable, trustworthy, and well intentioned. They develop close relationships with others easily and feel comfortable depending on others and having others depend on them. Secure people also are comparatively free of worries about either being abandoned or about others becoming too intimate (Hazan & Shaver, 1987). Their romantic relationships are characterized by positive affect (Simpson, 1990); high levels of trust, commitment, satisfaction, and interdependence (Collins & Read, 1990; Simpson, 1990); and positive and trusting styles of love (Hazan & Shaver, 1987; Hendrick & Hendrick, 1989; Levy & Davis, 1988).

Anxious–ambivalent adults have negative working models of themselves and positive, yet guarded, models of significant others (Bartholomew & Horowitz, 1991). They see themselves as misunderstood and underappreciated, and they view others as undependable and either unwilling or unable to pledge themselves to intimate, committed relationships. Ambivalent adults report that their partners are reluctant to get as close as they would like, they worry that their partners do not truly love them or might leave them, and they desire to become deeply intertwined with their partners (Hazan & Shaver, 1987). As a rule, their relationships contain more negative affect (Simpson, 1990); low levels of trust, commitment, satisfaction, and interdependence (Collins & Read, 1990; Simpson, 1990); and obsessive, enmeshed, and jealous forms of love (Hazan & Shaver, 1987; Hendrick & Hendrick, 1989; Levy & Davis, 1988).

Avoidant adults may exhibit one of two different underlying motives (see Bartholomew, 1990). Dismissing–avoidants have a positive view of self and a negative, often cynical, view of others. They tend to be aloof, emotionally distant, and skeptical, and they consider significant others to be either unreliable or overly eager to make long-term commitments. Fearful–avoidants, on the other hand, have a negative view of both themselves (as unworthy of love) and others (as not likely to be loving). Both dismissing– and fearful–avoidant persons are uncomfortable being intimate with others, they find it difficult to completely trust and depend on others, and they become apprehensive when a partner gets too close (Hazan & Shaver, 1987). Similar to ambivalent persons, both dismissing– and fearful–avoidant individuals tend to be involved in relationships containing frequent negative affect (Simpson, 1990) and lower levels of trust, commitment, satisfaction, and interdependence (Collins & Read,

1990; Simpson, 1990). The negative character of their relationships, however, originates from either an acute fear of intimacy (fearful–avoidants) or a strong disdain for intimacy (dismissing–avoidants). Although different motivational sources can underlie avoidant attachment, the behavioral strategies that fearful– and dismissing–avoidants use to regulate negative affect may often be similar.

THE PRESENT STUDIES

Two studies were conducted to examine how dating partners interact in stressful situations that should activate behaviors prototypical of the avoidant or ambivalent attachment orientations.

Study 1

In Study 1, the female partner in heterosexual dating relationships was made to feel anxious about an impending event, and her male partner was given the opportunity to provide emotional support. Based on Bowlby's work, we hypothesized that anxiety would activate the attachment system in the women and that their need for comfort and support would activate the caregiving component of the attachment system in their partners. Consequently, we expected women who were more secure to seek support and men who were more secure to provide it. We expected more avoidant women, on the other hand, to resist the "distance reduction" that support seeking involves and more avoidant men to refrain from giving support. Finally, we expected more ambivalent women to seek support strongly and more ambivalent men to be very willing to provide support.

Eighty-three couples who had dated for an average of 18 months took part in the study (see Simpson, Rholes, & Nelligan, 1992). Participants first completed a version of the Adult Attachment Questionnaire (AAQ; see Simpson et al., 1996). This measure contains 17 items, most of which are sentences from Hazan and Shaver's (1987) three attachment vignettes. Similar to other self-report measures (see Griffin & Bartholomew, 1994a, 1994b, for reviews), two orthogonal dimensions underlie the AAQ. The first measures high versus low levels of avoidance. People who score high on this dimension tend to classify themselves as avoidant on the Hazan and Shaver measure, whereas people who score low tend to classify themselves as secure. The second dimension reflects high versus low ambivalence. People who score high on this dimension tend to categorize themselves as anxious–ambivalent on the Hazan and Shaver measure. On the AAQ, prototypically secure persons should score low on both dimensions (i.e., they should be neither ambivalent nor avoidant). Several studies using the AAQ have verified the reliability and predictive validity of both dimensions (see Griffin & Bartholomew, 1994b; Rholes, Simpson, & Blakely, 1995; Simpson et al., 1992, 1996).

After completing the AAQ and a battery of other questionnaires, the woman in each couple was escorted to a waiting room, where an anxiety induction procedure was administered. The experimenter first took the woman's pulse to accentuate the stressful nature of the "impending" event, and then said: "In the next few minutes, you are going to be exposed to a situation and set of experimental procedures that arouse considerable anxiety and distress in most people. Due to the nature of these procedures, I cannot tell you any more at the moment. Of course, I'll answer any questions or concerns you have after the experiment is over."

The experimenter then led the woman to a room used for psycho-physiological research. She opened a heavy metal door to a dark, windowless room resembling an isolation chamber that contained what appeared to be psychophysiological equipment. After each woman saw the equipment, the experimenter told her that the equipment was not fully set up and led her back to the waiting room. The male partner was then taken to the waiting room, and the couple was left alone for 5 minutes. The man was told he was waiting to complete additional questionnaires. Thus, he had no reason to be anxious. The experimenter said nothing to the man about his partner's impending experience. During the 5-minute wait, the couple's interaction was unobtrusively videotaped. The experimenter then reentered the room and explained that the woman's remaining part of the experiment could not be conducted due to malfunctioning equipment. After a few more minutes, each couple was debriefed and informed that they had been videotaped. The reason for the deception was explained, and couples were given an opportunity to erase their videotapes. None chose to do so.

Three independent raters then viewed the videotapes and evaluated the behavior of both members of each couple. Raters evaluated each woman on adjectives that assessed her level of anxiety and the extent to which she sought comfort and support from her partner. Raters evaluated each man on adjectives that indexed the extent to which he offered his partner reassurance and emotional support. The content of the partners' conversations was rated for the extent to which each woman discussed her feelings about the impending situation, along with the extent to which each man made supportive comments, tried to avoid or downplay his partner's anxiety, or made comments that seemed to calm her. Finally, raters coded physical "approach" behaviors as well as behaviors indicative of resistance to the partner's attempts to initiate physical contact.

Results

In contrast to our expectations, there were no significant findings involving ambivalence. Avoidance, on the other hand, was significantly related to a number of theoretically relevant behaviors. First, as expected, less avoidant women, particularly those who were rated by observers as more anxious, sought greater support from their partner. Among more avoidant women, the higher their level of anxiety, the less they sought support. Women scoring high on avoidance were not higher in anxiety than women who scored low; thus, attachment orientation and anxiety were not confounded. The findings for men were complementary to those for women. The more distressed their female partners were, the more support and reassurance was offered by men scoring low on avoidance. More avoidant men, in contrast, were less likely to be supportive, especially if their partners were highly distressed. Interestingly, the amount of support that women sought did not correlate with the amount they received. Men's supportiveness, in other words, was contingent on their partners' emotional state rather than their partners' efforts to solicit support.

Turning to the content of the conversations, men made more supportive comments if their partners discussed their feelings about the impending event more extensively. This effect, however, was significantly stronger for less avoidant men. Women were rated as calmer if their partners offered more supportive comments. Intriguingly, such comments had a stronger impact on highly avoidant women. In contrast to conversational support, support offered in the form of close body contact (e.g., a hug) elicited considerable resistance from highly avoidant women. Finally, discriminant validation analyses showed that all findings remained significant when each partner's score on the Relationship Closeness Inventory (RCI; Berscheid, Snyder, & Omoto, 1989) and Rubin's (1970) Love Scale were partialed out. Hence, the effects are not due to covariation between attachment orientations and closeness or love.

Support Seeking, Reactions to Support, and Support Giving

In some ways, the behavior of participants in this study is reminiscent of behavior in the Strange Situation. Avoidant women were less likely to seek support from their partners if they were upset. In fact, they often attempted to distract themselves by thumbing through magazines in the waiting room. Such behavior is analogous to the tendency of avoidant infants to turn toward the world of objects and away from their attachment figure in order to regulate and control their emotional distress in the Strange Situation. Regardless of their level of avoidance, women appeared calmer if their partners made supportive comments during the waiting period. Highly avoidant women, however, were more responsive to their partner's comments than were less avoidant women. This indicates that avoidant persons do respond to some forms of social support, even though they seek it less actively. Their self-imposed isolation during times of distress, therefore, does not imply that they do not appreciate support when it is offered in a form with which they are comfortable. Support expressed through physical contact, however, may be less welcomed by highly avoidant persons than support offered via more distal modes of interaction, such as reassuring comments.

The fact that less avoidant men offered greater reassurance and support is consistent with previous research showing that men who are more secure tend to be warmer (Collins & Read, 1990), more constructive in difficult situations (Pistole, 1989), and better facilitators of communication (Kobak & Hazan, 1991). Phillips, Simpson, Lanigan, and Rholes (1995) recently have found that highly avoidant men and women report feeling uncomfortable about offering emotional support to others and feel less obliged to do so. They also regard persons who need their help, including friends, as psychologically weak and immature.

In well-functioning relationships, both partners should serve as sources of support (or as secure bases) for one another. The results of Study 1 suggest that this ideal, however, is likely to hold primarily for couples in which neither member has an avoidant attachment orientation. Avoidant persons are less likely to turn to their partner when they are upset and less inclined to offer support when their partner is upset. In the absence of stress, couples in which one or both partners are avoidant may experience relatively high levels of satisfaction and exhibit low levels of dysfunctional behavior. However, when faced with significant stress, avoidant partners may be less capable of supporting one another, resulting in decreased satisfaction and more dysfunctional behavior.

In both the present study and Phillips et al. (1995), the ambivalent orientation was unrelated to both support seeking and support giving. To understand these results, one must understand the working models of ambivalent persons. Returning to the Ainsworth quotation that introduced the chapter, ambivalent persons desire support from attachment figures yet, given their attachment history, remain uncertain about whether they will receive it. Therefore, activation of the attachment system in such persons may generate complex, even contradictory, behavioral responses that are not easily captured by the relatively simple, unidimensional behavioral ratings that were used in this study. One important task for future research, therefore, is to develop rating scales that more adequately "capture" the kinds of support seeking and support giving characteristic of ambivalent persons.

Study 2

Conflict with attachment figures has several properties that make it well suited for testing principles of attachment theory. It can raise questions about the attachment figure's availability, particularly among ambivalent persons; it can test partners' skill at sustaining a cooperative relationship; and finally, it can provide an occasion for partners to evaluate and perhaps revise feelings and beliefs about the current partner and relationship (Simpson & Rholes, 1994).

Only a handful of studies have examined how adults' attachment orientations relate to conflict resolution. Securely attached persons report using integrating resolution strategies more often than both their avoidant and ambivalent counterparts, and they are more willing to compromise than ambivalent persons (Pistole, 1989). Moreover, when discussing intimate topics, secure persons engage in more self-disclosure than avoidant persons and show more disclosure flexibility and topical reciprocity than both avoidant and ambivalent persons (Mikulincer & Nachshon, 1991). During problem-solving interactions, spouses with more secure working models regulate their emotions in a more constructive fashion (Kobak & Hazan, 1991). Finally, secure teenagers display less dysfunctional anger, remain more constructively engaged, and show less avoidance of the issue under discussion during problem-solving conversations with their mothers than insecure teenagers (Kobak, Cole, Ferenz-Gillies, Fleming, & Gamble, 1993).

Kobak and Duemmler (1994) suggest that conflict increases an individual's need for emotional support from his or her attachment figure. This need, however, produces a psychological bind in which individuals require support from the persons with whom they are in conflict, and this, in turn, should make working models more accessible. Under such circumstances, individuals who have positive perceptions of self and others (i.e., secure persons) should engage in direct and open communication in which their partner's perspective in the conflict is recognized and discourse remains constructive and coherent. Individuals with ambivalent or avoidant orientations should follow different trajectories, however. In conflictual situations, avoidant persons, who wish to skirt attachment-related issues and depress activation of their attachment system, should divert attention away from the conflict. If successful in this effort, they should become disengaged from the partner and the conflict and, therefore, experience little anxiety or distress. They also should be less supportive toward the partner, and their interactions should be less constructive.

Conflict should activate the working models of ambivalent persons as well, leading them to feel heightened anxiety about loss of control over the partner and about separation or abandonment. In response to these feelings, ambivalent persons often may become angry with their partners (Bowlby, 1973). Thus, because conflict can cause them to feel anxious and angry simultaneously, ambivalent persons may often fail to reach adequate conflict resolutions.

In Study 2, both partners in 123 heterosexual dating relationships (average length = 21 months) initially completed questionnaires assessing their attachment orientation (the AAQ), their personality traits on measures of introversion, neuroticism, and agreeableness, and the nature of their current relationship (see Simpson et al., 1996). One week later, the couples returned for the second phase of the study, during which half of them were randomly assigned to identify and discuss a major problem in their relationship and half were assigned to identify and discuss a minor problem. Each partner first nominated three to five issues that had been a recent source of disagreement. Partners in the major problem condition then jointly identified the most significant unresolved problem. They were asked to remember the last major disagreement they had about the issue, and then were told to try their best to resolve it. The instructions were: "Remember what you were arguing about and why you were upset with your partner. Remember what you were thinking about and how you felt during the argument. After remembering these things, we would like you to discuss this issue with each other. We'd like each of you to tell the other what it is about his or her attitudes, habits, or behaviors that bothers you. Please discuss the issue in detail." Partners in the minor problem condition went through the same procedures, but they were told to identify and discuss a minor problem. The experimenter informed each couple that their discussion would be videotaped and subsequently rated by observers. The discussions lasted 7–10 minutes.

Following the discussion, each partner completed self-report measures that assessed the amount of distress they felt during the discussion, changes in their perceptions of the partner or relationship, and the amount of anger and hostility they felt at the end of the discussion. During the debriefing, the experimenter emphasized that all relationships involve problems and disagreements, and that points of contention can be a healthy feature of strong, committed relationships. No couple was allowed to leave until the experimenter was convinced that both partners felt good about their experience in the study.

Raters evaluated the behavior of men and women separately. Their ratings assessed two dimensions relevant to successful conflict resolution (Gottman, 1979): the extent of each partner's observable stress and anxiety, and the extent of each partner's warmth and supportiveness. Ratings of the extent to which the discussion was constructive and was moving toward successful conflict resolution also were made.

Hypotheses and Results

Five major hypotheses were tested: three concerning ambivalence and two concerning avoidance. First, more ambivalent persons who discussed a major problem were expected to view their partner and relationship less positively after the discussion. Specifically, we expected them to report lower levels of love and commitment, supportiveness and open communication, and mutual respect for their partner. Second, more ambivalent persons who discussed a major problem were expected to report more anger and hostility and to display greater stress and anxiety (rated by observers). Third, conversations about major problems that involved more ambivalent persons were expected to be poorer in quality (rated by observers). Specifically, their conversations should have less interpersonal synchrony, remain farther from problem resolution, involve less emotional closeness, be less constructive, be more strained, and involve more talking to (rather than with) the partner.

We predicted that the discussions of more avoidant persons also would be lower in quality. However, given their tendency to retreat from emotional experiences, avoidant persons were not expected to display negative affect or devalue their partner or relationship, even when discussing a major problem. Finally, given the findings of Study 1, we expected avoidant men to be less warm and supportive, particularly when discussing a major problem with their partner. Because previous attachment research has examined support giving only in men, it was unclear whether avoidant women also would be less supportive.

Most of the results confirmed these predictions. More ambivalent men and women reported feeling more distressed during their conversations than did less ambivalent men and women. They also displayed greater stress and anxiety, and they reported feeling greater anger and hostility, especially when they discussed a major problem.[2] The conversations of more ambivalent men and women were rated as lower in quality, and this was especially true for highly ambivalent women who discussed a major problem. More ambivalent men and women who discussed a major problem also reported more negative perceptions of their partner or relationship after the discussion. Interestingly, these decrements in perception were *not* mediated either by the quality of the interaction or the degree to which the conversation had moved toward problem resolution.

Consistent with expectations, more avoidant men exhibited less warmth and supportiveness and their interactions were rated as lower in quality, particularly when they discussed a major problem. More avoidant women, however, did not show these effects. Indeed, no significant effects involving avoidance emerged for women in Study 2.

Finally, discriminant validation analyses confirmed that these effects remained significant once trait measures of introversion, neuroticism, and agreeableness, as well as relationship measures of love, liking, commitment, satisfaction, trust, and subjective closeness were partialed out. The effects, therefore, appear to be specific to attachment orientations per se.

Ambivalence and Conflict Resolution

In many respects, ambivalent women in Study 2 resemble the distressed wives described in previous marital interaction studies. In these studies, women have been found to initiate, guide, and control conflict resolution discussions, usually adopting a more direct, confrontational, and negative demeanor than their husbands (Gottman, 1979). They often do so because their husbands withdraw from conflict (Levenson & Gottman, 1985; Locke, 1951) and because women usually assume greater responsibility for the maintenance and well-being of relationships (Cancian & Gordon, 1988; Surra & Longstreth, 1990). Either or both explanations could account for why the quality of interactions in the present study were particularly poor in couples that included an ambivalent woman and had the task of resolving a major problem.

Although it seems reasonable to believe that the negative tenor of ambivalent persons' interactions led them to report less positive perceptions of their partners or relationships, the data provide little support for this interpretation. When ratings of the quality of interaction and the degree of problem resolution were partialed out, ambivalence was still significantly associated with less positive perceptions of the partner or relationship. Using a similar problem-solving task, Kobak and Hazan (1991) also found that the link between marital partners' marital satisfaction and their agreement about each other's working models was not mediated by the quality of their problem-solving discussions. Thus, the perceptions of the partner or relationship reported by ambivalent persons immediately following conflict resolution may stem directly from the nature of their working models rather than from frustrations generated by difficult interactions.

Ambivalent persons who discussed a major problem also felt greater anger and hostility toward their partners after the interaction. As discussed previously, anger can be used functionally to reproach the partner in the interest of maintaining the relationship, or it can emerge dysfunctionally as malice and spite (Bowlby, 1973). We were unable to differentiate these types of anger in Study 2.

Avoidance and Conflict Resolution

Because of their discomfort with intimacy and their belief that attachment figures cannot be counted on to alleviate distress, highly avoidant persons should try to minimize involvement in interpersonal conflicts, opting to maintain a safe emotional distance from the partner and topic of disagreement. This can be accomplished in several ways, such as downplaying the significance of the topic for the partner or relationship or ignoring the partner's feelings. Strategies such as these, however, should discourage constructive conflict resolution. Presumably because they are adept at using these strategies (see Main et al., 1985), avoidant persons in Study 2 did not experience heightened distress, greater anger, or less positive perceptions of their partner or relationship.

Avoidance and Warmth / Supportiveness

Avoidant men were rated as less warm and supportive than less avoidant men, particularly when they discussed a major problem. Nevertheless, they did *not* display greater anger and hostility. Nonsupportiveness often is accompanied by anger during conflict resolution (Levenson & Gottman, 1983). However, anger requires involvement in the issue being discussed. To the extent that avoidant people successfully limit their involvement, nonsupportiveness should not—and did not—covary with their level of anger. However, this is not to say that anger and support would not be correlated positively in other circumstances.

The findings for warmth and supportiveness in men conceptually replicate those reported in Study 1. Both studies reveal that situations relevant to attachment issues elicit less supportive responses from more avoidant men. Study 2 extends Study 1, however, by documenting an unanticipated sex difference: Avoidant women did *not* display less warmth and support toward their partners. Since only men were given the chance to provide support in Study 1, Study 2 is the first investigation to reveal this gender difference. Traditional female sex roles encourage the expression of greater warmth and supportiveness (Gilligan, 1982), better listening skills (Miller, Berg, & Archer, 1983), and more interpersonal sensitivity (Hall, 1978). Women also take greater responsibility for maintaining relationships (Cancian & Gordon, 1988; Surra & Longstreth, 1990). Thus, sex roles may override the prototypical interaction style associated with the avoidant orientation, particularly for avoidant women confronted with situations that could strain their relationship. Avoidance also was associated with less effective conflict resolution behavior among men, but not women. This finding bolsters the premise that sex roles may differentially affect how avoidant men and women behave, at least in conflict resolution settings.

Changing Perceptions of Partners or Relationships

Anxious–ambivalent infants (Ainsworth et al., 1978) and children (Main et al., 1985), and preoccupied adults (Main & Goldwyn, in press) display a wide and highly variable range of positive and negative responses toward their attachment figures when they are upset, sometimes exhibiting both approach and avoidance tendencies in the same setting. As adults, ambivalent persons experience pronounced vacillations in relationship happiness and satisfaction over relatively short periods of time (Tidwell, Reis, & Shaver, 1996). Little is known, however, about why their relationships are so turbulent. Study 2 indicates that the way in which ambivalent persons react to conflict might partially explain this phenomenon.

Conflict elicits a cascade of unpleasant feelings in ambivalent persons, and it should raise doubts about the quality and viability of their current partner and relationship. Moreover, if fears of abandonment become salient, ambivalent persons ought to derogate the partner and relationship to minimize or "prepare for" potential loss. Persons who are not ambivalent, in contrast, may not experience conflict as aversive, but as an occasion in which open communication and the joint, constructive sharing of feelings can occur (cf. Holmes & Rempel, 1989). As a consequence, attempts to resolve conflict may give less ambivalent persons the opportunity to engage in behaviors they value and allow them to confirm—and perhaps even strengthen—their confidence in their partner and relationship (Simpson & Rholes, 1994).

CONCLUSIONS

The present studies investigated situations that, according to attachment theory, should "release" behaviors prototypical of avoidant and ambivalent attachment orientations. In both studies, distress served as the releasing factor. The specific source of distress, however, differed in the two studies. In Study 1, anxiety about an impending event that was *external* to couples' relationships was the releaser. In terms of the categories proposed by Kobak and Duemmler (1994), Study 1 focused on the willingness and capacity of partners to seek or provide a "safe haven." In Study 2, distress mainly emanated from *within* couples' relationships. During the conflict resolution task, partners were compelled to confront both their own feelings about their partner and their partner's feelings about them. In doing so, they had an opportunity to assess weaknesses in their partner or relationship and to contemplate the prospect of relationship dissolution. In addition, the conflict resolution task allowed for the expression of psychological intimacy or for partners to reject bids for intimacy. Thus, couples in Study 2 faced the task of trying to maintain what Kobak and Duemmler called a "cooperative partnership." In Study 1, external distress led highly avoidant and less avoidant people to behave very differently, but it did not lead to differences in the behavior of persons with high versus low levels of ambivalence. In Study 2, however, when distress originated from problems internal to the relationship, numerous behavioral differences were observed as a function of both ambivalence and avoidance.

The central findings of Study 1 were that highly avoidant women sought less support from their partners if they were more distressed, and more avoidant men were less likely to provide support if their partners were more distressed. Such behavior, however, was observed only when women were highly distressed. If the female partner was less distressed, the behavior of avoidant men and women was indistinguishable from their less avoidant counterparts, and little or nothing in their actions fit the description of avoidance in the theoretical literature (Bowlby, 1973, 1980). The major findings of Study 2 were that more ambivalent persons felt greater distress and anger during the conflict resolution discussions, had discussions that were rated as lower in quality, and perceived their partner or relationship in a more negative light following the discussions. The study also found that avoidant men engaged in discussions of lower quality and were rated as being less warm and supportive.

Of all these findings, two stand out as particularly important. First, in both studies, highly avoidant persons were less likely to provide emotional support to others (see also Phillips et al., 1995). Simpson and Rholes (1994) recently have suggested that the depth of a relationship (i.e., its degree of closeness, commitment, and emotional bonding) may be determined in large part by the way partners handle stressful events (e.g., a child's serious illness or serious financial difficulties). Relationships in which partners successfully support each other through times of crisis should grow closer and become stronger, in essence forging "secure" attachment relationships. Conversely, relationships in which partners fail to provide support should become comparatively dysfunctional or disturbed. Finally, relationships which are free of major life stress may remain relatively superficial because partners lack the opportunity to provide support to one another. According to this perspective, relationships in which avoidant persons are involved should either remain superficial (if little stress is encountered) or should be damaged by the avoidant person's inability to provide comfort and support during difficult times.

Interestingly, Study 2 revealed that the association between avoidance and the provision of support differed for men and women. Traditional male sex roles tend to be more congruent with the prototypical emotional and behavioral features of the avoidant orientation. As a result, highly avoidant men may experience few barriers to enacting their basic inclination to distance themselves from others. The desire to establish distance, however, is at odds with the traditional female sex role of "relationship maintainer." Therefore, avoidant women should experience strong conflict between sex-role requirements and their avoidant tendencies, particularly in situations that call for relationship maintenance.

The sex differences found in Study 2, however, must be interpreted in the context of two other studies. First, a number of differences were discovered between highly avoidant and less avoidant women in Study 1. Thus, the findings of Study 2 should not be interpreted to mean that sex-role pressures invariably override avoidant propensities in women. Second, Phillips et al. (1995) found that both avoidant men and women feel uncomfortable about giving support to close friends, and are less likely to actually do so. Therefore, the findings of Study 2 must be interpreted cautiously. Sex differences in attachment-related behavior may emerge in a relatively narrow range of situations.

The second noteworthy result is the link between ambivalence and perceptions of the partner or relationship following the conflict resolution discussion in Study 2. More ambivalent persons were considerably less positive about their partner or relationship following conflict resolution. We believe this occurs because of two complementary tendencies. First, ambivalent persons may devalue their partner or relationship for defensive purposes if they think their relationship may be in jeopardy. Second, ambivalent persons may be easily disappointed in their partner because their working models accentuate doubts about the commitment and underlying motives of attachment figures. Any behaviors displayed by partners that fall below their rigorous evaluative standards may be interpreted by ambivalent persons as signs of untrustworthiness or lack of true commitment.

Study 2 also revealed that negative perceptions of the partner or relationship in the postdiscussion phase were not mediated by the quality of the conflict resolution interaction. This implies that working models may play a direct role in generating negative evaluations and that relationship satisfaction may reside as much "in the head" of ambivalent persons as it does in the reality of their interactions. If this is true, insight-oriented forms of therapy may produce better and more lasting changes in ambivalent people than behavioral therapies (see Dozier & Tyrrell, Chapter 9, this volume). Kobak, Ruckdeschel, and Hazan (1994) have speculated that symptoms of marital distress often are reactions to attachment-related fears and expectations, and they recommend treatments that directly address these concerns. Behavioral therapies aim to produce immediate change in a couple's interactions by enhancing communication and problem-solving skills. In contrast, insight-oriented therapies attempt to uncover beliefs, expectations, and feelings that spouses have about themselves, their partner, and their relationship and, at the same time, to restructure emotional processes. This type of therapy should help partners understand their feelings more fully and cope with them more effectively. Consistent with this view, Snyder, Wills, and Grady-Fletcher (1991) found that couples who were treated with insight-oriented marital therapy were less likely to have divorced 4 years later in comparison to couples who received behavioral marital therapy. We believe that insight-oriented therapy may be particularly important for couples in which at least one partner is highly ambivalent.

In summary, our program of research helps confirm a fundamental tenet of attachment theory: namely, that the cardinal behavioral features of secure, avoidant, and ambivalent attachment orientations are most likely to be witnessed in situations that activate the attachment system and individuals' internal working models. Studies 1 and 2 were designed to elicit distress from different sources. The procedure used in Study 1 generated environmentally based fear and anxiety, providing partners with different attachment orientations the opportunity to give or receive support. The procedure used in Study 2, on the other hand, generated relationship-based distress, allowing us to examine the way partners with different attachment orientations handle difficulties internal to their relationship. The fear induction procedure of the first study should have activated concerns about only one issue, intimacy versus independence. The conflict resolution paradigm, in comparison, probably evoked a wider range of concerns, and this might explain why effects were found for both the avoidant and the ambivalent orientation in Study 2. It should have elicited fears of loss and abandonment (in ambivalent people) as well as concerns about intimacy and independence (in avoidant people). The different results of these studies, thus, suggest that researchers must be careful to consider which kinds of stressful situations relate to which aspects of working models when investigating situations that activate the attachment system.

ACKNOWLEDGMENTS

This research was supported by National Institute of Mental Health Grant No. MH49599 to Jeffry A. Simpson and W. Steven Rholes, who contributed equally to this chapter.

NOTES

1. Within each AAI category, respondents are also categorized as either resolved or unresolved with respect to death of attachment figures or other traumatic experiences involving attachment figures, if either of these events have occurred.

2. These findings were stronger for women than men. See Simpson et al. (1996).

REFERENCES

Ainsworth, M. D. S., Blehar, M. C., Waters, E., & Wall, S. (1978). *Patterns of attachment: A psychological study of the Strange Situation.* Hillsdale, NJ: Erlbaum.

Bartholomew, K. (1990). Avoidance of intimacy: An attachment perspective. *Journal of Social and Personal Relationships, 7,* 147–178.

Bartholomew, K., & Horowitz, L. M. (1991). Attachment styles among young adults: A test of a four-category model. *Journal of Personality and Social Psychology, 61,* 226–244.

Berscheid, E., Snyder, M., & Omoto, A. M. (1989). The Relationship Closeness Inventory: Assessing the closeness of interpersonal relationships. *Journal of Personality and Social Psychology, 57,* 792–807.

Bowlby, J. (1969). *Attachment and loss: Vol. 1. Attachment.* New York: Basic Books.

Bowlby, J. (1973). *Attachment and loss: Vol. 2. Separation: Anxiety and anger.* New York: Basic Books.

Bowlby, J. (1980). *Attachment and loss: Vol. 3. Loss: Sadness and depression.* New York: Basic Books.

Cancian, F., & Gordon, S. L. (1988). Changing emotional norms in marriage: Love and anger in U.S. women's magazines since 1900. *Gender and Society, 2,* 308–342.

Collins, N. L., & Read, S. J. (1990). Adult attachment, working models, and relationship quality in dating couples. *Journal of Personality and Social Psychology, 58,* 644–663.

Feeney, J. A., Noller, P., & Callan, V. J. (1994). Attachment style, communication, and satisfaction in the early years of marriage. In K. Bartholomew & D. Perlman (Eds.), *Attachment processes in adulthood* (pp. 269–308). London: Jessica Kingsley.

George, C., Kaplan, N., & Main, M. (1996). *Adult Attachment Interview* (3rd ed.). Unpublished manuscript, University of California, Berkeley.

Gilligan, C. (1982). *In a different voice: Psychological theory and women's development.* Cambridge, MA: Harvard University Press.

Gottman, J. M. (1979). *Marital interaction: Experimental investigations.* London: Academic Press.

Griffin, D., & Bartholomew, K. (1994a). The metaphysics of measurement: The case of adult attachment. In K. Bartholomew & D. Perlman (Eds.), *Attachment processes in adulthood* (pp. 17–52). London: Jessica Kingsley.

Griffin, D., & Bartholomew, K. (1994b). Models of the self and other: Fundamental dimensions underlying measures of adult attachment. *Journal of Personality and Social Psychology, 67,* 430–445.

Hall, J. A. (1978). Gender effects in decoding nonverbal cues. *Psychological Bulletin, 85,* 845–857.

Hamilton, C. E. (1995, March). *Continuity and discontinuity of attachment from infancy through adolescence.* Paper presented at the biennial meeting of the Society for Research in Child Development, Indianapolis, IN.

Hazan, C., & Shaver, P. (1987). Romantic love conceptualized as an attachment process. *Journal of Personality and Social Psychology, 52,* 511–524.

Hazan, C., & Shaver, P. (1994). Attachment as an organizational framework for research on close relationships. *Psychological Inquiry, 5,* 1–22.

Hendrick, C., & Hendrick, S. S. (1989). Research on love: Does it measure up? *Journal of Personality and Social Psychology, 56,* 784–794.

Holmes, J. G., & Rempel, J. K. (1989). Trust in close relationships. In C. Hendrick (Ed.), *Review of personality and social psychology: Vol. 10. Close relationships* (pp. 187–220). Newbury Park, CA: Sage.

Kobak, R. R., Cole, H. E., Ferenz-Gillies, R., Fleming, W. S., & Gamble, W. (1993). Attachment and emotion regulation during mother–teen problem solving: A control theory analysis. *Child Development, 64,* 231–245.

Kobak, R. R., & Duemmler, S. (1994). Attachment and conversation: Toward a discourse analysis of adolescent and adult security. In K. Bartholomew & D. Perlman (Eds.), *Attachment processes in adulthood* (pp. 121–149). London: Jessica Kingsley.

Kobak, R. R., & Hazan, C. (1991). Attachment in marriage: Effects of security and accuracy of working models. *Journal of Personality and Social Psychology, 60,* 861–869.

Kobak, R. R., Ruckdeschel, K., & Hazan, C. (1994). From symptom to signal: An attachment view of emotion in marital therapy. In S. M. Johnson & L. S. Greenberg (Eds.), *The heart of the matter: Perspectives on emotion in marital therapy* (pp. 46–71). New York: Brunner/Mazel.

Levenson, R. W., & Gottman, J. M. (1983). Martial interaction: Physiological linkage and affective exchange. *Journal of Personality and Social Psychology, 45,* 587–597.

Levenson, R. W., & Gottman, J. M. (1985). Physiological and affective predictors of change in relationship satisfaction. *Journal of Personality and Social Psychology, 49,* 85–94.

Levy, M. B., & Davis, K. E. (1988). Lovestyles and attachment styles compared: Their relations to each other and to various relationship characteristics. *Journal of Social and Personal Relationships, 5,* 439–471.

Locke, H. J. (1951). *Predicting adjustments in marriage: A comparison of a divorced and a happily married group.* New York: Henry Holt.

Main, M. (1981). Avoidance in the service of attachment: A working paper. In K. Immelmann, G. Barlow, L. Petrinovich, & M. Main (Eds.), *Behavioral development: The Bielefeld interdisciplinary project* (pp. 651–693). New York: Cambridge University Press.

Main, M., & Goldwyn, R. (in press). Interview-based adult attachment classifications: Related to infant–mother and infant–father attachment. *Developmental Psychology.*

Main, M., Kaplan, N., & Cassidy, J. (1985). Security in infancy, childhood, and adulthood: A move to the level of representation. In I. Bretherton & E. Waters (Eds.), Growing points in attachment theory and research. *Monographs of the Society for Research in Child Development, 50,* 66–104.

Mikulincer, M., & Nachshon, O. (1991). Attachment styles and patterns of self-disclosure. *Journal of Personality and Social Psychology, 61,* 321–331.

Miller, L. C., Berg, J. H., & Archer, R. L. (1983). Openers: Individuals who elicit intimate self-disclosure. *Journal of Personality and Social Psychology, 44,* 1234–1244.

Phillips, D., Simpson, J. A., Lanigan, L., & Rholes, S. W. (1995). *Providing social support: A study of adult attachment styles.* Paper presented at the joint meetings of the European Association of Social Psychology and the Society of Experimental Social Psychology, Washington, DC.

Pistole, M. C. (1989). Attachment in adult romantic relationships: Style of conflict resolution and relationship satisfaction. *Journal of Social and Personal Relationships, 6,* 505–510.

Rholes, W. S., Simpson, J. A., & Blakely, B. (1995). Adult attachment styles and mothers' relationships with their young children. *Personal Relationships, 2,* 35–54.

Rubin, Z. (1970). Measurement of romantic love. *Journal of Personality and Social Psychology, 16,* 265–273.

Simpson, J. A. (1990). Influence of attachment styles on romantic relationships. *Journal of Personality and Social Psychology, 59,* 971–980.

Simpson, J. A., & Rholes, W. S. (1994). Stress and secure base relationships in adulthood. In K. Bartholomew & D. Perlman (Eds.), *Attachment processes in adulthood* (pp. 181–204). London: Jessica Kingsley.

Simpson, J. A., Rholes, W. S., & Nelligan, J. S. (1992). Support seeking and support giving within couples in an anxiety-provoking situation: The role of attachment styles. *Journal of Personality and Social Psychology, 62,* 434–446.

Simpson, J. A., Rholes, W. S., & Phillips, D. (1996). Conflict in close relationships: An attachment perspective. *Journal of Personality and Social Psychology, 71,* 899–914.

Snyder, D. K., Wills, R. M., & Grady-Fletcher, A. (1991). Long-term effectiveness of behavioral versus insight-oriented marital therapy: A four year follow-up study. *Journal of Consulting and Clinical Psychology, 59,* 138–141.

Sroufe, L. A., & Waters, E. (1977). Attachment as an organizational construct. *Child Development, 48,* 1184–1199.

Surra, C. A., & Longstreth, M. (1990). Similarity of outcomes, interdependence, and conflict in dating relationships. *Journal of Personality and Social Psychology, 59,* 501–516.

Tidwell, M. O., Reis, H. T., & Shaver, P. R. (1996). Attachment, attractiveness, and social interaction: A diary study. *Journal of Personality and Social Psychology, 71,* 729–745.

van IJzendoorn, M. H. (1995). Adult attachment representations, parental responsiveness, and infant attachment: A meta-analysis on the predictive validity of the Adult Attachment Interview. *Psychological Bulletin, 117,* 387–403.

Waters, E., Merrick, S. K., Albersheim, L. J., & Treboux, D. (1995, March). *Attachment security from infancy to early adulthood: A 20-year longitudinal study.* Paper presented at the biennial meeting of the Society for Research in Child Development, Indianapolis, IN.

8

Adult Attachment and Relationship-Centered Anxiety

Responses to Physical and Emotional Distancing

JUDITH A. FEENEY

Hazan and Shaver's (1987) innovative work attempted to explain adult romantic relationships from the perspective of attachment theory. According to this perspective, romantic relationships are similar in important respects to infant–caregiver bonds, and the major attachment styles described in the infant literature (secure, avoidant, and anxious–ambivalent) are also manifested in romantic love. Using a simple forced-choice measure of these three attachment styles, Hazan and Shaver found clear differences between adult attachment groups in reports of early family background, mental models of relationships, and adult love experiences.

Researchers have subsequently used both categorical and continuous measures to study adult attachment. Some measures have been based on a four-group model of attachment that identifies two forms of avoidance: fearful, involving pervasive distrust and fear of rejection, and dismissing, involving a sense of independence and a defensive denial of attachment needs (Bartholomew, 1990; Bartholomew & Horowitz, 1991). Irrespective of the particular measures used, research has established reliable relations between attachment style and indices of the quality and stability of romantic relationships (see Shaver & Hazan, 1993, for a review).

Until recently, researchers into adult attachment have largely ignored the role of stress and anxiety in eliciting attachment behavior. Yet Bowlby's (1969, 1973, 1980) attachment theory, on which adult attachment work is based, proposes that attachment behavior is most likely to be activated under conditions of stress or threat. Bowlby (1969) argued that conditions of apparent threat which activate attachment behavior in young children are of three types: conditions of the child, such as fatigue and pain; environmental conditions, such as alarming events; and absence or discouraging of proximity on the part of attachment figures. Consistent with the claim that attachment-style differences are most pronounced under stressful conditions, the laboratory procedure commonly used to assess infant attachment style (the Strange Situation) was designed to enable observation of infants' behavior under such conditions. The research described in this chapter focuses on the link between attachment and what will be referred to as "relationship-centered anxiety"—that is, anxiety stemming from absence or discouraging of proximity on the part of attachment figures.

Within attachment theory, the concept of affect regulation highlights the importance of behavior under stressful conditions. Attachment styles are thought to develop from individuals' experiences of regulating distress with attachment figures; hence, these styles reflect strategies that have been learned as ways of dealing with negative affect. If attachment figures are available and responsive to the child's signals of distress, distress can be acknowledged and regulated with strategies that involve seeking comfort and support; such a constructive approach to affect regulation is characteristic of secure attachment. If attachment figures are insensitive or rejecting, the child learns to inhibit displays of distress and to restrict attempts to seek comfort and support; this pattern of compulsive self-reliance is characteristic of avoidant attachment. If attachment figures are inconsistent or inept in responding to the child's signals, the child becomes hypervigilant in attending to and expressing distress; this pattern of dependency typifies anxious–ambivalent attachment (Kobak & Sceery, 1988; Sroufe & Waters, 1977).

Thus, attachment styles reflect the extent of negative feelings in distressing situations, and also the methods that individuals use to cope with that distress (Mikulincer, Florian, & Tolmacz, 1990). Adult attachment researchers have not fully appreciated that attachment theory is primarily a theory of affect regulation, and have tended to treat attachment style as a traitlike construct that influences behavior in all settings, irrespective of variables such as stress and anxiety.

Recent experimental work by Simpson, Rholes, and Nelligan (1992) was the first to address this issue with an adult sample. In a study of dating couples, Simpson et al. assessed the effects of attachment style and experimentally manipulated anxiety on attachment-related behaviors. Female subjects were told that they were to participate in an experiment that most people experience as distressing. During the purported waiting time, couples were videotaped to allow observers to rate females' anxiety and their support-seeking behavior, as well as male partners' support-giving behavior.

Using items derived from the original forced-choice measure of adult attachment, Simpson et al. reported two major underlying dimensions of attachment: Secure–Avoidance (a bipolar factor) and Anxious Attachment. Behavior in the experimental situation was related to Secure–Avoidance, but not to Anxious Attachment. Secure women sought more support from their partners as their level of anxiety (observer-rated) increased, whereas avoidant women sought less support as their anxiety increased. Moreover, secure men offered more support as their partners' level of anxiety increased, whereas avoidant men offered less support as partners' anxiety increased. These results support the argument that attachment-style differences are more pronounced in stressful situations. They also suggest that researchers, in describing the "typical" behavior displayed by attachment groups, need to specify the context in which the behavior occurs; for example, avoidant persons' tendency to act in a distant manner seems to be confined to stressful situations (Simpson et al., 1992).

Mikulincer, Florian, and Weller (1993) studied the implications of attachment for responses to stress in a more "naturalistic" setting: missile attacks occurring during the Gulf War. Attachment groups (secure, avoidant, and ambivalent) differed in their emotional reactions to the attacks: Avoidant and ambivalent individuals reported higher levels of hostility and somatization than secure individuals, and ambivalent subjects also reported high levels of anxiety and depression. The attachment groups also differed in the strategies used to cope with the threat: Secure individuals tended to seek support from others, avoidant individuals tended to distance themselves from the situation, and ambivalent individuals focused on their negative feelings about the situation. These results support the proposition that secure attachment facilitates constructive attitudes and approaches to stressful situations.

In focusing on attachment and responses to stressful situations, the studies by Simpson et al. (1992) and Mikulincer et al. (1993) represent an important development in adult attachment research. Furthermore, these studies complement each other in useful ways. The approach adopted by Simpson et al. involved the experimental induction of stress, and allowed for multiple dependent measures (conversation ratings, physical behavior) to be taken by outside observers. By contrast, the work reported by Mikulincer et al. involved a real-life situation, but was limited by the fact that all measures were obtained retrospectively and at a single point in time.

These studies leave unanswered questions, however, concerning the influence of stress and anxiety on the emotions and behaviors associated with attachment style. In terms of Bowlby's analysis of the conditions that activate attachment behavior, both studies focused on "environmental conditions." There are several reasons why it is crucial for researchers to study the link between attachment and relationship-centered anxiety.

First, it is clear that focusing on any one set of threatening conditions cannot provide a complete picture of the implications of stress and attachment style for adults' relationship behavior. Further, relationship-centered anxiety may be more relevant to adult relationship behavior than are environmental stressors. The attachment system in adults is likely to be activated only by relatively extreme environmental threats, whereas many such situations cause young children to seek the protection of attachment figures. Finally, the amount of anxiety elicited by partners' absence or discouraging of proximity is likely to be related to attachment dimensions, and these relations are of interest in their own right. For example, individuals who are highly anxious about their attachment relationships are likely to respond with greater anxiety to situations involving physical or emotional separation from romantic partners. Thus it is important to study attachment style differences in the *extent* of relationship-centered anxiety, as well as in the responses to such anxiety. Insecure attachment has been linked with greater distress in response to missile attacks (Mikulincer et al., 1993), but not in response to a stress-induction paradigm (Simpson et al., 1992). The lack of association between attachment style and anxiety in the latter study simplifies the interpretation of focal relations, but is unlikely to generalize to contexts in which the relationship itself is the source of anxiety.

The only published work to address the issue of attachment style and relationship-centered anxiety is that of Cafferty, Davis, Medway, O'Hearn, and Chappell (1994). The context for this research, like that of Mikulincer et al., was the Gulf War. Rather than assessing the effects of the wartime environment on the individual, however, Cafferty et al. studied the impact of separation on the relationships of couples in which the male spouse was deployed overseas during the war. Subjects completed self-report questionnaires 4 months after being reunited with their partners. For the deployed men, secure attachment was associated with reports of more positive and less negative affect during reunion; secure men also reported less postreunion conflict and higher marital satisfaction than preoccupied men. For the nondeployed wives, results for conflict and satisfaction replicated those for the men, but no link was observed between attachment style and affect during reunion. In explaining these results, Cafferty et al. (1994) suggest that some separations are more likely than others to activate attachment dynamics. The stronger results observed among the deployed men may reflect the fact that, for them, separation involved an unfamiliar and highly stressful environment.

The research presented by Cafferty et al. points to the importance of studying separation and reunion responses in adult attachment relationships, but much further work needs to be done in this area. Cafferty and colleagues focused on reunion following war-related separation; they did not explore the actual experience of separation, and their data did not permit comparisons with more routine instances of separation. Further, the study dealt with physical separation, rather than with partners' discouraging of proximity; again, important comparisons remain to be made between these two types of relationship-centered anxiety. Finally, their sample comprised couples in long-term marriages. In less established romantic relationships, issues of physical and emotional distancing may be more salient, in terms of the future of the developing relationship.

This chapter presents research from our laboratory exploring the links between attachment style and relationship-centered anxiety in a sample of dating couples. In Task 1, subjects provided retrospective, open-ended descriptions of their responses to physical distancing in their current relationship. In Task 2, couples were videotaped during three conflict-based interactions: two that focused on issues of distance and closeness between relationship partners, and one that involved a more concrete goal conflict.

This research is based on theoretical and empirical work suggesting that working models of attachment are activated in conversations in which one partner's concerns about the other's availability are an implicit or explicit topic (Kobak & Duemmler, 1994). Kobak and Duemmler argue that such "goal conflicts" provide a better means of studying adult attachment than do fear-eliciting (or stressful environmental) situations: Fear-eliciting situations may activate the attachment system to such high levels that there is an emphasis on physical contact rather than psychological support. For this reason, and because of the dearth of research into attachment and relationship-centered anxiety, the present research focused on couples' goal conflicts concerning separation, distance, and closeness.

These goal conflicts can be studied in different ways. Subjects may be asked to talk about actual situations in which partners have been unavailable or unresponsive to them; alternatively, they may be exposed to standardized laboratory paradigms designed to elicit concerns about partners' availability and responsiveness. To provide a more complete picture of the link between attachment and relationship-centered anxiety, the present research employed both of these methods (Tasks 1 and 2, respectively).

Subjects for this research were 72 heterosexual couples who had been dating their current partners for at least 12 months. One member of each couple was enrolled in an introductory psychology course at the University of Queensland, and received course credit for participation. Subjects were between ages 17 and 37, although most were under 22 years of age. Length of current dating relationships ranged from 12 to 77 months, with a mean of 23.4 months. Approximately half of the sample were full-time students, with the remainder spread fairly evenly across occupational categories.

TASK 1

This task focused on subjects' open-ended reports of their experiences of separation from their current dating partners. The eliciting of open-ended reports offers a relatively unobtrusive method of data collection, and minimizes response sets such as social desirability and experimenter demand (Lolas, 1986). Because there are few constraints on responses, this technique can provide rich and complex data concerning subjects' own interpretations of their experiences (Feeney & Noller, 1991). Consistent with previous research, three aspects of the separation experience were assessed: coping strategies, emotional reactions, and perceived effects on the dyadic relationship.

Hypotheses

Previous research supports the distinction between problem-focused and emotion-focused coping (although some coping strategies, notably support seeking, can serve both problem- and emotion-focused functions). There is also evidence that, in most situations, problem-focused coping is positively related to adjustment; for example, Folkman, Lazarus, Gruen, and DeLongis (1986) found that planful problem solving was associated with fewer psychological symptoms. Hence, it was expected that secure attachment would be associated with greater use of support seeking and problem-focused coping, and with less use of emotion-focused coping.

In terms of effects on the dyadic relationship, it should be noted that securely attached individuals advocate open communication between relationship partners (Feeney, Noller, & Callan, 1994). In dating relationships, periods of physical separation are likely to raise issues concerning the goals of individual partners and the future of the relationship. Hence, it was expected that secure attachment would be linked with reports that partners had actively renegotiated their relationships following separation (i.e., that they had discussed what each partner wanted from the relationship, or how much time they were able to devote to the relationship). It was expected that secure attachment would also be associated with perceptions that the separation had a positive effect, serving to bring the partners closer.

Given the open-ended nature of this research, and the lack of a clear framework for classifying emotional reactions to separation, it was considered important to allow the major themes to emerge from the data.

Hence, no specific predictions were made concerning the link between attachment and emotional reactions to separation.

Measures and Procedure

Subjects completed the four-group forced-choice measure of attachment style (Bartholomew & Horowitz, 1991), in which subjects categorize themselves as secure, preoccupied (anxious–ambivalent), dismissing, or fearful. This categorical measure was used to compare the attachment characteristics of the present sample with those of samples previously reported in the literature; the focal analyses, however, employed continuous measures of attachment.

The continuous measures were derived from a set of 15 items based on Hazan and Shaver's (1987) original measure of adult attachment. Responses to these items were used to form the two scales of Comfort with closeness (referred to as Comfort) and Anxiety over relationships (referred to as Anxiety) obtained with a different sample (see Feeney et al., 1994), and reported independently by other researchers (Fitzpatrick, Fey, Segrin, & Schiff, 1993; Simpson et al., 1992). The Comfort scale consisted of eight items, including "I find it relatively easy to get close to others"; and "I find it difficult to depend on others" (reversed). The Anxiety scale consisted of five items, including "I find that others are reluctant to get as close as I would like"; and "I often worry that my partner won't want to stay with me." The Comfort factor essentially contrasts secure and avoidant attachment, and Anxiety corresponds closely to anxious–ambivalent attachment. These scales showed good internal consistency, with alpha coefficients exceeding .70. Because the items used a 5-point response format (1 = not at all like me, to 5 = very much like me), scores could range from 8 to 40 for Comfort, and from 5 to 25 for Anxiety.

Before completing the attachment measures, subjects described their experiences of separation. (The tasks were completed in this order, because it was important that the open-ended reports be uncontaminated by exposure to the content of the attachment measures.) The dating partners were taken to separate rooms to avoid interaction, and were asked to think about a time when they had been physically separated from their current partner. They were asked to talk for 5 minutes about this experience: how they felt about the situation and how they coped with it, how their partner had reacted, and how the situation had affected their relationship as a couple. Subjects' descriptions were tape recorded and later transcribed for content analysis.

Content Coding

Content coding was used to explore the three major aspects of the separation experience: coping strategies, emotional reactions, and perceived effects on the relationship (see Table 8.1 for examples of the major content codes). Only those strategies and reactions that were mentioned by at least 15 subjects were retained. For all variables, an independent rater coded a sample of 30 transcripts in order to establish interrater reliability.

Coping Strategies

First, coping strategies were defined using the broad categories described by previous researchers: support seeking (using resources of the social network), problem-focused coping (directed toward management of the problem), and emotion-focused coping (dealing with the associated emotional distress). The categories of problem- and emotion-focused coping were subdivided to provide more fine-grained information, consistent with the coping scales reported by Folkman, Lazarus, Dunkel-Schetter, DeLongis, and Gruen (1986). Problem-focused coping was subdivided

TABLE 8.1. Examples of Content Coding (Task 1)

Variable	Example
Coping strategies	
Support seeking	"What I did was to socialize with my friends, talk to them on the phone, and tell them about what was happening."
Problem-focused	"We wrote a lot to each other, and told how we felt, and promised each other that we would be there."
Emotion-focused	"Because of my anxiety about maybe her being unfaithful, I went and did the same! And I got drunk a lot."
Emotional reactions	
Loneliness	"I missed him, and I felt quite lonely."
Despair	"When I was apart from him, I felt hollow, in pain—insecure inside. I felt physically sick without him."
Perceived effects	
Closer together	"Separation has been quite good for us, in that we've developed into ourselves, while also being able to communicate with each other—so it's brought us closer together."
Ongoing problems	"How these events affected us—well, we're still trying to resolve these problems, about him wanting to spend more time alone—I'm not sure I want to continue the relationship."
Mixed effects	"On my part, after, there was a lot of mistrust, a lot of bitterness. But we are a little more independent, and that has improved the relationship."

into three categories: confrontive coping (active discussion and negotia-tion of the situation with the relationship partner), maintaining contact with the partner (by writing and telephoning), and engaging in activities related to personal or couple goals (together, the latter two themes comprise "planful problem-solving," as reported by Folkman, Lazarus, Dunkel-Schetter, et al., 1986). Emotion-focused coping was also divided into three categories: positive reappraisal, escape–avoidance, and mini-mizing (the latter combines distancing and self-controlling, as reported by Folkman, Lazarus, Dunkel-Schetter, et al., 1986).

For each broad category (support seeking, problem-focused coping, and emotion-focused coping), subjects received a score of 1 if they reported using that strategy; otherwise, a score of zero. Similarly, the fine-grained categories within problem- and emotion-focused coping were scored as 1 (applicable) or zero (not applicable). Interrater reliability (assessed using kappa coefficients) ranged from .58 (positive appraisal) to .90 (escape) for the fine-grained categories, and exceeded .80 for each broad category.

Finally, the number of coping strategies used by each subject was calculated by tallying the different types of strategies (e.g., confrontive, support-seeking) reported; hence, scores could range from 1 to 7. This measure provides information about the variety of coping methods adopted. It is widely recognized that the coping process typically involves a combination of strategies (Folkman & Lazarus, 1985); moreover, because the problem of separation is one over which partners usually have limited control, it is unlikely that any single strategy will be entirely successful in minimizing the negative effects of the problem.

Emotional Reactions

Two broad types of negative emotional reactions emerged from the reports of separation. "Loneliness" was defined by explicit references to feeling "lonely" or "alone," and was reported by 91 subjects; "despair" was defined by references to more extreme negative feelings, such as "depression," "worthlessness," and "pain" (reported by 45 subjects). Subjects received a score of 1 if they reported experiencing the particular reaction, otherwise, a score of zero. Interrater reliability analyses of these categories yielded kappa coefficients of .79 (loneliness) and .88 (despair). Transcripts were also rated for the extent to which subjects reported missing the partner during separation. Scores ranged from 1 ("not at all") to 4 ("a great deal"). Ratings made by the two coders showed adequate interrater reliability ($r = .72$).

Perceived Effects on the Relationship

Comments concerning the effects of the separation were classified into three mutually exclusive categories: The separation was seen as bringing the two partners closer together, as creating ongoing problems, or as having mixed effects. Interrater reliability of this trichotomous variable was high (kappa coefficient = .78). A dichotomous variable was also coded to tap reports of renegotiation of the relationship upon reunion. If such renegotiation was explicitly mentioned, a score of 1 was given; otherwise, zero. A kappa coefficient of .70 indicated adequate interrater reliability.

Results and Discussion

In the following sections, the attachment characteristics of the sample are first described. The focal analyses, relating attachment to reports of separation, are presented next. In these analyses, the attachment dimensions (of both self and partner) were correlated with subjects' reports of responses to separation, separately by gender.

Attachment Characteristics of the Sample

The numbers of males and females endorsing each description of the forced-choice attachment measure were as follows: secure, 38 and 27 respectively; preoccupied, 8 and 16; dismissing, 15 and 10; and fearful, 11 and 19. Thus, almost half of the subjects described themselves as secure, with the remainder spread fairly evenly across the three insecure styles. These results are similar to those reported by other researchers using similar measures (e.g., Scharfe & Bartholomew, 1994). The association between gender and attachment style approached significance, with males tending to endorse the dismissing and secure styles, and females tending to choose the preoccupied and fearful styles. The sex differences in endorsement of the preoccupied and dismissing styles are consistent with those reported by Bartholomew and Horowitz (1991), although it is unusual to find an association between gender and endorsement of the secure style.

The two attachment scales were roughly normally distributed: Scores on Comfort ranged from 12 to 39, with a mean of 27.44, and scores on Anxiety ranged from 5 to 24, with a mean of 11.46. The two scales were negatively intercorrelated, $r = -.20$. The forced-choice attachment measure was related in theoretically meaningful ways to the two attachment scales. Secure subjects reported the highest levels of Comfort, followed by preoccupied, then by dismissing subjects; fearful subjects reported the least Comfort. Preoccupied subjects reported the greatest Anxiety, followed by fearful subjects; both dismissing and secure groups reported relatively low Anxiety.

There was no evidence of partner matching on attachment characteristics. All possible attachment combinations (based on the forced-choice measure) were represented in the sample, and subjects' and partners' responses to the attachment measures were not reliably related. A number of researchers have reported that secure subjects tend to be paired with secure partners, and that anxious–ambivalent individuals tend to be paired with avoidant partners (Collins & Read, 1990; Feeney, 1994; Kirkpatrick & Davis, 1994; Senchak & Leonard, 1992). On the other hand, Hammond and Fletcher (1991) studied couples in long-term dating relationships (a sample similar to the present one), and reported no association between partners' attachment ratings. It is not yet clear why patterns of partner matching vary widely across studies.

Reports of Separation

All subjects in the sample were able to describe an experience of physical separation from the partner. Some subjects described a single episode of separation; these ranged in length from 2 weeks to 12 months. Other subjects described periods of time that involved repeated separations, such as where partners saw each other only once or twice per month. All reported instances of separation arose from changes to one partner's work or living arrangements. Importantly, security of attachment was not confounded with type of separation. Specifically, attachment style was not related to the nature of the separation experience (single episode vs. repeated), or to length of separation.

Strategies for Coping with Separation

All three broad classes of coping strategies were related to own attachment dimensions. Support seeking was associated with attachment security for both males and females ($r = .24$ with males' Comfort, and $r = -.31$ with females' Anxiety). Problem-focused and emotion-focused coping were linked with security of attachment for males only ($r = -.25$ between problem-focused coping and male Anxiety, and $r = -.23$ between emotion-focused coping and male Comfort). With regard to the subdivisions within problem-focused and emotion-focused coping, links with own attachment dimensions were again confined to males: males' Comfort was directly related to their use of confrontive coping ($r = .33$), and inversely related to their use of escape–avoidance ($r = -.24$). Finally, the number of different coping strategies used was inversely related to own Anxiety for both males ($r = -.23$) and females ($r = -.24$).

The coping strategies adopted by male subjects were unrelated to the attachment dimensions of their partners. By contrast, females' reports of emotion-focused coping were positively related to their partners' Anxiety ($r = .29$).

In summary, secure attachment was linked with more constructive patterns of coping with separation. Males high in Comfort were more likely than others to engage in support seeking, and less likely to rely on emotion-focused coping. Females low in Anxiety reported more support seeking; males low in Anxiety reported more problem-focused coping, and their partners reported less emotion-focused coping. Both males and females low in Anxiety reported a greater variety of coping strategies in response to separation. This finding suggests that individuals low in Anxiety are likely to be more adaptable and less adversely affected by the experience of physical separation. More generally, the present results are largely consistent with those of Mikulincer et al. (1993), relating attachment style to responses to environmental threats.

Interestingly, the link between males' attachment security and their coping strategies was strongest for confrontive coping and escape coping. Of the three forms of problem-focused coping assessed in this study, confrontive coping appears to be the most adaptive; certainly it represents the most direct attempt to manage the problem. (In contrast to confrontive coping as defined by Folkman, Lazarus, Dunkel-Schetter, et al., 1986, the instances of this strategy in the present study emphasized open communication, but not hostility or risk taking.) Conversely, of the three forms of emotion-focused coping, escape–avoidance appears to be the most maladaptive; positive appraisal and minimizing involve primarily cognitive approaches to regulating emotion, whereas escape involves destructive behaviors such as reliance on alcohol and drugs. Hence, attachment security seems to be most strongly related to those coping strategies that are clearly constructive or destructive.

Emotional Reactions to Separation

Reports of loneliness were unrelated to attachment dimensions of self and partner, for both genders. By contrast, males' reports of despair were related positively to their own Anxiety ($r = .23$), and negatively to that of their partners ($r = -.28$); females' reports of despair were related positively to their own Anxiety ($r = .29$), and negatively to their own Comfort ($r = -.23$). Males' reports of the extent of "missing the partner" were unrelated to attachment dimensions of self and partner, but females' reports of missing the partner were directly related to males' Comfort ($r = .24$), and inversely related to males' Anxiety ($r = -.28$).

In summary, reports of loneliness in response to separation were unrelated to the attachment dimensions. This null result may reflect the relatively widespread occurrence of feelings of loneliness, with almost two-thirds of the sample reporting these feelings. Further, the extent of "missing the partner" was only weakly related to attachment. The partners of secure males, however, were more likely to endorse such feelings, a tendency that presumably reflects the greater satisfaction and intimacy and the lower ambivalence and conflict in relationships with secure partners. The most consistent finding for emotional responses to separation was that feelings of despair were associated with insecure attachment and, in particular, with Anxiety over relationships.

Effect of Separation on the Relationship

As noted earlier, reports of the effect of separation were classified into three categories: The separation was seen as bringing the partners closer, as creating ongoing problems, or as having mixed effects. Most subjects (80%, $n = 115$) reported that the separation had brought them closer. Because of the small numbers in the remaining categories, these categories were combined. Hence two groups of subjects were formed: those who saw the separation as creating some problems, and those who saw it as bringing only increased closeness.

The link between attachment dimensions and reported effect of separation was analyzed using t-tests. Two tests were performed for each gender, relating the dichotomous measure of "effect of separation" to scores on Comfort and Anxiety. For males, Comfort was associated with reported effect of separation; males who reported problems following separation were lower in Comfort than those who reported no such problems. For females, Anxiety was associated with effect of separation, with females who reported postseparation problems being higher in Anxiety than those who did not.

It is interesting to note that the perceived effect of separation was related to Comfort for males, but to Anxiety for females. These results fit with those of several previous researchers, in pointing to the negative effects of males' lack of comfort with intimacy, and of females' anxiety about basic relationship issues (e.g., Collins & Read, 1990; Kirkpatrick & Davis, 1994). Moreover, "perceived effect on the relationship" is of central importance in studying separation from romantic partners, because this variable is likely to be a marker of how the relationship ultimately fares. Males who are uncomfortable with intimacy may make less active efforts to maintain the relationship with the absent partner, especially given that males are generally not seen as the makers or maintainers of relationships (Surra & Longstreth, 1990). Similarly, females who worry a lot about their partners' feelings toward them may react to periods of separation with greater anxiety, jealousy, and conflict (Feeney et al., 1994); hence, it is not surprising that separation can lead to serious relationship difficulties for these females.

The effect of separation was also considered in terms of whether subjects mentioned having renegotiated the relationship upon reunion. Males' reports of renegotiation were unrelated to the attachment dimensions of self and partner. Females' reports of renegotiation, however, were related directly to own Comfort ($r = .32$) and inversely to own Anxiety ($r = -.29$). The latter result is relevant to the finding that females high in Anxiety reported more negative effects of separation on their relationships. It seems that these females, while likely to experience jealousy and anxiety over separation, may be reluctant to discuss these issues directly with their partners.

TASK 2

The unstructured reports of separation experiences obtained in Task 1 offer important advantages in terms of ecological validity. This approach can be usefully complemented, however, by more experimental methods that allow researchers to standardize the situations to which couples are exposed. Task 2 was designed to achieve this aim.

As mentioned earlier, goal conflicts can be studied using standardized laboratory paradigms. This research employed three such interaction scenes involving explicit conflict of interests between partners, based on the work of Raush, Barry, Hertel, and Swain (1974). Two scenes were "relationship-based," involving issues of psychological distance and closeness. In one of these scenes, the male was instructed to act in a cold and distant manner toward his partner, and the female partner was instructed to reestablish closeness; in the other scene, the roles of the male and female were reversed. The third scene was "issue-based." That is, it involved a concrete issue rather than the relationship itself, allowing for important comparisons with the other scenes. Attachment differences in response to conflict may be widespread, because any form of conflict may raise concerns about the quality and future of the relationship; however, such differences should be more pronounced in situations that focus on the partner's availability and responsiveness.

It is important to note that in the two scenes involving issues of psychological distance and closeness, the focus was on *responses to the partner's distancing behavior,* because the overall aim of this research was to study responses to distancing and separation. To maintain this focus, these scenes were reconceptualized as "self-distant" and "partner-distant" (rather than the original conceptualization of male-distant and female-distant). As the term implies, the self-distant condition includes males in the male-distant scene and females in the female-distant scene; the "partner-distant" condition includes males in the female-distant scene and females in the male-distant scene. By reconceptualizing the scenes in this way, it is possible to focus directly on behavior in response to partners' distancing (i.e., the "partner-distant" condition).

The self-distant scene was clearly essential, as it allowed both males and females to adopt the roles of pursuer and of distancer. Behavior in this scene was not of direct interest, however, and was not expected to show important links with attachment dimensions. The behavior of the partner who is asked to act "distant" serves as the background for the ensuing interaction, in which the pursuer is likely to perceive some threat to the attachment relationship; further, the partner who acts in a distant manner essentially controls the interaction. In fact, in assessing responses to partner distancing, it would be ideal if subjects who were instructed to act distant behaved in a standardized manner, rather than in ways reflecting their own characteristics (such as their attachment style). It was considered important to check this possibility, however, as detailed later.

Hypotheses

Questionnaire Measures

It was expected that secure attachment would be associated with greater relationship satisfaction and with more positive expectations of the partner's behavior and motives. Secure attachment was also expected to be associated with less discomfort in conflict interactions, and with greater satisfaction. However, it was expected that these proposed correlates of security would be most strongly related to attachment in the partner-distant scene.

Behavior in Conflict Interactions

It was expected that secure attachment would be associated with less negative affect in the conflict situations, with more approach and less avoidance behavior, and with constructive conversational patterns. Again, it was expected that these proposed correlates of security would be most strongly related to attachment in the partner-distant scene.

Measures and Procedure

The same couples completed Task 1 and Task 2. The measures for Task 2 were completed on the same day as the verbal reports were obtained, but at a later point. The measures and experimental procedures employed in Task 2 are detailed in the following sections.

Preinteraction Questionnaire

Before taking part in the interaction scenes, couples independently completed a preinteraction questionnaire. This questionnaire included a measure of relationship satisfaction, the Quality Marriage Index (QMI; Norton, 1983). The QMI consists of six items assessing the overall quality of dyadic relationships. Because these items do not describe specific behaviors occurring within the relationship, the measure does not overlap with other variables of interest to this research (e.g., communication). The QMI is highly reliable (Cronbach's alpha for this sample = .91).

The preinteraction questionnaire also informed subjects that they were about to take part in three short interactions that focused on their relationship as a couple and on how they dealt with relationship issues. Subjects were asked to rate their expectations for their partner's behavior and motives in these interactions. For each aspect of expectations (behavior and motives), seven semantic differential scales were employed to tap the evaluative dimension (e.g., for behavior, disagreeable to agreeable, pleasant to unpleasant; for motives, negative to positive, considerate to self-centered). Each scale ranged from 1 to 7, with high scores indicating more favorable expectations. Ratings were summed to yield a total score for expected behavior and one for expected motives, each with a possible range from 7 to 49. These scales showed high internal consistency (.86 and .87, respectively).

Interaction Scenes

Couples then took part in the interaction scenes. As noted earlier, two of the scenes involved issues of psychological distance and closeness. In one scene, the male was instructed to act in a cold and distant manner toward his partner. To facilitate this distancing behavior, the male was first asked to recall an experience in which he had found someone's presence intolerable, and had wanted nothing at all to do with that person. He was then asked to imagine feeling that way about his partner, and to focus on some incident or quality about the partner which would disturb him intensely. The research assistant spent several minutes with the male partner, inducing and reinforcing this mood of coldness and irritability (see Raush et al., 1974, for details). In the same scene, the female partner was instructed to try to reestablish closeness with her partner. The scene began with the male staring out of the window, and the female entering the room. The second scene was the reciprocal of the first, with the female acting distant and the male attempting to reestablish closeness.

The third interaction scene involved goal conflict that was "issue-based," rather than "relationship-based." Because the issue-based scenes employed by Raush et al. were unsuitable for dating couples, a new scene was devised in which partners discussed leisure activities. In this ("leisure") scene, a conflict of interests was established by asking each partner to advocate pursuing a different leisure activity, to be undertaken during a period of time that the couple had already agreed to spend together.

The three scenes were counterbalanced to minimize order effects. For each scene, the research assistant established the goal conflict by talking to the relationship partners separately, and priming each partner to pursue his or her particular goal throughout the coming interaction. Each interaction was videotaped for 5 minutes.

Postinteraction Questionnaire

Immediately after each scene, the partners were taken to separate rooms to complete a brief postinteraction questionnaire. Subjects used 7-point Likert scales to rate three aspects of the interaction: how typical it was of the couple's usual interactions (based on a single rating), how much discomfort they had experienced (summed across ratings of "how comfortable" [reversed] and "how upsetting"), and how satisfied they were with the interaction (summed across ratings of "satisfaction with outcome" and "satisfaction with process"). Both scales formed by summing Likert ratings were highly reliable, with alpha coefficients exceeding .80. After completing the postinteraction questionnaire, subjects were debriefed about the nature and purpose of the study. They were told that if the session had raised issues concerning their relationship, these could be discussed with the researcher.

Observer Ratings

An independent observer rated three aspects of behavior in the interaction scenes: affect, nonverbal behavior, and conversational patterns. For all of these measures except conversational patterns (described later in this chapter), interrater reliability was established by having a second coder rate a sample of 30 videotapes.

Global ratings of affect were made for each partner in each interaction, using 7-point scales. Five emotions were rated: anger, anxiety, sadness, disgust, and happiness. Because attachment theory emphasizes the link between attachment and negative affect, the main focus was on ratings of negative affect (anger, anxiety, sadness, and disgust). Although the number and nature of discrete emotions is the subject of debate, theoretical and empirical work support the inclusion of anger, anxiety (or fear), sadness, and disgust among the basic negative emotions (Chance, 1980). Happiness was assessed to check whether any observed link between insecure attachment and negative affect might simply reflect the tendency of insecure subjects to display greater levels of *all* types of affect. Correlations assessing interrater reliability of the affect ratings ranged from .69 (sadness) to .90 (happiness).

Fifteen nonverbal behaviors related to approach and avoidance tendencies were recorded, based on the work of Simpson et al. (1992): touching partner's body, touching partner's face, placing arm or hand on partner's shoulder, hugging, kissing, holding hands, resisting contact, leaning toward partner, moving toward partner, turning head or body toward partner, leaning away from partner, moving away from partner, turning head or body away from partner, smiling, and eye contact. To maximize objectivity, most of these behaviors were recorded using frequency counts (i.e., the number of discrete occurrences of each behavior in each scene). However, three behaviors (turning toward partner, turning away from partner, and eye contact) were recorded using global rating scales ranging from 1 to 6. Global ratings were more appropriate for assessing these behaviors: Some subjects, for example, gazed almost continuously at their partners, and the low score for eye contact which would result from a count of discrete occurrences would not reflect the extent of the behavior. Correlations assessing interrater reliability ranged from .79 (moving toward partner) to .97 (touching partner's face). Behaviors recorded using frequency counts were later recoded as 6-point scales, based on their frequency distributions; this recoding made these behaviors comparable in scale with those initially recorded as global ratings.

Conversational patterns were coded using the six-category system developed by Raush et al. (1974): cognitive, resolution of conflict, interpersonal reconciliation, appeals, rejection, and coercion (see Table 8.2 for definitions and examples). This coding system was considered the most appropriate because it was derived from the specific conflict interactions in which the couples engaged. Each conversational turn was first coded into one of the 36 "action categories" detailed by Raush et al. (1974). Because of the fine discriminations required in this coding task, two coders worked together to achieve consensus coding. In a minority of instances, a single conversational turn involved elements of more than one conversational category; in these cases, the dominant theme in the turn was used to define the category. Following consensus coding, the 36 discrete categories were "lumped" into the six major groups (see Raush et al., 1974). For each scene, subjects were given scores on the six categories, derived by summing the number of turns coded in each category.

Results and Discussion

The focal analyses (linking attachment with responses to conflict) involved correlating the two attachment dimensions with ratings by participants and observers, separately by gender. For participants' (questionnaire) ratings, correlations were calculated with both own and partners' attachment dimensions. For observers' ratings, correlations were calculated with own attachment dimensions only. This decision was made for two interrelated reasons: First, the large number of dependent variables made it important to limit the number of statistical tests, and second, the central focus was on the link between own attachment dimensions and responses to the partner's "primed" distancing behavior. As discussed earlier, the distancing behavior was elicited by specific instructions from the researcher, and was not of direct interest. However, because this behavior may have been influenced by characteristics of the individual (such as his or her attachment style), additional analyses addressed the possibility that any links between own security of attachment and responses to partner's distancing could be explained in terms of the behavior of the distancer.

Preinteraction Questionnaire

For the measure of *relationship satisfaction* (QMI), individuals' scores ranged from 10 to 42. Scores were generally high, with a mean of 37.42 (a

TABLE 8.2. Definitions and Examples of Six Conversational Patterns (Task 2)

Category	Definition	Examples
Cognitive	Neutral acts; suggestions; rational arguments	"I'll phone them and see if they can come over another time." "I'm using that as an example of what might happen."
Resolution of conflict	Attempts to defuse conflict; accepting other's plans, feelings; compromising, collaborating	"I think we should make a special effort to spend more time together." "We should talk about the problem and hopefully we can sort it out."
Interpersonal reconciliation	Apportioning responsibility; showing concern for other's feelings; seeking or offering reassurance	"That's my insensitivity coming out there." "I need you to tell me how you feel about me now."
Appeals	Appealing to fairness, to love or to other's motives; pleading, coaxing	"I don't think that would be fair to either of us." "Can't you give me a little bit of attention once in a while?"
Rejection	Leaving the field; challenging other's move as a strategy; personal rejection of other	"Stop it—I'm disgusted! I don't want to hear it." "I just don't want to be around you right now."
Coercion	Commanding, demanding; disparaging or threatening other; inducing guilt	"You think you're just perfect." "You'd better stop acting like that, or I won't want to be with you."

typical finding in samples of dating and married couples). For both genders, QMI scores were linked with Comfort of both self and partner (r's ranged from .32 to .42). Although all correlations between the QMI and Anxiety were negative, they were not statistically significant.

Correlations were also calculated between attachment dimensions and *expectations of partner's behavior and motives* in the conflict interactions. These correlations were calculated separately by gender, by attachment dimension (Comfort, Anxiety), by individual (self/partner), and by dependent variable (behavior, motives), giving a total of 16 correlations. Four of these were significant: males' expectations of their partner's motives were inversely related to their own Anxiety ($r = -.25$) and directly related to their partner's Comfort ($r = .27$), and females' expectations of their partner's behavior and motives were both directly related to their own Comfort ($r = .35$ and $r = .23$, respectively). The strongest finding in this set of results is that own security of attachment is associated with more favorable expectations of partners. It is important to note that when subjects were asked to rate their partners' behavior and motives, they knew very little about the nature of the forthcoming interactions. Hence, it appears that secure attachment is linked with generalized expectations of relationship partners.

Postinteraction Questionnaire

Before turning to the focal analyses, it is important to consider subjects' perceptions of the *typicality* of the conflict interactions. The overall mean rating was 3.53 (1 = not at all typical; 7 = completely typical), suggesting that subjects generally perceived the interactions as reasonably typical of behavior occurring within their relationships. The leisure scene was rated as more typical (*M* = 4.57) than either the self-distant or partner-distant scenes (*M* = 3.02 and *M* = 2.98, respectively). There were very few reliable links between ratings of typicality and attachment dimensions. Females' Anxiety, however, was associated with higher typicality ratings for the leisure and the partner-distant scenes (*r* = .24 and *r* = .23, respectively). These correlations are consistent with previous research, in pointing to the link between females' Anxiety and high levels of relationship conflict. It is not surprising that this finding did not extend to the self-distant scene; the behavior of females high in Anxiety would be expected to be typified by proximity seeking and dependence, rather than by distancing.

Ratings of *discomfort* (which could range from 2 to 14) were greatest for the partner-distant scene (*M* = 7.81) and least for the leisure scene (*M* = 4.41). To obtain a broad look at the link between attachment dimensions and discomfort in the interactions, discomfort ratings were first averaged over the three scenes. Correlations with these averaged ratings were calculated separately by gender, by attachment dimension (Comfort, Anxiety), and by individual (self/partner). Three of the eight correlations were significant. Specifically, males' discomfort was associated directly with males' Anxiety (*r* = .34) and inversely with females' Comfort (*r* = −.24); females' discomfort was associated directly with females' Anxiety (*r* = .28). Hence, for both genders, own Anxiety was linked with greater reported discomfort. More fine-grained analyses showed that this link between own Anxiety and discomfort applied to the leisure scene and to the partner-distant scene, but not to the self-distant scene.

Mean ratings of *satisfaction* (which could also range from 2 to 14) were greater for the leisure scene (*M* = 10.18) than for either the self-distant or partner-distant scenes (*M* = 8.08 and *M* = 7.97, respectively). Again, a broad look at the link between attachment dimensions and satisfaction was first obtained by averaging ratings of satisfaction over the three scenes, and correlating these averaged ratings with the attachment dimensions. Four of the eight correlations were significant. Males' satisfaction was associated directly with males' Comfort ($r = .26$) and inversely with males' Anxiety ($r = -.29$); females' satisfaction was associated inversely with both females' and males' Anxiety ($r = -.24$ and $r = -.34$, respectively). Hence, as for discomfort, the most consistent link was with own Anxiety, which was related to less satisfaction with the conflict interactions. More fine-grained analysis indicated, once again, that the correlations between attachment and satisfaction applied only to the leisure scene and the partner-distant scene.

As noted earlier, the attachment dimensions were associated with relationship satisfaction (but not with relationship length). Hence, the greater satisfaction with conflict interactions reported by secure individuals might simply reflect the higher levels of general satisfaction within these relationships. To check this possibility, the correlational analyses reported in this section were repeated, with relationship satisfaction partialed out. The link between males' Comfort and their satisfaction with the conflict interactions was no longer significant, but all three correlations with the Anxiety dimension remained reliable. Thus, the effects of anxious attachment on satisfaction with conflict interactions cannot be attributed to more global differences in relationship satisfaction.

Observer Ratings: Preliminary Analyses

In the focal analyses, discussed in the next section, the attachment dimensions were correlated with observer ratings of affect, nonverbal behavior, and conversation. Prior to these analyses, factor analyses were performed on the affect ratings and on the ratings of nonverbal behavior, for the purpose of data reduction. In each case, the principal components method was used.

As noted earlier, the present research focused primarily on negative affect (anger, anxiety, sadness, disgust). Happiness was measured to check whether any links between attachment and negative affect might be explained in terms of general affective expression; happiness ratings were not strongly correlated with the other ratings of affect, however, and were not included in the factor analysis of affect measures. Factor analysis of the four ratings of negative affect revealed two major factors, accounting for 80% of the variance. The first factor was defined by fear and sadness (with factor loadings of .85 and .92, respectively); the second was defined by anger and disgust (with factor loadings of .81 and .89, respectively). These two factors were labeled Worry and Hostility, respectively. Scores were obtained for each factor by summing the relevant ratings of affect.

Factor analysis of the ratings of nonverbal behavior also revealed two major factors, accounting for 32% of the variance. The first factor, labeled "touch," was defined by five behaviors: touching partner's body, touching partner's arm, touching partner's face, hugging, and kissing. The second factor was a bipolar factor marked by positive factor loadings on turning away, moving away, and leaning away from partner, and by negative loadings on eye contact and moving toward partner; this factor was labeled "avoidance." Scores on the factors of touch and avoidance were derived by summing the ratings on the relevant nonverbal behaviors (using the 6-point scales).

Observer Ratings: Correlations with Attachment Dimensions

Overview. As outlined earlier, the leisure scene was included in order to assess behavior in response to a concrete conflict issue; compared to issues of distance and closeness, concrete issues may not be seen as so threatening to the future of the relationship. In the self-distant scene, it was expected that the primed "distancing" behavior would be largely unrelated to attachment dimensions, but it was considered important to check this expectation. The main focus was on behavior in the *partner-distant* scene, in which subjects responded to the cold and distant behavior shown by their partners. In this section, the three scenes are discussed in that order (leisure, self-distant, partner-distant); correlations between attachment dimensions and the three types of observer data (affect, nonverbal behavior, and conversation ratings) are presented within each scene.

The ratings of happiness, which were included as a control measure, were not reliably related to attachment dimensions for either gender in any conflict scene; these ratings are not discussed further. Hence for each scene, the focal analyses involved a total of 40 correlations; for males and females separately, each attachment dimension was correlated with each of the 10 dependent variables (two affect factors, two nonverbal factors, and six conversation ratings).

Leisure Scene. In this scene, only one significant correlation was obtained. This correlation will not be discussed further; given the number of statistical tests performed, it is likely to have occurred by chance.

Self-Distant Scene. Four of the 40 correlations in this set were significant. Three of these correlations involved measures of conversational behavior: For males, both Comfort and Anxiety were positively associated with verbal appeals ($r = .25$ and $r = .27$, respectively), and for females, Comfort was positively associated with interpersonal reconciliation ($r = .26$).[1] The remaining significant correlation involved

nonverbal behavior, with males high in Comfort showing less avoidance
($r = -.24$).

It is important to acknowledge that the number of significant correlations in this set was slightly greater than expected by chance, suggesting
the possibility that own attachment dimensions may be confounded with
behavior as "distancer." In other words, there is weak evidence that secure
subjects, when instructed to act in a cold and distant manner toward their
partners, may show somewhat less negativity, verbally and/or nonver-
bally. At the same time, any confounding between attachment dimensions
and behavior as "distancer" is clearly weak, especially given that no
significant correlation accounted for more than 8% of the variance in the
particular measure of behavior.

Partner-Distant Scene. Of the 40 correlations in this set, 11 were
statistically significant. These results are detailed in Table 8.3. Both the
Comfort and Anxiety dimensions of attachment were related to observers'
ratings, although the associations were specific to gender and to the
particular dependent variable. Males' Comfort was associated with more
touching and less avoidant nonverbal behavior, and with less verbal
rejection and more interpersonal reconciliation. Males' Anxiety was
associated with more coercion and less resolution of conflict. For females,
Comfort was associated with less negative affect (both Worry and
Hostility), and with more cognitive statements; Anxiety was associated
with less touching and more avoidant nonverbal behavior. Note that the

TABLE 8.3. Significant Correlations between Own Attachment and Responses
to Partners' Distancing Behavior (Task 2)

Focal variables	Simple r	Partial r, controlling for corresponding partner behaviors
	Males	
Comfort—touch	.23*	.18
Comfort—avoidance	−.30**	−.27*
Comfort—rejection	−.24*	−.37**
Comfort—reconciliation	.24*	.23*
Anxiety—coercion	.38***	.33**
Anxiety—resolution	−.46***	−.43***
	Females	
Comfort—hostile affect	−.23*	−.25*
Comfort—worried affect	−.30**	−.16
Comfort—cognitive	.24*	.23*
Anxiety—touch	−.23*	−.23*
Anxiety—avoidance	.38***	.36**

*$p < .05$; **$p < .01$; ***$p < .001$.

number of significant correlations in this set is considerably greater than that expected by chance. Further, in contrast to the previous set, several of these correlations were significant at well beyond the .05 level, with the attachment dimensions accounting for up to 22% of the variance in the dependent variables.[2]

In order to assess whether the 11 significant correlations could be attributed to systematic differences in partner characteristics, the correlational analyses were repeated twice, controlling for two different sets of variables. First, partners' attachment characteristics (i.e., Comfort and Anxiety) were partialed out. Second, partners' behavior as distancer was partialed out, using observers' ratings. For example, in exploring the link between *own attachment* and *own affect* in the partner-distant scene, the two ratings of *partner affect* were controlled. Similarly, in exploring the link between own attachment and own nonverbal behavior, the two ratings of partner's nonverbal behavior were controlled, and so on.

Controlling for partners' attachment characteristics did not substantially alter any of the significant correlations (hence these results are not tabulated). Controlling for partners' observer-rated behaviors also made little difference to the results, although 2 of the 11 partial correlations failed to reach significance (see final column of Table 8.3). These analyses suggest that the link between own security of attachment and more positive responses to partners' distancing cannot be attributed simply to differences in partner behavior. This potential confound cannot be ruled out completely, however, given that it is impossible to control for all aspects of partner behavior.

The links between own security of attachment and more positive responses to partners' distancing showed some interesting patterns (again, see Table 8.3). For males, high Comfort was associated with positive nonverbal responses to distancing (more touching, less avoidance), and both high Comfort and low Anxiety were associated with constructive patterns of verbal behavior. Note that for males, attachment was not related to ratings of affect in response to partner's distancing. This result might stem from a "floor" effect in the measures of male affect, given previous evidence of greater emotional expressivity on the part of females (Noller, 1993). Post hoc analyses of the present data confirmed that females displayed more affect than males, particularly in the partner-distant scene; mean ratings of negative affect in this scene were around 1.8 for males, and 2.3 for females. Hence, any link between males' security of attachment and negative affect may have been obscured by the low means and reduced variability on ratings of affect.

For females, links between own attachment and responses to distancing occurred for all three sets of dependent measures, although the findings for verbal behavior were weak. The most consistent findings were that females' Comfort was associated with less negative affect (both worry and hostility), and that females' Anxiety was associated with negative nonverbal responses (less touching, more avoidance).

The gender differences in these results are worth noting. Females' lack of Comfort with closeness was linked with high levels of negative affect; by contrast, males' lack of Comfort with closeness was reflected in verbal and nonverbal behaviors. Females' Anxiety about relationships was linked with nonverbal behavior, whereas males' Anxiety about relationships was reflected verbally. It has already been suggested that the overall low levels of male affect may be responsible for the gender difference in results for affect. Reasons for the other gender differences are less clear, but sex-role socialization may be involved. For example, consider the case of individuals who are high in Anxiety, and who are thus likely to be particularly distressed by partners' discouraging of proximity. Males high in Anxiety may show such distress via attacking and self-centered verbalizations, because overt displays of negativity and aggression tend to be seen as more acceptable from men than from women. Anxious females, on the other hand, may try (either consciously or otherwise) to avoid overt displays of negativity, but may manifest their distress through gestures and facial expressions. Of course, further research is required to replicate these results.

Participants' and Observers' Perspectives Compared

As noted earlier, observers' ratings supported the link between attachment security and constructive approaches to conflict resolution, *when the partner acted distant.* In the self-distant scene, in which the subject tended to be in control of the interaction, there were fewer links between attachment dimensions and observer ratings of behavior. Further, in the leisure scene, there were virtually no reliable links between attachment dimensions and observer ratings of behavior. In other words, observable attachment differences were much more marked for the scene in which the partner seemed to be threatening the future of the relationship.

Participants' ratings (from the questionnaires) indicated that prior to the conflict interactions, when only vague information about the impending tasks had been provided, secure individuals (and those with secure partners) held more favorable expectations of their partners than did insecure individuals. Furthermore, secure individuals reported less discomfort and greater satisfaction with the interactions. This finding held for both the concrete (leisure) scene, and for the partner-distant scene. In other words, participants' ratings provided little evidence that attachment differences might become more pronounced under conditions of greater stress.

In summary, the proposition that attachment differences are stronger under conditions of greater stress received considerable support from observers' ratings, but not from participants' ratings. It appears that, for participants themselves, attachment security is associated with fairly global, positive perceptions of the partner and the relationship. These perceptions may be driven primarily by general mental models of others, or by experiences specific to the relationship; in either case, these perceptions appear to have pervasive effects. This proposition is supported by the fact that, in the absence of specific information concerning the forthcoming interactions, secure couples held more favorable expectations of their partner's motives than insecure couples.

GENERAL DISCUSSION

The two tasks reported here clarify the implications of attachment for the experience of physical and emotional separation from relationship partners. The open-ended reports of physical separation provided in Task 1 showed that secure subjects were less likely to respond to physical separation with feelings of insecurity. In addition, they were more likely to use a variety of coping strategies in dealing with the separation, and to try to confront the problem directly by negotiating with the partner. Secure subjects also reported more favorable relationship outcomes following periods of physical separation: They tended to recognize the need to renegotiate the relationship, and were more likely than insecure subjects to report that physical separation actually brought the relationship partners closer together. These results support the perspective outlined by Mikulincer and Florian (Chapter 6, this volume), in which secure attachment is seen as a resilience factor that fosters constructive responses to distress.

Task 2 explored the link between attachment and experiences of distancing (or emotional separation). The overall pattern of results supports what may appear, superficially, to be two contradictory views of adult attachment. On the one hand, to outside observers, attachment differences in behavior are more pronounced in situations in which the relationship itself seems to be under threat. In other words, attachment differences cannot be fully described without referring to the nature of the situation. On the other hand, for the attached individual, security exerts pervasive effects on perceptions of the relationship across a range of variables and conflict situations. It seems that both of these views of adult attachment have credence, and that which view is empirically supported depends largely on the nature of the tasks and measures employed by the researcher.

A comparison of the present results with those of previous researchers suggests that not all stressful situations are similar in their effects on attachment behavior. First, note that insecure attachment was associated with greater negative affect in both tasks described in this chapter. This finding contrasts with that of Simpson et al. (1992), who used a laboratory-based stress-induction paradigm, but is consistent with the work of Mikulincer et al. (1993) on responses to missile attacks, and Rholes, Simpson, and Grich Stevens (Chapter 7, this volume) on couple conflict. It is not surprising that situations which are extremely stressful, or which threaten the relationship itself, elicit greater anxiety in insecure individuals. This finding supports the proposition that insecure individuals tend to appraise life stressors as more threatening and less controllable (Mikulincer & Florian, Chapter 6, this volume).

Second, note that both of the major attachment dimensions (Comfort and Anxiety) were associated with behavior in response to distancing and separation. Again, this finding contrasts with that of Simpson et al. (1992), who found no links between Anxiety and responses to the stress-induction paradigm. However, the present finding is similar to that reported by Rholes et al. (Chapter 7, this volume) for couple conflict. There seems little doubt that relationship conflict is a salient issue for those individuals who are highly anxious about their relationships, particularly when questions of distance and separation are at stake.

The present findings emphasize the importance of considering gender differences when studying the activation of attachment behavior. Together with the findings reported by Rholes et al. (Chapter 7, this volume), these results suggest that there are important gender differences in the link between attachment dimensions and responses to stress. These differences are only poorly understood at this stage, however, and require clarification by future studies employing comprehensive sets of measures of affect and behavior.

The present results extend those of Cafferty et al. (1994), who focused on attachment as a predictor of reunion responses following separation. Specifically, it appears that attachment differences can also be observed in responses to the experience of separation itself. Further, it seems that even relatively brief instances of separation from romantic partners can elicit attachment concerns, especially when partners have not made a clear commitment to the future of the relationship. In fact, the open-ended reports of Task 1 suggest that physical separation may bring to a head unresolved issues within the individual, and also within the relationship. This situation is clearly illustrated in the following extract, in which a preoccupied female describes her experience of being separated from her dismissing partner.

> I felt physically sick without him. I kept repeating "God loves me, and he loves me," every time the pain came on. How did he react? I don't know. I have this feeling that all the things I went through are not mutual. I don't think he cares about me the same way as I do for him. We haven't had a chance to get closer in our relationship—something is keeping us back, although in my heart I want to get closer. I guess

it's mainly the fact that we both don't want to get hurt. And we don't express our feelings very well. Well, he doesn't, and I don't want to tell him. The reason why I don't tell him is I'm afraid that if I do, we'll get closer—although I do want to get closer.

An important direction for future research is to replicate these tasks with larger samples. Longitudinal studies are also needed, both to overcome the problems inherent in retrospective reports, and to compare the links between attachment and responses to stress and conflict across the course of relationships. These issues are clearly important; it seems that insecure individuals are most likely to behave in counterproductive ways when their relationships are threatened by stress or conflict, but it is at these very times that relationships are most vulnerable.

NOTES

1. The finding that verbal appeals were more common among males high in Comfort *and* males high in Anxiety is difficult to interpret, given that Comfort is an index of security, whereas Anxiety is an index of insecurity. This finding may reflect the complex nature of the "appeals" category, which includes both straightforward appeals to fairness, and more plaintive approaches.

2. Even using Bonferroni adjustment, resulting in an extremely conservative alpha rate of .001, most of the correlations with the Anxiety scale remained significant.

REFERENCES

Bartholomew, K. (1990). Avoidance of intimacy: An attachment perspective. *Journal of Social and Personal Relationships, 7*, 147–178.

Bartholomew, K., & Horowitz, L. M. (1991). Attachment styles among young adults: A test of a four-category model. *Journal of Personality and Social Psychology, 61*, 226–244.

Bowlby, J. (1969). *Attachment and loss: Vol. 1. Attachment.* New York: Basic Books.

Bowlby, J. (1973). *Attachment and loss: Vol. 2. Separation: Anxiety and anger.* New York: Basic Books.

Bowlby, J. (1980). *Attachment and loss: Vol. 3. Loss.* New York: Basic Books.

Cafferty, T. P., Davis, K. E., Medway, F. J., O'Hearn, R. E., & Chappell, K. D. (1994). Reunion dynamics among couples separated during Operation Desert Storm: An attachment theory analysis. In K. Bartholomew & D. Perlman (Eds.), *Advances in personal relationships* (Vol. 5, pp. 309–330). London: Jessica Kingsley.

Chance, M. R. A. (1980). An ethological assessment of emotion. In R. Plutchik & H. Kellerman (Eds.), *Emotion: Theory, research, and experience* (pp. 81–111). New York: Academic Press.

Collins, N. L., & Read, S. J. (1990). Adult attachment, working models, and relationship quality in dating couples. *Journal of Personality and Social Psychology, 58,* 644–663.

Feeney, J. A. (1994). Attachment style, communication patterns and satisfaction across the life cycle of marriage. *Personal Relationships, 1,* 333–348.

Feeney, J. A., & Noller, P. (1991). Attachment style and verbal descriptions of romantic partners. *Journal of Social and Personal Relationships, 8,* 187–215.

Feeney, J. A., Noller, P., & Callan, V. J. (1994). Attachment style, communication and satisfaction in the early years of marriage. In K. Bartholomew & D. Perlman (Eds.), *Advances in personal relationships* (Vol. 5, pp. 269–308). London: Jessica Kingsley.

Fitzpatrick, M. A., Fey, J., Segrin, C., & Schiff, J. L. (1993). Internal working models of relationships and marital communication. *Journal of Language and Social Psychology, 12,* 103–131.

Folkman, S., & Lazarus, R. S. (1985). If it changes it must be a process: Study of emotion and coping during three stages of a college examination. *Journal of Personality and Social Psychology, 48,* 150–170.

Folkman, S., Lazarus, R. S., Dunkel-Schetter, C., DeLongis, A., & Gruen, R. J. (1986). Dynamics of a stressful encounter: Cognitive appraisal, coping, and encounter outcomes. *Journal of Personality and Social Psychology, 50,* 992–1003.

Folkman, S., Lazarus, R. S., Gruen, R. J., & DeLongis, A. (1986). Appraisal, coping, health status, and psychological symptoms. *Journal of Personality and Social Psychology, 50,* 571–579.

Hammond, J. R., & Fletcher, G. J. O. (1991). Attachment styles and relationship satisfaction in the development of close relationships. *New Zealand Journal of Psychology, 20,* 56–62.

Hazan, C., & Shaver, P. (1987). Romantic love conceptualized as an attachment process. *Journal of Personality and Social Psychology, 52,* 511–524.

Kirkpatrick, L. A., & Davis, K. E. (1994). Attachment style, gender, and relationship stability: A longitudinal analysis. *Journal of Personality and Social Psychology, 66,* 502–512.

Kobak, R. R., & Duemmler, S. (1994). Attachment and conversation: Toward a discourse analysis of adolescent and adult security. In K. Bartholomew & D. Perlman (Eds.), *Advances in personal relationships* (Vol. 5, pp. 121–149). London: Jessica Kingsley.

Kobak, R. R., & Sceery, A. (1988). Attachment in late adolescence: Working models, affect regulation, and representations of self and others. *Child Development, 59,* 135–146.

Lolas, F. (1986). Behavioral text and psychological context: On pragmatic verbal behavior analysis. In L. A. Gottschalk, F. Lolas, & L. L. Viney (Eds.), *Content analysis of verbal behavior* (pp. 11–28). Berlin: Springer-Verlag.

Mikulincer, M., Florian, V., & Tolmacz, R. (1990). Attachment styles and fear of personal death: A case study of affect regulation. *Journal of Personality and Social Psychology, 58,* 273–280.

Mikulincer, M., Florian, V., & Weller, A. (1993). Attachment styles, coping strategies, and posttraumatic psychological distress: The impact of the Gulf War in Israel. *Journal of Personality and Social Psychology, 64,* 817–826.

Noller, P. (1993). Gender and emotional communication in marriage: Different cultures or differential social power? *Journal of Language and Social Psychology, 12,* 132–152.

Norton, R. (1983). Measuring marital quality: A critical look at the dependent variable. *Journal of Marriage and the Family, 45,* 141–151.

Raush, H. L., Barry, W. A., Hertel, R. K., & Swain, M. A. (1974). *Communication, conflict and marriage.* San Francisco, CA: Jossey-Bass.

Scharfe, E., & Bartholomew, K. (1994). Reliability and stability of adult attachment patterns. *Personal Relationships, 1,* 23–43.

Senchak, M., & Leonard, K. E. (1992). Attachment styles and marital adjustment among newlywed couples. *Journal of Social and Personal Relationships, 9,* 51–64.

Shaver, P. R., & Hazan, C. (1993). Adult romantic attachment: Theory and evidence. In D. Perlman & W. Jones (Eds.), *Advances in personal relationships: Vol. 4. Adult attachment relationships* (pp. 29–70). London: Jessica Kingsley.

Simpson, J. A., Rholes, W. S., & Nelligan, J. S. (1992). Support seeking and support giving within couples in an anxiety-provoking situation: The role of attachment styles. *Journal of Personality and Social Psychology, 62,* 434–446.

Sroufe, L. A., & Waters, E. (1977). Attachment as an organizational construct. *Child Development, 48,* 1184–1199.

Surra, C. A., & Longstreth, M. (1990). Similarity of outcomes, interdependence, and conflict in dating relationships. *Journal of Personality and Social Psychology, 59,* 501–516.

PART IV
Clinical Applications

9

The Role of Attachment in Therapeutic Relationships

MARY DOZIER
CHRISTINE TYRRELL

Bowlby (1988) suggested that the most fundamental therapeutic change involves revisions to clients' internal working models of attachment. According to attachment theory, the client has developed internal working models of others that affect expectations of, and behaviors toward, others. For the client to reformulate working models, these models must be examined and modified through psychological and behavioral exploration. In therapy, the client is encouraged to explore expectations of the therapist, expectations of significant others, and memories of earlier attachment figures. Through this process of exploration, working models of the self and other are challenged, and presumably modified.

Suggesting that working models of attachment are central to the treatment of relationships is far from a new idea. Only recently, however, have attachment researchers begun to make necessary empirical connections, connections that we will explore in this chapter. Attachment researchers' attention to the development of sound methodology for assessing internal working models of attachment (Main & Goldwyn, in press) and for assessing attachment to romantic partners (Hazan & Shaver, 1987) has been key to the surge in research activity in this area. Research using these methodologies suggests that working models affect how people interact with others generally (Kobak & Sceery, 1988) and with their therapists more specifically (Dozier, 1990; Dozier, Cue, & Barnett, 1994; Korfmacher, Adam, Ogawa, & Egeland, in press). In this chapter, we review the various approaches used to conceptualize and assess attachment in adulthood, including both self-report and interview methodologies. We provide an overview of empirical findings that relate working models to self-presentation and interpersonal behaviors, and consider the particular effects of differential attachment strategies.

A MODEL OF THERAPEUTIC CHANGE

From an attachment theory perspective, the therapist's work with a client is similar to, yet more difficult than, the mother's with her infant. In either case, a primary task is to provide a secure base that promotes safe exploration. The mother's task is easier than the therapist's because she need not compensate for the failures of other attachment figures. The infant's expectations of the mother originate out of his or her own experiences of the mother's availability. The task of therapy is often made more difficult because of the client's previous experiences with unavailable or rejecting caregivers. Clients' working models frequently lead to expectations that are rigid and inconsistent with reality, as when an available, empathic therapist is perceived as judgmental and rejecting. The client must rework the model so as to be able to establish the therapist as a secure base. Thus, exploration of prior working models cannot wait until after a secure base is established; rather, the processes occur in tandem. According to Bowlby (1988), the client's exploration of his or her model of the therapist is a critical task of therapy.

A second therapeutic task indicated by Bowlby is exploration of current interpersonal relationships. This aspect of therapy focuses on such issues as how the client chose particular relationship partners, feelings toward and thoughts about significant others, and interpersonal behaviors. The therapist helps the client explore how current feelings, thoughts, and behaviors relate to earlier experiences with attachment figures. The exploration of working models of earlier attachment figures and attachment experiences is a third therapy task. Memories and conceptualizations of earlier attachment experiences are recalled and explored with the therapist's help, and the client is encouraged to examine how previous conceptualizations have affected current functioning. The client is gently helped to explore and rework these models of attachment figures.

Our conceptualization of the therapeutic change process is presented in Figure 9.1. We suggest that change in the client's working model of the therapist, of attachment figures, and of specific others in his or her world are prerequisites to more fundamental change in working models of the generalized self and other. The client enters therapy with expectations of

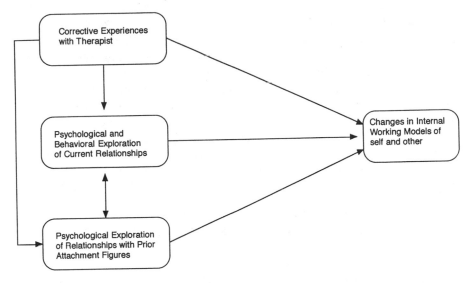

FIGURE 9.1. Our model of therapeutic change.

the therapist that are based at least partly on previous experiences with caregivers. As the therapist behaves in ways that call the model into question, the client gradually explores alternative models. At the same time, the therapist encourages the client to explore different approaches to significant others, at both psychological and behavioral levels. This exploration of interpersonal relationships is facilitated by the client's having experienced some success in developing a more accurate and positive working model of the therapist. The therapist helps the client explore how relationships with attachment figures affect current approaches to the therapist and to significant others. Bowlby (1988) emphasized the need to intervene in each of these areas to promote maximum exploration. We expect that, when treatment is directed toward one aspect of the model, change may be specific to that component. For example, if therapy focused very specifically on changing the client's behavioral approaches to significant others, relatively little change in working models of attachment figures would be expected. Conversely, if the intervention focused on relationships with attachment figures, relatively little change in behavioral strategies in current relationships would be expected. At least one outcome study supports this specificity hypothesis (Foa, Rothbaum, Riggs, & Murdock, 1991).

These experiences of more openly and fully exploring relationships with the therapist, attachment figures, and significant others provide fertile ground for the exploration of working models of the self and other more generally. We propose that these generalized models of self and other are the last to change, however. This conceptualization of change has at least some indirect empirical support. For example, Pearson, Cohn, Cowan, and Cowan (1994) found that women who had apparently revised their working models of attachment figures were behaviorally responsive and attentive to their infants, but their generalized models of self and other remained negative. Thus, fundamental change to generalized models is probably a long process, which may not be affected by time-limited psychotherapies. Target and Fonagy (1994) found that children with serious emotional disorders showed greater improvement as treatment length and intensity increased, suggesting that long-term intensive therapy may be required to effect more fundamental change.

ATTACHMENT IN ADULTHOOD: ALTERNATIVE CONCEPTUALIZATIONS

Many researchers and theoreticians have contributed to the study of adult attachment in recent years. This interdisciplinary approach to attachment in adulthood has led to the development of many different conceptualizations of this construct, as well as to the development of a variety of assessment methods. Although a number of authors have attempted to review these different approaches to adult attachment (Berman & Sperling, 1994; Fishler, Sperling, & Carr, 1990), there is a continued need for more specificity and clarity in defining these various approaches. Before discussing research that relates attachment in adulthood to clinical intervention, we attempt to address a few key considerations about the definition and measurement of adult attachment as a construct.

Main, Kaplan, and Cassidy (1985) proposed that the working model of attachment is "a set of conscious and/or unconscious rules for the organization of information relevant to attachment and for obtaining or limiting access to that information" (p. 66). Thus, central to this definition are unconscious rules, including but not limited to defensive exclusion of information from awareness. Because of the role that unconscious rules and defensive exclusion are thought to play, this conceptualization of adult attachment does not lend itself to assessment through self-report. Rather, as described later, working models are assessed through discourse analysis of subjects' discussion of their early attachment relationships. The analysis considers the role of unconscious processes in the recall and manipulation of attachment-related information.

Hazan and Shaver (1987) hypothesized that adults' romantic love can be conceptualized as an attachment process, and proposed the concept of attachment styles in adulthood. Attachment style is assumed to be accessible to conscious awareness, thus allowing assessment through self-report. Hazan and Shaver conceptualize adult attachment style in a way suggested to be functionally equivalent to Ainsworth's (Ainsworth, Blehar, Waters, & Wall, 1978) original three categories of infant attachment.

The Hazan and Shaver one-item measure has subjects read three descriptions of approaches to relationships (termed, secure, avoidant, and anxious–ambivalent, à la Ainsworth et al.) and indicate which of the three best characterizes their own approach. Other approaches ask subjects to rate each of the three descriptions on a continuum (Shaver & Brennan, 1992), or to complete a questionnaire that includes items relevant to the three approaches (Collins & Read, 1990; Simpson, 1990). Bartholomew and Horowitz (1991) proposed that attachment style reflects two independent dimensions, including the internalized model of self and the internalized model of other. These internalized models can either be positive (self is worthy of love; other is trustworthy and available) or negative (self is unworthy of love; other is unreliable and rejecting). These two dimensions form a 2 × 2 matrix, resulting in four categories of adult attachment style: secure, preoccupied, fearful–avoidant, and dismissing–avoidant. In contrast to most research on attachment styles that uses self-report measures, Bartholomew and Horowitz use a semistructured interview to assess their four attachment styles. Interviews are audiotaped and coders rate the subject on four 9-point scales that assess the extent to which the individual fits each of the four attachment style prototypes. Despite being interview based, the Bartholomew measure fits better with attachment styles than with working models because ratings of attachment style are based on subjects' report of their feelings and behaviors, rather than on analysis of the discourse.

Although the constructs of attachment styles and internal working models share a conceptual framework, there are key differences that lead to different operationalizations. Specifically, assessments of internal working models are made through discourse analysis as subjects talk about thoughts and feelings regarding attachment figures. Attachment style is assessed through subjects' self-report of relationships with currently important figures in their lives. Additionally, internal working models are assessed in relation to earlier attachment figures whereas attachment styles are assessed in relation to current significant others. One might expect that there would be a strong relationship between the two variables, but this expectation has not been supported by the empirical literature (Waters, Merrick, Albersheim, & Treboux, 1995). Thus, it seems important to distinguish between internal working models and attachment style. However conceptually similar, the two seem to measure something different. Two differences key to our examination of therapy relationships involve the assessment of unconscious versus conscious process and the attachment figure that is the target, that is, earlier attachment figure versus current significant other.

In this chapter, we focus on literature relevant to internal working models rather than attachment styles for several reasons. First, we see the role of unconscious processes as central to the work of psychotherapy. For example, we expect that individuals who habitually defensively exclude attachment-related information from consciousness approach treatment providers differently and use treatment differently than those who do not habitually exclude such information. Second, we see internal representations of earlier attachment figures as more pivotal to approaches to treatment providers than representations of current significant others. In adulthood, current significant others may not always be attachment figures. Bowlby (1977) suggested that a true attachment figure must be perceived as "stronger and/or wiser" (p. 203). This definition clearly applies to attachment figures during infancy and childhood, when caregivers provide protection and a sense of security. However, friends, spouses, and romantic partners may or may not meet these criteria in adulthood. The therapist is perhaps a prototypical example of an attachment figure in adulthood. The relationship is caretaking and nonreciprocal, and the client typically perceives the therapist as stronger and wiser. Thus, we expect that internalized representations of earlier attachment figures are central to approaches to the therapist.

INTERNAL WORKING MODELS

Main and Goldwyn (in press) conceptualize adult attachment as the individual's "state of mind with regard to attachment." Different states of mind are associated with different patterns of processing attachment-related thoughts, feelings, and memories. Individuals characterized by an autonomous or coherent state of mind are "free to evaluate attachment experiences" (Main & Goldwyn, in press). They employ information processing strategies that allow ready access to, and flexible manipulation of, attachment-related thoughts, memories, and feelings. Presumably, having had appropriately available caregivers or having reformulated experiences with less available caregivers, attachment-related information can be processed nondefensively. Persons with an autonomous state of mind are neither enmeshed in earlier conflicts, such that they have little perspective on their experiences, nor do they try to remain distant and detached from the impact of earlier attachment experiences, such that they must defensively exclude important information. Rather, they are able to conceptualize attachment experiences freely and fully.

Main (1990) has described autonomous strategies as primary because they allow the biologically based attachment system to achieve the intended outcome of providing protection to the organism. The biological basis of the attachment system is clearer in infancy and childhood, when physical protection from danger is afforded. For example, it is easy to see the evolutionary value of an infant's moving quickly and unhesitantly toward the caregiver when threatened. However, even in adulthood, when attachment is best reflected by representational processes, autonomous strategies might be seen as primary because they involve a nondefensive valuing of attachment.

According to Main (1990), secondary strategies are developed when autonomous strategies fail to produce desired outcomes. In infancy, this can be seen in the infant's adopting avoidant or resistant behavioral strategies for coping with relatively unavailable caregivers. Such infants employ secondary strategies that involve the deactivation or hyperactivation of the attachment system, rather than directly seeking out and obtaining comfort from the caregiver. The deactivation of the attachment system is characterized by attempts to turn attention away from the caregiver when the infant is distressed or needy, times when other infants would seek out the caregiver. Hyperactivation of the attachment system is characterized by excessive vigilance and preoccupation with the caregiver, thus compromising the infant's exploratory behavior.

Adults' secondary strategies parallel these infant behavioral strategies. Hyperactivating strategies are associated with enmeshment in attachment issues and deactivating strategies are associated with attempts to devalue or dismiss the importance of attachment.

ASSESSMENT OF ATTACHMENT STATE OF MIND

The Adult Attachment Interview (AAI; George, Kaplan, & Main, 1985) is used to assess adults' state of mind with regard to attachment. The interview is semistructured; questions are asked in a set order, but with flexibility allowed in following up responses. The interview usually lasts about an hour, ranging from about 45 to 75 minutes. In the interview, subjects are asked to describe their childhood relationships with their parents, to recall incidents of distress, and to conceptualize relationship influences. They describe their relationships with parents by choosing several descriptive adjectives and then generating specific memories that instantiate the adjectives. The incidences of distress they are asked to recall include memories of being separated from or rejected by their parents, and of being emotionally upset, physically hurt, and sick. They are asked to reflect upon their attachment experiences, considering how they were affected by the way they were raised and how their parents became the sort of parents they were.

Classification of State of Mind

Main and Goldwyn's (in press) classification system requires that verbatim transcriptions of the audiotaped interviews are used. It is vital that careful, verbatim transcriptions be available because some coding (particularly with regard to the unresolved classification) can hinge on indices of disorganization or disorientation in a single section of the interview. Coders are expected to have attended a 2-week training workshop offered by Mary Main and to have satisfactorily completed the reliability test, agreeing with Main and Erik Hesse on at least 80% of the test cases. (These are newly specified criteria and have not been fully met in most of the studies described.)

Coders read the transcript at least twice, to assess probable early experiences with attachment figures and the subject's state of mind. Probable early experiences are scored on five scales (loving, rejecting, involving, pressuring to achieve, and neglecting) for each significant attachment figure. Subject's state of mind is scored on six scales (idealizing of, anger at, and derogation of mother and father, insistence on lack of memory, metacognition, passivity). Two additional scales rate the extent to which subjects are unresolved with regard to a trauma or abuse, and two scales rate coherency. Main and Goldwyn suggest reliance on state of mind scales for the derivation of attachment classifications.

Interviews are then classified as autonomous, preoccupied, dismissing, or unresolved. When an unresolved classification is given, a secondary classification (of autonomous, preoccupied, or dismissing) is also given. Results are often reported using the four-group coding scheme (including unresolved) and the three-group coding scheme (forcing unresolved subjects into the best fitting secondary classification).

The interviews of persons who are free to evaluate attachment are characterized especially by the valuing of attachment, as well as the openness with which they recall and integrate experience. Main and Goldwyn argued that such interviews meet Grice's (1975) conversational maxims, including maxims of quality, quantity, relation, and manner. The most important maxim of quality, or truthfulness, is met by the prototypically autonomous subject, who is a cooperative collaborator in the interview process, providing credible data regarding attachment experiences. The maxim of quantity is met by the autonomous subject who presents enough detail to document generalizations, but not so much as to suggest that the subject has lost him- or herself in the account. Interviews with autonomous subjects also tend to meet the last two conversational maxims. The maxim of relation is met when relevant information is provided, and the maxim of manner is met when the presentation is "clear and orderly" (Main & Goldwyn, in press).

Subjects classified as preoccupied are enmeshed in earlier attachment issues. They seem to deal with the anxiety associated with attachment-related memories by hyperactivating their attachment systems. They have ready access to attachment-related memories but are unable to present them in a coherent manner. They tend to be characterized by a rambling style in which they shift topics frequently and seem caught up in their experiences. There is often evidence that these individuals have unresolved conflict with their earlier attachment figures. They have difficulty when asked to reflect upon relationship influences because they have so little perspective on their relationships. In terms of Grice's conversational maxims, they tend to particularly violate maxims of quality, by "oscillating between viewpoints," quantity, because they are not concise, and relevance, in that they get off the conversational track (Main & Goldwyn, in press).

In contrast, subjects classified as dismissing tend to devalue, or dismiss, the importance of earlier attachment experiences. They rely on defensive exclusion to manage the anxiety associated with the consideration of attachment-related topics. More specifically, they often have limited access to memories of times when attachment systems may have been activated (such as when they were frightened or hurt as children). Indeed, they may claim such unlikely things as "I was never really sick as a child" or "I never seemed to get hurt." If they do have access to such memories, they nonetheless maintain a sense of personal invulnerability, such as by indicating that they were not affected adversely by problematic circumstances. This defensive exclusion is associated with the idealization of parents. For example, parents may be described as perfect or wonderful, but no behavioral evidence is presented that supports this characterization. Dismissing individuals violate, most importantly, the conversational maxims of quality, in that they present information that is not credible, and quantity, in that they present inadequate detail (Main & Goldwyn, in press). Overall, these individuals show a deactivation of the attachment system and a devaluing of attachment relationships.

Individuals classified as unresolved with regard to loss or trauma usually show some disorganization of speech and thought when discussing specific traumatic incidents, such as abuse or the loss of a loved one. Indices of unresolved state of mind include lapses in monitoring of reasoning or discourse during the discussion of the loss. For example, unusual attention to detail or prolonged silences suggest lapses in monitoring of discourse, whereas confusing time periods, or speaking as if a death had not occurred, suggest lapses in reasoning (Main & Goldwyn, in press). Less frequently, unresolved status results from very disorganized behavioral responses at the time of the loss or abuse.

Kobak's *Q*-Set

Based on Main and Goldwyn's (in press) classification system, Kobak (1989) developed a Q-set for coding the AAI. Kobak's Attachment Q-set consists of 100 items that were derived from Main's conceptualization of adult attachment. The Q-sort methodology requires that the rater sort the 100 cards into nine categories from most characteristic to least characteristic of the subject. The items are forced into a normal distribution, with fewer items in the more extreme categories (5, 8, 12, 16, 18, 16, 12, 8, and

5 items in the categories from most to least descriptive of the subject). The resulting Q-sort for a subject is then correlated with criterion Q-sorts that have been generated for secure (vs. insecure) and deactivating (vs. hyper-activating) states of mind (Kobak, Cole, Ferenz-Gillies, Fleming, & Gamble, 1993). In the one study comparing the Main and Goldwyn categorical system with the Q-set, discriminant function analysis revealed a 89% concordance rate for subjects classified as autonomous, 94% for subjects classified as dismissing, and 88% for subjects classified as preoccupied (Kobak et al., 1993). Items have not yet been developed that allow assessment of unresolved status.

In this chapter, we will be presenting studies that have used either the Main and Goldwyn classification system or the Kobak Q-set. There are several important differences in these systems that are important to highlight. The greatest conceptual and methodological difference is that Main and Goldwyn's system yields categorical distinctions, whereas the Q-set yields quantitative distinctions. Main (personal communication, August 1994) argued that a categorical system best captures the phenomenon because different attachment categories represent qualitatively different states of mind. Kobak (personal communication, June 1996) suggested that reliability is enhanced when a quantitative system is used, particularly one involving a composite score derived from the ratings of multiple raters. A second key difference between the systems is that unresolved status is not assessed using the Q-set, and recently has taken on increased importance in the Main and Goldwyn classification system. Despite these differences, it is also important to note again that the two systems use the same AAI data for coding, and that Kobak's Q-set derives largely from Main and Goldwyn's conceptualization of attachment in adulthood. In the studies described in this chapter, when interviews were coded using Main and Goldwyn's system, classifications will be referred to autonomous, dismissing, preoccupied, and unresolved states of mind. When interviews were coded using Kobak's Q-set, subjects' scores will be referred to as reflecting secure versus insecure strategies, and deactivating versus hyperactivating strategies. Dismissing states of mind and deactivating strategies are parallel terms, as are preoccupied states of mind and hyperactivating strategies.

ATTACHMENT AND APPROACHES
TO RELATIONSHIPS

Therapy is a context in which a number of relationship issues are played out. Therefore, it is important to first consider how working models of attachment affect approaches to relationships. Secure or autonomous working models of attachment are characterized by open, flexible, and nondefensive deployment of attention to attachment-related issues, allowing the individual access to past and current relationship issues. It would make sense if this nondefensive approach to one's own intrapsychic and interpersonal issues translated into approaches to others that seemed open, receptive, and collaborative. Indeed, this seems to be the case. For example, Kobak et al. (1993) found that teenagers with secure working models showed less avoidance and less dysfunctional anger than other teens while solving an interpersonal problem with their mothers. Significant others seem to perceive persons with secure working models as open and flexible, as evidenced by Kobak and Sceery's (1988) finding that peers rated college students who were rated as secure as more ego resilient than college students rated as insecure.

Preoccupied states of mind are characterized by vigilant attention to evidence of caregiver availability. Not surprising, then, are findings that hyperactivating college freshmen appeared dependent and vulnerable to others (Kobak & Sceery, 1988). Dismissing states of mind involve attempts to turn attention away from attachment-related issues, often manifested as a cold devaluing of attachment. Again consistent with this attachment strategy, deactivating freshmen were perceived by their peers as more hostile than others (Kobak & Sceery, 1988). Similarly, Kobak et al. (1993) found that teens using more deactivating strategies showed more dysfunctional anger than teens using hyperactivating strategies in problem-solving interactions with their mothers.

SYMPTOM REPORTING

The self-report of symptomatology might best be seen as reflecting self-presentational issues, in addition to symptomatology. At times self-reports of psychiatric symptomatology and psychological distress have been handled as if they represented objective indices of psychopathology. However, Shedler and colleagues (Shedler, Mayman, & Manis, 1993) have presented convincing, empirically based arguments that the self-report of low levels of symptomatology tells little about how symptomatic individuals actually are. Low levels are reported both by those that appear unsymptomatic by other assessments, and by those that appear highly symptomatic; on the other hand, high levels are reported primarily by those that appear symptomatic by other assessments. Shedler et al. argued that defensive exclusion among some truly symptomatic individuals leaves them indistinguishable from unsymptomatic others. Thus, self-report of symptomatology reflects a willingness to acknowledge vulnerability to oneself and others. Symptom reporting, then, could be expected to be related to attachment organization. Given that individuals with autonomous states of mind are expected to be relatively healthy psychologically, they should be expected to report lower levels of symptomatology than preoccupied individuals. Because dismissing individuals are expected to defensively exclude information regarding their own distress from awareness, they should be indistinguishable from autonomous individuals in self-reported symptomatology. Preoccupied individuals should be comfortable feeling and acknowledging distress, thus reporting high levels of symptomatology.

Level of Symptomatology

Consistent with these expectations, Kobak and Sceery (1988) found that hyperactivating college freshmen reported more psychological symptoms on the Hopkins Symptom Checklist-90 (Derogatis, 1977) than did deactivating or secure women. Although mean differences between secure and deactivating women were in the direction of secure women reporting less symptomatology, the differences did not approach significance.

Pianta, Egeland, and Adam (1996) administered the Minnesota Multiphasic Personality Inventory-2 (MMPI-2; Butcher, Dahlstrom, Graham, Tellegen, & Kaemmer, 1989) and the AAI to 110 high-risk pregnant women. Using Main and Goldwyn's (in press) three-group classification scheme (autonomous, dismissing, preoccupied), results showed that preoccupied women tended to report more symptomatology than other women. In particular, preoccupied women reported significantly more psychopathic deviance, more paranoia, and more schizophrenia-like symptoms, than other women. The only other difference (on the clinical scales) resulted from dismissing women reporting less hysteria than other women.

Pianta et al.'s (1996) findings suggest that persons with preoccupied internal working models report more symptomatology than persons with dismissing working models. This is consistent with Kobak and Sceery's finding that women rated as hyperactivating on the AAI reported more symptoms than did women rated as deactivating or secure. The question remains whether these two samples of women using hyperactivating strategies were truly more symptomatic than others or whether they were relatively more comfortable reporting distress.

We investigated differences related to working models in symptom reporting, and the convergence of these self-reports with the reports of interviewers and clinicians (Dozier & Lee, 1995). Participants were 76 subjects with serious psychopathological disorders who were part of a longitudinal investigation of case management effectiveness. Most (62%) of the subjects were diagnosed with schizophrenia, with a large minority (36%) diagnosed with bipolar disorder. All completed the AAI and the Brief Symptom Inventory (BSI; Derogatis & Spencer, 1982). The BSI is a self-report inventory consisting of 54 items, which yields nine clinical scale scores. One set of interviewers completed ratings of subjects' symptomatology following the AAI, and a second set following a separate

Quality of Life Interview. In addition, the clinician who worked most closely with each subject rated symptomatology.

AAI's were coded using the Kobak Q-set, yielding two scores for each subject, one for primary attachment strategies (secure vs. insecure), and a second for secondary attachment strategies (deactivating vs. hyperactivating). Differential reliance on primary attachment strategies was unrelated to the self-report of symptoms. However, the three sets of expert raters assessed clients with higher scores on security as less symptomatic than clients with lower scores on security.

Consistent with Pianta et al. (1996) and Kobak and Sceery (1988), greater reliance on hyperactivating secondary strategies (rather than deactivating strategies) was associated with the self-report of more symptomatology across virtually all psychiatric symptoms. The question of interest was whether this increased tendency to report vulnerability among persons with preoccupied strategies reflected a bias in reporting or a perception shared by others. Expert raters' data suggested the former; across all three sets of raters, deactivation was associated with expert ratings of greater psychopathology. These findings suggest that, although hyperactivating strategies are associated with greater self-report of symptomatology, they are not associated with greater symptomatology as observed by others.

Type of Symptomatology

Given that hyperactivating strategies are associated with the felt experience of distress, and deactivating strategies are associated with the defensive exclusion of distress, the form symptoms take should also be different for different attachment classifications. More specifically, hyperactivating strategies should be associated with disorders in which distress is felt, such as anxiety or depression, whereas deactivating strategies should be associated with disorders in which symptoms are experienced external to the self, such as substance abuse and eating disorders (Cole-Detke & Kobak, 1996). A host of studies have been conducted recently investigating the type of symptomatology associated with secondary attachment strategies (Allen, Hauser, & Borman-Spurrell, 1996; Cole-Detke & Kobak, 1996; Patrick, Hobson, Castle, Howard, & Maughn, 1994; Rosenstein & Horowitz, 1996). With some exception (Patrick et al., 1994), the findings are relatively consistent in suggesting that hyperactivating strategies are associated with the felt experience of distress, such as depression (Cole-Detke & Kobak, 1996) or borderline personality disorder (Patrick et al., 1994), whereas deactivating strategies are associated with more externalized indices of distress, such as eating disorders (Cole-Detke & Kobak, 1996), conduct disorders (Rosenstein & Horowitz, 1996), and hard-drug use (Allen et al., 1996).

ATTACHMENT AND USE OF TREATMENT

Given these different self-presentational strategies, it follows that different working models of attachment should be associated with characteristically different reliance on treatment providers. Investigations by Egeland, Adam, Ogawa, & Korfmacher (1995), as well as by our group (Dozier, 1990; Tyrrell & Dozier, 1997b) have examined these associations.

STEEP Project

Korfmacher et al. (in press) looked at the effectiveness of the STEEP (Steps toward Effective, Enjoyable Parenting) intervention for high-risk pregnant women. Mothers were provided with home visits and group sessions (with other mothers) from the time they were about 6 months pregnant until their babies were 12 months of age. The interventions were weekly, alternating between home visits and group sessions, with crisis intervention provided as needed. Although the intervention was intended to affect working models of attachment through the mothers' exploration of their own issues, the living tasks facing these high-risk mothers gave low priority to insight-oriented interventions. Thus, even though the intervention did not proceed as intended, the data of greatest interest concerned differences in how women with different internal working models made use of the available support. In a later section, we will discuss findings regarding the intervention's effectiveness. At this point, we look at how women with different working models of attachment used treatment differently.

Internal working models were assessed using the four-category coding scheme of Main and Goldwyn (in press). In the intervention group, 16% had primary classifications of dismissing, 47% had primary classifications of autonomous, 2% had a primary classification of preoccupied, and 34% had primary classifications of unresolved. The preoccupied category was not included in analyses because of inadequate sample size.

The home visitors for mothers regularly reported the types of treatment in which mothers engaged. Interventions were categorized as insight oriented, secondary ego support, parenting problem solving, other problem solving, crisis intervention, supportive therapy, or companionship. Significantly more of the autonomous mothers (69%) engaged in parenting problem solving at some point during the year's intervention than dismissing mothers (33%) or unresolved mothers (21%). Significantly more autonomous mothers (84%) also engaged in supportive therapy than dismissing mothers (33%) or unresolved mothers (65%). Significantly more unresolved mothers (40%) received crisis intervention than dismissing mothers (0%) or autonomous mothers (3%).

Home visitors also rated the level of the mother's participation in therapy, the mother's emotional commitment to the project, their own positive regard for the mother, the mother's relationship to the group of mothers, and the number of treatment "roadblocks." Autonomous mothers were rated as higher (more involved, better liked, fewer roadblocks) than unresolved mothers on each of these variables. They were also rated as more emotionally committed to the project than dismissing mothers.

Thus, autonomous mothers appeared to be the most willing collaborators in the psychotherapy venture, a finding consistent with expectations. Dismissing mothers were the most distant, relying on their home visitors more than other mothers for companionship and less for supportive therapy. Unresolved mothers appeared to live the most chaotic lives. They were less able to use home visitors to solve problems so as to avoid crises, and thus used home visitors much more than did others for crisis intervention.

Texas Case Management Project

We have examined differences related to attachment organization in how case management services are used by persons with serious psycho pathological disorders. Persons with serious psychopathological disorders are an interesting population to study for several reasons. First, many such persons are *assigned* to treatment. Therefore, the self-selection factor affecting the decision to enroll in treatment is probably less important than among persons without debilitating psychiatric disorders. Clients may be assigned to case management (Dozier et al., 1994) or to residential care (Dozier, 1990), or some other treatment. Second, clients often need help in a range of areas, and treatment providers often have some latitude in deciding how to intervene. For example, such individuals may have needs for help with housing, obtaining benefits, and dealing with interpersonal conflicts and emotional issues. Therefore, it is possible to investigate the type of intervention provided, which could be related to both clinician and client attachment. A wide range of services was also offered in the Korfmacher et al. (in press) study, allowing an investigation of a similar issue in that study. Populations consisting of persons who need a range of services allow examination of the type of intervention in which the treatment dyads engage. The range of interventions provided in more traditional psychotherapy is quite small. Thus, investigations of more traditional psychotherapy rarely afford examination of the range of interventions.

In our first study relating attachment organization to the use of treatment, 42 persons from one of two community-based residential treatment facilities were included as participants (Dozier, 1990). All participants had serious psychopathological disorders that prevented them from living independently in the community. All had a history of at least two psychiatric hospitalizations, and had diagnoses of thought or affective disorders.

The clinician with whom each participating client worked most closely completed a rating of the client's use of treatment. The clinician had at least daily contact with the client, usually in a psychotherapylike interaction, and had known the client for at least a month. Cooperation with treatment was assessed as the extent to which clients showed up for appointments and took medication as prescribed. The extent to which clients sought out versus rejected help, the extent to which they talked about problems and acknowledged difficulties, and their general use of treatment were also rated by clinicians.

Clients' scores for security–insecurity and deactivation–hyperactivation were correlated with the ratings obtained from clinicians, yielding associations between clinician ratings and attachment organization. Security–insecurity was positively correlated with clinicians' ratings of cooperation. More specifically, clients rated as less secure were less cooperative with treatment. We note that this finding primarily reflects variability within the insecure range, that is, from a little insecure to very insecure. Deactivation was negatively correlated with help seeking, self-disclosure, and general treatment use, with correlations with compliance in the same direction, although the latter were nonsignificant (see Table 9.1). Thus, persons rated as more deactivating were rated by their clinicians as less likely to seek out help, less likely to talk about their problems, and as poorer users of treatment than persons rated as more preoccupied (or hyperactivating).

Despite using different populations, different treatment modalities, and different coding schemes for working models of attachment, these findings regarding secure working models of attachment converge well with the findings from the STEEP project to suggest that secure working models are associated with a more collaborative approach to treatment. The association between deactivating attachment strategies and treatment rejection is consistent with Egeland's finding that dismissing mothers were the least emotionally involved in the project and engaged in supportive therapy less than other mothers. Because we relied on the Q-set, we were not able to examine relationships between unresolved status and

TABLE 9.1. Partial Correlations between Attachment Dimensions and Clinician Ratings

	Attachment dimensions	
	Security–Insecurity	Deactivation–Hyperactivation
Cooperation	.37[*]	−.23
Help-seeking	.18	−.55[**]
Self-disclosure	.16	−.50[**]
General treatment use	.03	−.32[*]

Note. From Dozier (1990). Copyright 1990 by Cambridge University Press. Reprinted by permission. The effects of diagnosis and gender were partialed out.
$*p < .05; **p < .01.$

treatment use. Korfmacher et al.'s (in press) finding that unresolved mothers were unable to avoid crises, however, is consistent with findings in very different contexts regarding maladaptiveness of persons with unresolved states of mind (e.g., Solomon, George, & De Jong, 1995). We anticipate that this finding will be replicated and extended by others.

INTERVENING TO CHANGE INTERNAL WORKING MODELS

Our findings (Dozier, 1990; Tyrrell & Dozier, 1997b) and the findings of Korfmacher et al. (in press) suggest that individuals' internal working models affect their approaches to therapy. In some ways, it seems that people approach therapists in much the same ways that they approach significant others in their lives. If they elicit the same responses from therapists that they elicit from others, or are allowed to interact in their customary way, it seems that therapy will not be successful in changing working models. For example, clients relying on deactivating strategies communicate to others that they do not want to engage in interpersonal problem solving (Dozier, 1990; Kobak et al., 1993). If others respond in complementary fashion to this message, discussion of interpersonal and intrapsychic issues will be avoided. Clients using hyperactivating strategies, on the other hand, communicate to others that they are dependent and in need of help. A complementary response would involve taking care of the client in some way.

In a very different context, social psychology researchers (Snyder, Tanke, & Bersheid, 1977) have provided empirical evidence of how very compelling it is to provide complementary responses to strong interpersonal messages. Snyder et al. have shown that individuals tend to elicit responses from others that are consistent with their own expectations. Given that internal working models are associated with characteristically different interpersonal behaviors, we suggest that others feel compelled to provide responses that are consistent with, and complementary to, individuals' internal working models.

The therapist's task is to resist the pull to respond in ways that are consistent with expectations and complementary to behavioral strategies, a pull termed "countertransference" in the psychotherapy literature. To be therapeutic, the therapist needs to provide an environment that promotes the exploration of working models—indeed, an environment that *challenges* the client's working models. Thus, for the client relying on deactivating strategies, the therapist needs to promote exploration of psychological issues, helping the client to think about why such work feels so unsafe. For the client relying on hyperactivating strategies, the therapist needs to avoid taking care of the client, but rather help the client to take charge of his or her life. We suggest that role constraints of the treatment context itself may be important in challenging clients' working models. In addition, some treatment providers are expected to be more effective than others at "using the countertransference." Several studies we have conducted (Dozier et al., 1994; Dozier, Lomax, & Tyrrell, 1997; Tyrrell & Dozier, 1997b), as well as a study conducted by Fonagy et al., 1996 suggest that treatment has the potential of providing different conditions that can challenge customary ways of relating.

In a study of client–therapist interactions (Dozier et al., 1996), persons with serious psychopathological disorders were observed interacting with their significant others, such as spouse, parent, or clinicians, on each of two tasks. The first was a low-involvement task that provided baseline data for observational and self-report measures. The second task was more involving interpersonally, requiring that participants and partners work through interpersonal problems. The videotaped interactions were coded for the extent to which participants were rejecting of their partners. In addition, the participants and significant others rated the extent to which they felt sad, disorganized, and anxious. In the highly involving task, participants' heavier reliance on deactivating strategies was associated with greater rejection of significant others. Further, participants who relied more heavily on deactivating strategies had significant others who reported greater increases in sadness than participants who relied more on hyperactivating strategies. These findings suggest that persons using deactivating strategies manage interactions with others by rejecting significant others who raise issues that activate their attachment systems.

However, the findings were very different when clinicians were considered as partners. Persons relying on deactivating strategies actually tended to reject clinicians *less* than persons relying on preoccupied strategies. We suggest that, because of the role constraints associated with being in treatment, persons relying on deactivating strategies did not feel free to use their customary behavior, that is, rejecting their partner, when interpersonal issues were raised. Therapy may provide the greatest challenge, and hence the greatest benefit, to dismissing clients. Indeed, Fonagy et al. (1996) found that psychiatric inpatients with dismissing working models were more likely than other inpatients to make significant improvements in functioning.

Although treatment can provide a context for challenging customary behavioral strategies associated with different working models of attachment, the characteristics of the treatment provider may be important in determining whether challenge actually occurs. We investigated the relationship between clinician attachment strategies and the ability to respond therapeutically to clients with serious psychopathological disorders (Dozier et al., 1994). Clinicians were contacted monthly regarding their most recent contacts with participating clients. Depth of intervention was coded for each intervention. Greater depth of intervention was expected to be more challenging for clients relying heavily on deactivating strategies than for those relying on hyperactivating strategies. Interestingly, secure versus insecure clinicians made very different decisions about how to intervene with clients. As can be seen in Figure 9.2, insecure clinicians intervened in greater depth with more hyperactivating clients, whereas secure clinicians tended to intervene in greater depth with more deactivating clients. Thus, insecure clinicians intervened in ways that failed to challenge customary interpersonal strategies. They responded to the most obvious presentation of needs, providing "treatment" that differed little from everyday encounters. However, secure clinicians responded in noncomplementary fashion to clients' interpersonal behaviors, perhaps providing a "corrective emotional experience" (Winnicott, 1971). We suggest that the secure case managers had the internal resources that allowed them to respond to clients in ways that, although possibly somewhat uncomfortable for them, were challenging of their clients.

The most recent study from our lab (Tyrrell & Dozier, 1997b) explored the effects of clinician and client attachment strategies on treatment outcome as well as process. Participants were clients with serious psychopathological disorders and their case managers, recruited from an intensive clinical case management program in Washington, DC. Clients and case managers were administered the AAI. The interviews were coded using both Main and Goldwyn's (in press) classification system as well as Kobak's (1989) Q-set. When Main and Goldwyn's categorical system was

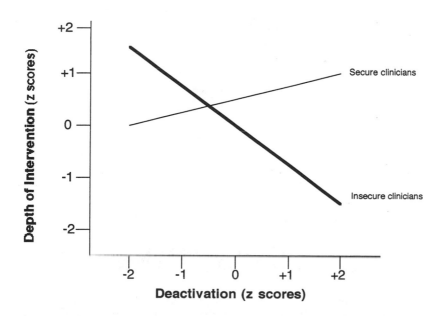

FIGURE 9.2. Depth of intervention as a function of client deactivation for secure and insecure clinicians.

used, 90% of clinicians were classified as autonomous and 83% of clients were classified as insecure. Thus, there was relatively little variability in *primary* strategies among clinicians or clients. However, as expected, there was considerable variability in secondary strategies for both groups. Using Main and Goldwyn's system, this variability was represented primarily as different subgroups within the autonomous group for clinicians, and as different subgroups spanning dismissing, autonomous, and preoccupied categories for clients. Kobak's continuous measure of deactivation–hyperactivation was used in analyses because it directly assesses the extent to which particular secondary strategies are used.

A client deactivation × clinician deactivation interaction emerged for several dependent variables. In particular, clients who were more deactivating had stronger alliances with their case managers, better quality of life, and higher levels of functioning when working with case managers who were less deactivating, whereas clients who were less deactivating had stronger alliances, better quality of life, and higher levels of functioning when working with case managers who were more deactivating. Therefore, results suggested that client–case manager dissimilarity on the deactivation–hyperactivation dimension of attachment was associated with the formation of stronger alliances and more therapeutic gains, as reported by both client and clinician. We argue that this pattern of results is due to a noncomplementary process. Case managers can more effectively challenge clients through their own interpersonal behavior when they are not concordant with clients for attachment strategies.

It is important to remember that nearly all clinicians in this study were classified as autonomous when using Main and Goldwyn's classification system. When clinicians' attachment strategies are best reflected by one of the insecure attachment categories, our previous findings suggest that this pattern of results will no longer hold. The clinician must have the ego strength and flexibility necessary to respond to the client in an noncomplementary manner, even if it is uncomfortable for the clinician at the time. Therefore, we argue that insecure clinicians are likely to have difficulty providing effective interventions, regardless of client attachment organization. Secure clinicians, on the other hand, are likely to work better with clients who differ from them with regard to deactivation–hyperactivation.

EFFECTIVENESS OF
ATTACHMENT-BASED INTERVENTIONS

Not surprisingly, interventions to emerge from within attachment theory have focused on affecting mothers' behavior with their children, as well as affecting mothers' working models of attachment. The connection between internal working models and parenting behavior is theoretically and empirically tight. Indeed, Main and Goldwyn's (in press) operationalization of working models actually emerged from investigation of similarities of mothers with babies sharing attachment classifications. For example, commonalities among the working models of secure babies' mothers were examined, as were commonalities among avoidant, resistant, and disorganized babies' mothers. The concordance between mother and child categories ranges from 69 to 85% (van IJzendoorn, 1992).

van IJzendoorn, Juffer, and Duyvesteyn (1995) provide a comprehensive review of studies that examine the effectiveness of attachment-based interventions aimed at increasing parental sensitivity and children's attachment security. In this section, we will overview a few of the well-documented and intensive therapeutic interventions. See van IJzendoorn et al. (1995) for a more complete review.

Lieberman, Weston, and Pawl (1991) assessed the effectiveness of an intervention for mothers that focused upon attachment issues relevant to the mother's feelings about parenting and to her own developmental history. A sample of poor, recently immigrated, Spanish-speaking Latino women were included in the sample because they were considered at high risk for developing attachment-related problems. Attachment security of infants to mothers was first assessed in the Strange Situation. Dyads were selected for the study from the 63% of the sample classified as insecure, and were randomly assigned to an intervention or control group.

Those mothers in the intervention group received weekly, individualized interventions specific to their needs and the needs of their children. The goal of the intervention was expressly to "promote secure attachment . . . by enhanc[ing] maternal empathy for the child's developmental needs and affective experience" (Lieberman et al., 1991, p. 200). Mothers and babies were present for the intervention, allowing the intervener access to the mother's report of, and observations of, conflicts she experienced in parenting. The intervener helped the mother reinterpret the child's behavior in ways that promoted more empathy, provided information about children's needs for comfort and nurturance, and helped the mother deal with her own unsettling feelings that interfered with her availability as a caretaker.

Differences between experimental and control group mothers and children were assessed in a nearly 2-hour laboratory session videotaped when the children were 24 months old. Intervention group mothers showed greater empathy for their children than did control group mothers. Intervention group toddlers were less angry, showed less restricted affect, less avoidance, and less resistance than control group toddlers. Following separation, the reunion behavior of the intervention group dyads was rated as better reflecting goal-corrected partnerships than that of the control group dyads. Differences in security of attachment for intervention and control group babies, as assessed by Q-sorts completed by home visitors, did not, however, approach significance. Lieberman et al. did not report that they assessed mothers' working models of attachment.

Perhaps because of the homogeneity of the dyads (all insecure) or because of the reasonably small sample size ($n = 30$ in experimental group), Lieberman et al. did not examine differences in the form that attachment insecurity took. Work by Korfmacher et al. (in press) and Dozier (1990) suggests that differences in secondary strategies may have been important in how these mothers used the treatment provided. Nonetheless, Lieberman et al. did examine the therapeutic process, or the extent to which the mother could connect her past experiences with her current feelings. Interestingly, mothers rated as better able to connect past experiences with current feelings had children who were rated more secure in the home observations. This finding could reflect differential effectiveness of the intervention for different dyads. However, given that no preintervention data are available, the possibility that these dyads were the highest functioning (and perhaps represented "unstable insecure" dyads) prior to the intervention cannot be ruled out.

Lieberman's intervention seems to have provided a secure base for mothers to explore their models of attachment relationships. Mothers' behaviors changed, as did child behaviors. Although reunion behavior suggested the development of more optimal goal-corrected partnerships for dyads in the intervention group, the absence of differences in security observed in home observations leaves it unclear whether the child's working model of the mother changed. If behaviors, even for children, are more readily changed than working models, these results could reflect the beginning of the change process; working models may require an intervention of longer duration or greater intensity.

Korfmacher et al. (in press) assessed the effectiveness of their intervention for high-risk first-time mothers. They sought to affect mothers' interactions with their babies via changing mothers' working models of attachment. Mothers were randomly assigned to an experimental intervention group or to a no-treatment control group. Mothers' working models were assessed with the AAI, which was administered following the intervention only. Differences between the working models of experimental and control group mothers following the intervention did not approach significance.

Although the intervention was intended to affect working models of attachment through the mothers' exploration of their own issues, the living tasks facing these high-risk mothers gave low priority to psychologically oriented interventions. For example, only 11% of the mothers ever engaged in insight-oriented therapy. Rather, most interventions concerned parenting help, problem solving regarding nonparenting issues, and support. Thus, it is not surprising that mothers receiving the experimental intervention did not differ from wait-listed mothers in terms of working models of attachment following the intervention. It seems that the interventions actually received by most parents (problem solving regarding parenting and other matters and supportive therapy) would have been expected to affect maternal *behavior* most directly. However, changes in maternal and child behavior were not reported by Egeland et al. Changes in maternal behavior might have then affected working models, but only indirectly. We suggest that insight-oriented therapy would have more directly affected working models of attachment figures. Fortunately, Korfmacher et al. assessed therapeutic process, that is, what home visitors were actually doing when they met with mothers. If the therapeutic process had not been assessed, the conclusion may errone-ously have been made that interventions directed toward changing ma-ternal working models do not lead to changes in internal representations.

Heinicke (in press) investigated the effectiveness of a relationship-based home visiting intervention for high-risk mothers. All mothers were pregnant with their first child. Mothers were randomly assigned to the home visiting intervention group or to a control group. Mothers in the intervention group were given the opportunity of weekly home visiting, a mother–infant group, and referrals to other social service agencies. The aim of the home visiting intervention was to provide mothers with a stable, trusting relationship in which the mother could enhance her communication skills, explore alternate approaches to her relationship with her child, and receive direct affirmation and support. The interven-tion attempted to enhance mothers' personal adaptation as well as the security of their relationships with their children.

All mothers were interviewed about their quality of partner and family support during the third trimester of their pregnancy. Levels of support for intervention and control mothers were essentially the same at this point in their pregnancies. For intervention mothers, their level of support remained stable during their infants' first year of life. In contrast, control mothers' level of support declined significantly over this same time period. When infants were approximately 14 months of age, attach-ment was assessed in the Strange Situation. Significantly more of the babies in the intervention group were assessed as secure than in the control group (74% and 45%, respectively). Thus, Heinicke's intervention enhanced both maternal adjustment and the quality of the mother–child relationship. Among other reasons, this intervention's positive effects were likely influenced by the fact that the intervention was of relatively long duration, approximately 27 months in length, and began early, when first-time mothers were in their third trimester of their pregnancies. The effects of this intervention on maternal working models were not as-sessed. Thus, we are unable to assess whether changes in mothers' behaviors with partners and with their babies were associated with changes in mothers' working models of their own attachment figures. We speculate that behavioral changes precede such changes in working models, however.

INTERVENING WITH FOSTER MOTHERS

To this point, we have been considering treatment in the more conventional sense of therapist (or case manager or home visitor) and client. We suggest, however, that foster mothers function as treatment providers for their foster infants. Infants placed in foster care have typically experienced problematic caregiving, including abuse and/or neglect, and have experienced disruptions in their relationships with caregivers. Whereas a therapeutic task may involve providing clients with experiences that cause them to explore their working models of attachment, the task of infants' foster parents may be to provide experiences that cause the infants to behaviorally explore alternative working models of caregiver availability.

When foster placement occurs after the beginning of the "attachment proper" phase, infants often develop coping strategies that serve to alienate caregivers (Tyrrell & Dozier, 1997a). Thus, children typically enter their relationships with foster parents with expectations that help them to cope with previously problematic experiences, but which are often inappropriate in the new context. If foster parents respond in complementary fashion to the infants' behaviors, expectations are perpetuated, just as it is if clinicians respond in complementary fashion to clients' behaviors. Therefore, we suggest that it is not enough for these children to have *sensitive* foster mothers. Rather, these children need foster mothers who are *therapeutic*; that is, mothers need to see their infants as needy even though the behavioral evidence might suggest otherwise. We are now assessing the effectiveness of an intervention designed to sensitize mothers to children's attachment strategies—to help them recognize foster infants' underlying needs for nurturance. We anticipate that foster mothers' working models affect the process and outcome of the intervention. Specifically, mothers with autonomous working models are expected to benefit most from the intervention, moving from sensitive to therapeutic more readily than others.

SUMMARY AND CONCLUSIONS

The studies discussed represent a first step in looking at how working models of attachment relate to treatment process and outcome. There has been a burgeoning interest in the clinical implications of attachment in recent years, and there will surely be much more research to follow. As of now, however, there is relatively little empirical work reported in the literature that examines how working models of attachment affect therapy process and outcome. Further, there is virtually no reported evidence of change in working models following treatment.

Direct evidence that working models of attachment affect approaches to treatment is limited (Dozier, 1990; Dozier et al., 1994, 1996; Korfmacher et al., in press; Fonagy et al., 1996; Tyrrell & Dozier, 1997b) . Nonetheless, these results are generally consistent with other findings regarding interpersonal behavior and are consistent with hypotheses. Results converge to suggest that autonomous clients are better collaborators in the treatment process, and that dismissing clients keep the greatest distance from treatment providers (Dozier, 1990; Korfmacher et al., in press). Nonetheless, the inherent challenge involved in therapy may lead to the greatest changes for dismissing clients (Dozier et al., 1996; Fonagy et al., 1996). In one study (Korfmacher et al., in press) persons with unresolved status were least able to collaborate with home visitors through problem solving and relied on home visitors more for crisis intervention than other clients. A number of investigations are finding more compelling differences between organized and disorganized (unresolved) strategies than between secure and insecure strategies (Solomon et al., 1995), particularly among infants and children. The Korfmacher et al. (in press) finding suggests that distinctions between organized and disorganized strategies may be critical to therapy process and outcome as well.

The effects of clinicians' working models on treatment have only begun to be explored. Our findings (Dozier et al., 1994; Tyrrell & Dozier, 1997b) are consistent with the relatively untested assumption that the clinician's own attachment issues influence therapeutic process. Clinicians relying on autonomous strategies appear best able to provide clients with experiences that challenge working models. We also have evidence that secondary strategies of clinicians interact with secondary strategies of clients in affecting treatment outcome.

We have proposed a model of psychotherapeutic change, in which exploration, such as that provided by autonomous clinicians, is critical. We expect that change in working models of the therapist, of attachment figures, or of significant others, can only occur if the client is challenged to explore these models. If there is no exploration, we anticipate that no change will occur. Thus, it is not enough to study the effectiveness of treatment. Taking into account the characteristics of the treatment providers, or the therapeutic process, is deemed critical to future investigations.

ACKNOWLEDGMENTS

The work in this chapter was supported by Grant Nos. MH44691 and MH52135 from the National Institute of Mental Health to Mary Dozier.

REFERENCES

Ainsworth, M., Blehar, M., Waters, E., & Wall, S. (1978). *Patterns of attachment: A psychological study of the Strange Situation.* Hillside, NJ: Erlbaum.

Allen, J., Hauser, S., & Borman-Spurrell, E. (1996). Attachment theory as a framework for understanding sequelae of severe adolescent psychopathology: An 11-year follow-up study. *Journal of Consulting and Clinical Psychology, 64*(2), 254–263.

Bartholomew, K., & Horowitz, L. (1991). Attachment styles among young adults: A test of a four-category model. *Journal of Personality and Social Psychology, 61*(2), 226–244.

Berman, W. H., & Sperling, M. B. (1994). The structure and function of adult attachment. In M. B. Sperling & W. H. Berman (Eds.), *Attachment in adults: Clinical and developmental perspectives* (pp.1–30). New York: Guilford Press.

Bowlby, J. (1977). The making and breaking of affectional bonds. I. Aetiology and psychopathology in the light of attachment theory. *British Journal of Psychiatry, 130,* 201–210.

Bowlby, J. (1988). *A secure base.* New York: Basic Books.

Butcher, J. N., Dahlstrom, W. G., Graham, J. R., Tellegen, A., & Kaemmer, B. (1989). *Minnesota Multiphasic Personality Inventory–2 (MMPI-2): Manual for administration and scoring.* Minneapolis: University of Minnesota Press.

Cole-Detke, H., & Kobak, R. (1996). Attachment processes in eating disorder and depression. *Journal of Consulting and Clinical Psychology, 64*(2), 282–290.

Collins, N., & Read, S. (1990). Adult attachment, working models, and relationship quality in dating couples. *Journal of Personality and Social Psychology, 58*(4), 644–663.

Derogatis, L. R. (1977). *SCL-90 administration, scoring, and procedures manual–I.* Baltimore, MD: John Hopkins University.

Derogatis, L. R., & Spencer, P. M. (1982). *Administration and procedures: BSI manual I.* Baltimore, MD: Clinical Psychometrics Research.

Dozier, M. (1990). Attachment organization and treatment use for adults with serious psychopathological disorders. *Development and Psychopathology, 2,* 47–60.

Dozier, M., Cue, K., & Barnett, L. (1994). Clinicians as caregivers: Role of attachment organization in treatment. *Journal of Counseling and Clinical Psychology, 62*(4), 793–800.

Dozier, M., & Lee, S. (1995). Discrepancies between self- and other-report of psychiatric symptomatology: Effects of dismissing attachment strategies. *Development and Psychopathology, 7,* 217–226.

Dozier, M., Lomax, L., & Tyrrell, C. L. (1997). *Therapeutic challenge for adults using deactivating attachment strategies.* Manuscript submitted for publication.

Egeland, B., Adam, E., Ogawa, J., & Korfmacher, J. (1995). *Adult attachment: Implications for the therapeutic process in a home visitation intervention.* Paper presented at the biennial meeting of the Society for Research in Child Development, Indianapolis, IN.

Fishler, P., Sperling, M., & Carr, A. (1990). Assessment of adult relatedness: A review of empirical findings from object relations and attachment theories. *Journal of Personality Assessment, 55*(3&4), 499–520.

Foa, E., Rothbaum, B., Riggs, D., & Murdock, T. (1991). Treatment of post-traumatic stress disorder in rape victims: A comparison between cognitive-behavioral procedures and counseling. *Journal of Consulting and Clinical Psychology, 59,* 715–723.

Fonagy, P., Leigh, T., Steele, M., Steele, H., Kennedy, R., Mattoon, G., Target, M., & Gerber, A. (1996). The relation of attachment status, psychiatric classification, and response to psychotherapy. *Journal of Consulting and Clinical Psychology, 64,* 22–31.

George, C., Kaplan, N., & Main, M. (1985). *Attachment interview for adults.* Unpublished manuscript, University of California, Berkeley.

Grice, H. (1975). Logic and conversation. In P. Cole & J. L. Moran (Eds.), *Syntax and semantics III: Speech acts* (pp. 41–58). New York: Academic Press.

Hazan, C., & Shaver, P. (1987). Romantic love conceptualized as an attachment process. *Journal of Personality and Social Psychology, 52,* 511–524.

Heinicke, C. (in press). Relationship-based intervention with at-risk mothers: Outcome in first year of life. In D. Cicchetti & S. Toth (Eds.), *Rochester Symposium on Developmental Psychology: Vol. X. Developmental approaches to prevention and intervention.* Rochester, NY: University of Rochester Press.

Kobak, R. R. (1989). *The Attachment Interview Q-set.* Unpublished document, University of Delaware.

Kobak, R. R., Cole, H. E., Ferenz-Gillies, R., Fleming, W. S., & Gamble, W. (1993). Attachment and emotion regulation during mother–teen problem solving: A control theory hypothesis. *Child Development, 64,* 231–245.

Kobak, R. R., & Sceery, A. (1988). Attachment in late adolescence: Working models, affect regulation, and representations of self and others. *Child Development, 59,* 135–146.

Korfmacher, J., Adam, E., Ogawa, J., & Egeland, B. (in press). Adult attachment: Implications for the therapeutic process in a home visitation intervention. *Applied Developmental Science.*

Lieberman, A., Weston, D., & Pawl, J. (1991). Preventive intervention and outcome with anxiously attached dyads. *Child Development, 62,* 199–209.

Main, M. (1990). Cross-cultural studies of attachment organization: Recent studies, changing methodologies, and the concept of conditional strategies. *Human Development, 33,* 48–61.

Main, M., & Goldwyn, R. (in press). Adult attachment classification system. In M. Main (Ed.), *Behavior and the development of representational models of attachment: Five methods of assessment.* Cambridge: Cambridge University Press.

Main, M., Kaplan, N., & Cassidy, J. (1985). Security in infancy, childhood, and adulthood: A move to the level of representation. In I. Bretherton & E. Waters (Eds.), Growing points in attachment theory and research. *Monographs of the Society for Research in Child Development, 50,* 66–104.

Patrick, M., Hobson, R., Castle, D., Howard, R., & Maughn, B. (1994). Personality disorder and mental representation of early social experience. *Development and Psychopathology, 6,* 375–388.

Pearson, J., Cohn, D., Cowan, P., & Cowan, C. P. (1994). Earned- and continuous-security in adult attachment: Relation to depressive symptomatology and parenting style. *Development and Psychopathology, 6,* 359–373.

Pianta, R., Egeland, B., & Adam, E. (1996). Adult attachment classification and self-reported psychiatric symptomatology as assessed by the Minnesota

Multiphasic Inventory-2. *Journal of Consulting and Clinical Psychology, 64*(2), 273–281.

Rosenstein, D., & Horowitz, H. (1996). Adolescent attachment and psychopathology. *Journal of Consulting and Clinical Psychology, 64*(2), 244–253.

Shaver, P., & Brennan, K. A. (1992). Attachment styles and the "Big Five" personality traits: Their connections with each other and with romantic relationship outcomes. *Personality and Social Psychology Bulletin, 18,* 536–545.

Shedler, J., Mayman, M., & Manis, M. (1993). The illusion of mental health. *American Psychologist, 48,* 1117–1131.

Simpson, J. (1990). Influence of attachment styles on romantic relationships. *Journal of Personality and Social Psychology, 59*(5), 971–980.

Snyder, M., Tanke, E. D., & Bersheid, E. (1977). Social perception and interpersonal behavior: On the self-fulfilling nature of social stereotypes. *Journal of Personality and Social Psychology, 35*(9), 656–666.

Solomon, J., George, C., & De Jong, A. (1995). Children classified as controlling at age six: Evidence of disorganized representational strategies and aggression at home and at school. *Development and Psychopathology, 7,* 447–463.

Target, M., & Fonagy, P. (1994). Efficacy of psychoanalysis for children with emotional disorders. *Journal of American Academy of Child and Adolescent Psychiatry, 33,* 361–371.

Tyrrell, C., & Dozier, M. (1997a). *Foster parents' understanding of children's problematic attachment strategies: The need for therapeutic responsiveness.* Manuscript submitted for publication.

Tyrrell, C., & Dozier, M. (1997b). *The role of attachment in therapeutic process and outcome for adults with serious psychiatric disorders.* Manuscript in preparation.

van IJzendoorn, M. (1992). Intergenerational transmission of parenting: A review of studies in non-clinical populations. *Developmental Review, 12,* 76–99.

van IJzendoorn, M., Juffer, F., & Duyvesteyn, M. (1995). Breaking the intergenerational cycle of insecure attachment: A review of the effects of attachment-based interventions on maternal sensitivity and infant security. *Journal of Child Psychology and Psychiatry, 36*(2), 225–248.

Waters, E., Merrick, S. K., Albersheim, L., & Treboux, D. (1995, April). *From the Strange Situation to the Adult Attachment Interview: A 20-year longitudinal study of attachment security in infancy and early childhood.* Paper presented at the meeting of the Society for Research in Child Development, Indianapolis, IN.

Winnicott, D. W. (1971). *Playing and reality.* New York: Basic Books.

10

Dismissing-Avoidance and the Defensive Organization of Emotion, Cognition, and Behavior

R. CHRIS FRALEY
KEITH E. DAVIS
PHILLIP R. SHAVER

In Bowlby's (1980) final volume on attachment and loss, a great deal of theoretical attention was devoted to mechanisms that might result in the partial or complete deactivation of the attachment system. Bowlby was particularly interested in such defensive mechanisms because he and others in the field of child psychoanalysis (Freud & Burlingham, 1974; Heinicke & Westheimer, 1966), had noticed that children's attempts to ignore or avoid painful thoughts of an absent attachment figure were often sprinkled with intrusions indicative of unconscious longing and despair. In his discussion of Robertson's (1952) film, *A Two-Year-Old Goes to Hospital*, Bowlby (1980) noted that Laura's apparent detachment from her missing mother was, at times, betrayed by subtle slips:

> [Laura would] sometimes let concealed feelings come through in songs and, apparently unknown to herself, substitute the name of "Mummy" for that of a nursery-rhyme character. On one occasion she expressed an urgent wish to see the steam-roller which had just gone from the roadway below the ward in which she was confined. She cried, "I want

to see the steam-roller, I want to see the steam-roller, I want to see my *mummy*, I want to see the steam-roller." (p. 11)

Similarly, researchers using Ainsworth's Strange Situation procedure (Ainsworth, Blehar, Waters, & Wall, 1978) have argued that infants who exhibit a tendency to avoid their mothers after a brief separation are not simply unaffected by the separation, but rather are defensively turning away from an attachment figure who has been unavailable on other occasions of need (Main & Weston, 1982; Sroufe & Waters, 1977). For instance, a common avoidant strategy used by infants is gaze aversion—looking away from the parent after a separation. Although gaze aversion could be interpreted as a simple indifference to the attachment figure's whereabouts, Waters, Matas, and Sroufe (1975) showed that infants' simple shifts in gaze often involve transitory blinking, whereas blinking rarely occurs when infants avert their gaze from attachment figures.

Such observations suggest that defensive attempts to suppress attachment-related thoughts and feelings are only partially successful, and even then are successful only for brief periods of time. It is worth noting, however, that most observations leading to this conclusion have involved infants and young children only. An individual's defensive strategies for regulating uncomfortable thoughts and feelings are likely to become more sophisticated and efficient as he or she matures (Cramer, 1987). Hence, defensive processes that are at first only partially successful have the potential, over time, to develop into strategies that maintain a more or less complete state of emotional detachment.

In the present chapter we outline a hypothesis about the development, structure, and dynamics of the psychological mechanisms that allow an individual to maintain the attachment system in a relatively complete state of deactivation. We will focus our discussion specifically on the psychological organization of *dismissing–avoidant adults*—adults theorized to devalue emotional attachments and to strive for self-reliance (Bartholomew, 1990). We begin by reviewing research that demonstrates phenotypic similarities in the ways avoidant infants and dismissing–avoidant adults regulate their behaviors and emotions under circumstances (separation and loss) that would, for secure individuals, produce great anxiety and despair. Specifically, we will show that avoidant infants and adults exhibit a striking propensity to avoid seeking contact with an attachment figure following separation. However, we will argue that there are different mechanisms driving behavioral avoidance for adults and infants. In infancy, avoidance appears to be the result of an explicit attempt to conceal the expression of attachment-related distress (Sroufe & Waters, 1977). In contrast, for dismissing–avoidant adults, avoidance appears to be the result of the relative absence of attachment-related distress.

To explain why dismissing–avoidant adults are able to keep the attachment system in a relative state of deactivation we will address three major questions. First, how does the mind need to be structured to effectively suppress attachment-related thoughts and feelings? That is, are there specific ways that thought and memory need to be organized to facilitate detachment? Second, what kinds of social and cognitive mechanisms are necessary to maintain a defensive psychological organization? Third, what are some possible developmental pathways that may give rise to dismissing-avoidance? As we address these questions and outline possible answers, we will highlight critical issues that need to be examined empirically and suggest possible ways to do so. In the process, we hope to stimulate interest in the topic of defenses and attachment, encourage new lines of programmatic research, and contribute to the understanding of what we consider to be a fascinating issue in attachment theory and research. Because the construct of dismissing-avoidance is relatively new, we begin with a brief overview of its conceptualization.

THE CONCEPTUALIZATION OF DISMISSING-AVOIDANCE

Many researchers interested in the attachment dynamics of adult romantic relationships have recently adopted Bartholomew's (1990; Bartholomew & Horowitz, 1991) individual difference framework. According to that framework, variability in patterns of attachment can be located within a two-dimensional space defined by the dimensions of Avoidance (also called Model of Others) and Anxiety (also called Model of Self). As shown in Figure 10.1, dismissing-avoidance is marked by high levels of Avoidance and low levels of Anxiety. Dismissing individuals are described by themselves and their friends as somewhat introverted, cold, and emotionally inexpressive (Bartholomew & Horowitz, 1991). These qualities are illustrated by Bartholomew's theoretical description of dismissing-avoidance, typically used in contemporary self-report measures of attachment style: "I am comfortable without close emotional relationships. It is very important to me to feel independent and self-sufficient, and I prefer not to depend on others or have others depend on me" (Bartholomew & Horowitz, 1991, p. 244).

Because both dismissing and secure adults are characterized by positive self models, it is important to distinguish between two kinds of self-reliance or independence. Theoretically, secure adults' confidence derives from a belief that others will be available to support and comfort them if need be. In other words, secure adults possess a *secure base* from which to explore the world (Bowlby, 1969/1982). They view other people as dependable and supportive (Hazan & Shaver, 1987) and hence feel more confident about finding trustworthy relationship partners and succeeding in novel environments. On the other hand, the independence of

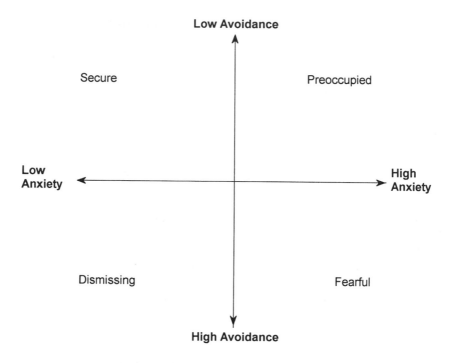

FIGURE 10.1. Bartholomew's (1990) theoretical model of adult attachment styles.

dismissing–avoidant adults is thought to stem from a reluctance to rely on others as a secure base and to count on them for emotional support.

To date there has been little published research on the psychological organization of dismissing adults. This is not surprising because the construct is relatively new (Bartholomew, 1990). Nevertheless, it is somewhat troubling that most published reports have not been able to identify variables that differentiate dismissing-avoidance from other attachment styles. To some extent, this failure can be attributed to reliance on categorical measurement models, which tend to yield only a small proportion of individuals who classify themselves as dismissing–avoidant (less than 20%), thereby reducing the statistical power of the test (see Fraley & Waller, Chapter 4, this volume). In addition to this problem, however, most of the published research has not explicitly tested hypotheses on dismissing-avoidance. To overcome some of these problems and advance our understanding of the psychology of dismissing-avoidance, in the present chapter we will focus on research conducted in our laboratories that (1) used dimensional measurement models and (2) explicitly tested hypotheses about the psychological organization of dismissing-avoidance.[1]

DEFENSIVE RESPONSES
TO SEPARATION AND LOSS

An observation that has received considerable attention in the literature on infant attachment is that some children do not seek the comfort of their attachment figures following brief separations (Ainsworth et al., 1978; Main & Weston, 1982). This relative absence of attachment behavior is particularly striking because the majority of infants who experience separation express intense distress and vigorously attempt to maintain or reestablish contact with their attachment figures. When a separation is pending, infants typically begin to cry and scream as a way to keep their attachment figures from leaving. Moreover, children may cling to an attachment figure or try to impede his or her departure (e.g., by grabbing onto an arm or leg). When a departed attachment figure returns, the majority of infants seek comfort and reassurance by moving closer and signaling a wish to be held (Ainsworth et al., 1978). In sharp contrast to infants who exhibit active contact-seeking responses, infants classified as *insecure avoidant* are more likely to avoid eye contact with the attachment figure, less likely to express distress when the attachment figure leaves, and less likely to seek the attachment figure's comfort following reunion (Ainsworth et al., 1978).

The behavior of dismissing–avoidant adults is conceptually similar to that of avoidant infants. Some of our recent studies illustrate this point. In one study, we examined adults' retrospective accounts of their reactions to the breakup of an exclusive romantic relationship (Fraley, Davis, & Shaver, 1995). We asked participants to write about the most recent experience in which someone they were dating in an exclusive romantic relationship broke up with them. We also asked participants to rate the extent to which their reactions to the breakup consisted of separation-protest behaviors of the kind generally observed in infancy (see Table 10.1). Consistent with observations of mother–infant separation in early childhood, the loss of a romantic attachment figure was associated with heightened attempts to reestablish contact with the former partner. These reactions included crying, calling, searching, and a general resistance to letting go. (Although none of our participants reported desperately grabbing onto the arms and legs of their partners, several reported clinging to old photos, shirts, and letters.) Consistent with the observations of infants classified as insecure–avoidant, scores on Griffin and Bartholomew's (1994) Relationship Styles Questionnaire (RSQ) measure of dismissing-avoidance were negatively correlated with these protest responses (see Table 10.1). Dismissing–avoidant adults were less likely to continue seeking the lost partner and less likely to pursue the affections of the lost partner.

In a second study we observed the attachment behavior of romantic partners separating from one another in local airports (Fraley & Shaver,

TABLE 10.1. Correlations between Dismissing-Avoidance and Self-Reported Attachment Behavior Following the Breakup of an Exclusive Romantic Relationship

Separation-protest item	Dismissing-avoidance
I felt angry at this person afterwards.	.01
I continued seeking this person afterwards by calling, visiting, etc.	−.34
I felt some denial, disbelief, or unwillingness to accept that my feelings were not reciprocated.	−.31
I cried over the experience.	−.04
I requested explanations from this person after the experience.	−.26
I disclosed my feelings to this person so he/she would know how I felt about him/her afterward.	−.23
I continued to try to win this person's heart after the experience.	−.24

$n = 56$, $SE = .14$

Note. Dismissing-avoidance was measured with Griffin and Bartholomew's (1994) Relationship Styles Questionnaire (RSQ).

1997a). Airport separations provide an interesting occasion for observing adult attachment dynamics because the environment is somewhat un-usual and unfamiliar, the separation is real, and there is a chance that the separation could be permanent. (In these ways, airport separations are an ideal analogue to the situation confronted by infants and young children in Ainsworth's Strange Situation.) We asked couples waiting in airport terminals to complete a one-page questionnaire containing attachment-style measures and simple demographic items. After each member of the couple independently filled out the questionnaire, our research team unobtrusively observed the couple until one of them boarded the plane or both boarded together. For couples who separated, we documented higher levels of separation protest, caregiving, and sexual intimacy than in couples who were flying together. Separating partners were more likely to hold hands, cry, vocally express their love for each other, and touch each other (both in caring ways, such as petting the other's head, and in sexually suggestive ways, such as petting the other's inner thigh). How-ever, these behaviors were less pronounced among individuals scoring high on Griffin and Bartholomew's (1994) measure of dismissing-avoidance. Dismissing–avoidant adults were more likely to turn away from their partners or try to hurry the separation.

Findings from both studies indicate that temporary or permanent separations from a romantic partner do not elicit attachment behavior as strongly for dismissing–avoidant adults as for other adults. Their behav-ior is phenotypically similar to that of infants classified as insecure–avoidant in the Ainsworth Strange Situation procedure, suggesting that the two attachment patterns may share a common psychological struc-ture.

AVOIDANCE: A RESULT OF CONCEALING DISTRESS OR CUTTING OFF DISTRESS?

Avoidant infants and dismissing–avoidant adults are similar in that both exhibit relatively low levels of attachment behavior following separation or loss. This relative absence of attachment behavior could be explained in either of two ways. One possibility is that avoidant individuals (infants and adults) may simply be unconcerned about, or indifferent to, their attachment figure's whereabouts and hence express little distress when separation occurs. Alternatively, avoidant individuals may be quite distressed under these conditions but attempt to conceal their distress by suppressing attachment-related behaviors and feelings. Because these two explanations have considerably different implications for understanding the organization of the attachment system, it is important to determine whether the relative absence of attachment behavior results from an explicit effort to suppress attachment behavior or from a relative inactivation of the attachment system itself.

Distinguishing between these two explanations can be tricky for two reasons. First, infants cannot tell researchers how they are feeling. If an infant exhibits low levels of attachment behavior, we cannot simply ask the child if he or she is concealing painful feelings or is truly unperturbed by the separation. Second, even if infants could provide a verbal description of their feelings, they might deliberately misrepresent their true feelings—particularly if the absence of emotional expression is due to defensive processes. This is also a major problem in the adult attachment literature, where the primary methods for studying psychodynamics rely on questionnaires. To determine whether defensive processes are at work in a given individual or sample it will be necessary to use indirect methods (see Greenwald & Banaji, 1995) that provide a way to prevent research participants from explicitly controlling the outcome (as with physiological measures) or second-guessing the way in which the outcomes are scored (as with implicit tests or between-subjects designs).

Historically, psychologists have used slips and intrusions as an indirect method for inferring the existence of latent psychological states (Wegner, 1989, 1994). For example, Freud examined his patients' free associations to their dreams in order to make inferences about latent anxieties and conflicts (Reiser, 1990). More recently, psychologists examining deception have sought to identify subtle clues, such as facial twitches and palmar sweating, that betray an individual's attempts to conceal mental states (DePaulo, Lanier, & Davis, 1983; Ekman & Friesen, 1975; Gross & Levenson, 1993; Harrigan, Harrigan, Sale, & Rosenthal, 1996). Such indirect methods can also be used to examine defensive processes in attachment.

The cool, aloof indifference of avoidant infants is often betrayed by subtle slips or indications of conflicting motives (Main & Weston, 1982), suggesting that these infants *are* distressed by separation despite their attempts to conceal their feelings. Sroufe and Waters (1977) monitored the heart rates of 12-month-old infants who were briefly separated from and reunited with their mothers in the laboratory (also see Spangler & Grossmann, 1993). These authors reported that infants who engaged in defensive strategies (e.g., moving away from, rather than toward, their mothers or suddenly engaging in play with a nearby toy) exhibited the same pattern of heart rate acceleration as infants who were overtly distressed by the separation and who explicitly sought comfort from their mothers following her return. Furthermore, heart rate patterns observed during defensive play activity were not marked by the same cardiac pattern of attentive engagement that characterized their play behavior before the separation. Also, as noted by Main and Weston (1982), there is a tendency for avoidant infants to direct their attention toward objects or activities that do not involve the attachment figure. For example, upon reunion an infant may turn to a specific toy and begin playing at some distance from the attachment figure. However, this play may be half-hearted, as indicated by the accidental dropping of puzzle pieces or the mechanical repetition of play motions. Such cues or slips suggest that avoidant infants experience attachment-related distress despite using defensive strategies to inhibit the expression of that distress.

It is also possible to use indirect methods to determine whether dismissing–avoidant adults are defensively trying to conceal their distress or are simply unaffected by separation from their partners. To distinguish between these two possibilities, we have conducted several studies using Wegner's thought-suppression paradigm (Wegner, Schneider, Carter, & White, 1987) as a way to make inferences about latent defensive processes. In Wegner's paradigm, participants are asked to try to suppress (i.e., ignore or inhibit) specific thoughts. Research on emotional and cognitive suppression has indicated that suppression generally leads to heightened physiological arousal (Gross & Levenson, 1993; Koriat, Melkman, Averill, & Lazarus, 1972) and increased vigilance with respect to the very idea a person is trying to suppress (Wegner, 1989, 1994). For example, Wegner and his colleagues (Wegner, 1989; Wegner et al., 1987) found that participants spent more time thinking about white bears when just previously they had been asked to suppress thoughts of a white bear than when they had not been so instructed. Wegner has argued that these *rebound effects* occur because the act of suppression ironically primes the very thought one is trying to suppress, thereby making it more accessible to consciousness at a later time. However, when participants are instructed to suppress thoughts they find personally intrusive (i.e., thoughts they have chronically suppressed in the past), the rebound effect reverses or disappears (Kelly & Kahn, 1994). Moreover, when participants are provided with effective cognitive strategies for avoiding unwanted thoughts, the rebound effect is substantially attenuated, making the thoughts considerably less accessible (Wegner et al., 1987).

The findings of Wegner and his colleagues indicate that suppression can have different effects depending on whether a person has the defensive strategies and experience necessary to redirect attention to unrelated thoughts. Specifically, in the absence of such strategies, attempts to suppress unwanted thoughts can result in increased activation of them (Wegner & Erber, 1992), leading to ironic slips and intrusions. However, with the development of defensive strategies for regulating attentional processes, the successful suppression of unwanted thoughts becomes possible and allows a person to decrease the accessibility of those thoughts (Kelly & Kahn, 1994; Wegner & Gold, 1995).

To determine whether dismissing–avoidant adults possess the strategies necessary to suppress their attachment systems successfully or are actually experiencing heightened covert distress, we adapted Wegner's paradigm to study the suppression of attachment-related thoughts in adults (Fraley & Shaver, 1997b, Study 1). We asked people involved in exclusive romantic relationships either to suppress or not to suppress thoughts of their partners leaving them for someone else—thoughts that should strongly activate the attachment system. Participants in the experimental group were asked to try their best *not* to think about their partners leaving them. Participants in the control group were not given these suppression instructions. To assess the effects of suppression on the subsequent accessibility of loss-related thoughts, participants were asked to perform a written stream-of-consciousness task. In this task, participants were instructed to think and write about what it would be like if their partner left them for someone else. If dismissing–avoidant adults have not acquired the defensive strategies necessary to disengage the attachment system, then attempts to suppress attachment-related thoughts and feelings should lead to a subsequent *rebound* in such thoughts in their stream-of-consciousness reports—an ironic indicator of latent distress or concern (Wegner et al., 1987). In contrast, if dismissing–avoidant adults do have the capacity to disengage the operation of the attachment system, then the suppression of attachment-related thoughts and feelings should result in a decrease in such thoughts (Kelly & Kahn, 1994).

The findings were more consistent with the latter explanation. Compared to dismissing–avoidant adults in the control condition, dismissing adults who were asked to suppress thoughts of separation and loss wrote *less* about abandonment in their subsequent stream-of-consciousness reports. That is, they had fewer ironic slips and intrusions than participants who were not dismissing. This finding suggests that dismissing–avoidant adults have the capacity to successfully disengage certain components of their attachment system by using defensive strategies.

This finding contrasts with the results from studies of infants. As noted earlier, Sroufe and Waters (1977) found that infants' defensive strategies did not successfully block the activation of the attachment system. Instead, avoidant infants continued to have high heart rate levels following separation and were not able to engage their attention completely in distracting toys. Hence, there appears to be a substantial difference in the psychological organization of avoidant infants and dismissing–avoidant adults despite similarities in their behavior. To pursue this finding further, we conducted a second study in which we asked participants involved in exclusive dating relationships to discuss aloud how they would act and feel if their romantic partner left them for someone else (Fraley & Shaver, 1997b, Study 2). As before, half of the participants were asked to spend 5 minutes suppressing the thought of their partner leaving them for someone else before being explicitly asked to discuss it. The control group was instructed to suppress a neutral thought (their partners leaving them temporarily to go to a restaurant). Participants' skin conductance levels (SCL) were monitored throughout the procedure to provide a measure of physiological arousal. If dismissing–avoidant adults have the capacity to disengage their attachment systems, then their attempts to suppress thoughts of separation and loss should result in decreases in SCL relative to control conditions. However, if defensive strategies are only partially successful in deactivating the attachment system for dismissing adults, then we should see an ironic increase in SCL relative to control conditions.

Again, the results were more consistent with the hypothesis that defensive suppression actually decreases the activation of the attachment system for dismissing adults. Dismissing–avoidants who suppressed attachment-related thoughts and feelings for 5 minutes had lower skin conductance when later instructed to think about separation than dismissing–avoidants who had suppressed a neutral thought.

These results indicate that the psychological organization of dismissing–avoidant adults differs substantially from that of avoidant infants. Both groups exhibit relatively low levels of attachment behavior following a separation or loss, but apparently for different reasons. The relative absence of attachment behavior on the part of avoidant infants appears to be due to a defensive effort to conceal troubling attachment-related thoughts and feelings. In contrast, the relative absence of attachment behavior on the part of dismissing–avoidant adults seems to be due to successful deactivation of the attachment system.

If dismissing–avoidant adults, unlike avoidant infants, are able to maintain a latent state of detachment during distressful situations, then several critical theoretical questions arise. For instance, what are the psychological mechanisms that allow dismissing adults to block their emotional responses? Are there unique ways in which memory, attention, goals, and social behavior need to be organized in order to keep the attachment system deactivated? What developmental processes may promote and maintain the psychological organization of dismissing-avoidance? In the remainder of this chapter, we will discuss these questions and outline some possible answers.

THE ARCHITECTURE OF DEFENSE AND THE ORGANIZATION OF ATTENTION, MEMORY, AND SOCIAL BEHAVIOR FOR DISMISSING INDIVIDUALS

In the previous section we argued that dismissing–avoidant adults fail to express attachment-related distress in situations involving separation or loss because they experience very little distress in these situations. In this section we attempt to identify the mechanisms that allow dismissing adults to maintain this state of detachment. We argue that dismissing–avoidant adults are able to keep the attachment system deactivated because of the way the systems mediating attention, social behavior, and memory are organized within these individuals. These systems appear to be centered on the implicit goal of avoiding attachment-related anxiety. This goal facilitates the development of attachment-related knowledge structures that are relatively isolated from or unconnected to structures representing significant aspects of the self. Furthermore, this goal diverts attention from attachment-related experiences, thereby preventing the incorporation of these experiences into a broadly connected memory system. In conjunction, these mechanisms reduce the likelihood that attachment-related knowledge structures will influence the processing of new information or become activated by new information that is being processed.

In addition to affecting the structure of memory, the motivation to avoid attachment-related anxiety also affects how the social environment becomes structured. Specifically, the way dismissing adults organize their attachment, caregiving, and sexual behavior appears to minimize experiences of anxiety and rejection. We will present data that show that dismissing adults are less likely to become attached to their partners—that is, to put themselves in a position where they have to rely on others more than they rely on themselves. As such, they reduce the likelihood that the attachment system will be strongly activated if the relationship falls apart. Furthermore, we will present data indicating that the caregiving and sexual behavior of dismissing adults serves the implicit goal of avoiding attachment and rejection. By avoiding attachment and intimacy, dismissing individuals create a cognitive and social environment for themselves that makes it relatively easy to keep the attachment system deactivated.

Derailing Attachment-Related Thoughts

How is it that dismissing–avoidant adults are able to deactivate the kinds of thoughts and feelings that should arise when a person is faced with separation or loss? Wegner's (1989, 1994) research indicates that a critical variable in successful thought suppression is the associative structure of the thoughts people use to distract themselves from unwanted thoughts. When those distracter thoughts are not associated with the thought being avoided, then suppression is relatively easy. However, when one is trying to avoid certain thoughts (e.g., cheese cake) by thinking about indirectly related thoughts (e.g., chocolate), it is more likely that suppression will lead to a rebound in the unwanted thought.

Wegner's research has demonstrated these points well. For example, he reported that when people were placed in an environment different from the one in which they had originally suppressed thoughts of a white bear, they were less likely to experience an ironic preoccupation with white bears (Wegner, 1989). Presumably, these participants were not being exposed to environmental cues that they had originally associated with the unwanted thought. Thus, they were able to focus their attention successfully on ideas that would not trigger white bear memories. In a related study, participants were told to distract themselves by thinking about red Volkswagens instead of white bears. These participants were less likely to experience a rebound in white bear thoughts following suppression than were participants who were not provided a focused way to distract themselves (Wegner et al., 1987). Apparently, when the mind is allowed to wander, it keeps returning to thoughts that have been prohibited.

For suppression to work successfully, it is necessary for the mind to have its own distracters—its own red Volkswagens. It needs to be able to focus attention on a set of thoughts or tasks that are unrelated to the idea one is trying to avoid. Research suggests that people learn how to do this, at least implicitly, when they repeatedly try to suppress unwanted thoughts (Kelly & Kahn, 1994; Wegner, 1994; Wegner & Gold, 1995). For example, Kelly and Kahn (1994) showed that when individuals were instructed to suppress thoughts they had found particularly bothersome in the past (and, hence, had practiced suppressing), they were able to decrease the accessibility of those thoughts, relative to control conditions. Presumably, with repeated attempts to suppress distressing thoughts, a person learns what kinds of distracting ideas or activities are likely to work.

This research serves as a good starting point for making inferences about the mechanisms that allow dismissing–avoidant individuals to suppress attachment-related thoughts and feelings. We hypothesize that dismissing individuals, like other individuals who have developed strategies for suppressing neutral thoughts (Wegner, 1989) or bothersome thoughts (Kelly & Kahn, 1994), have repeatedly tried to suppress their attachment systems in the past (see the next section) and hence have developed efficient and implicit strategies for doing so successfully. Thus, when faced with a situation that might activate attachment-related anxiety, dismissing adults are able to focus their attention on thoughts that are unrelated to attachment-related issues. Of course, in order for such attentional processes to be successful, it is necessary that these thoughts be relatively dissociated from other thoughts that might activate the attachment system. In the next section we discuss the ways in which memory needs to be structured if defensive suppression is to be successful.

The Structure of Defensive Memory Systems

The success of suppression is dependent upon the organization of the mental structures representing undesirable thoughts and desirable thoughts. When undesirable thoughts and feelings are diffusely spread throughout the representational structures of the mind, it should be more difficult to avoid activating them—particularly when they are linked to representations of the self, significant others, and life goals and experiences. This idea is illustrated in Figure 10.2. As depicted in Case A, when attention is focused on thoughts that are not directly linked to unwanted thoughts, but are *indirectly* linked to them, those thoughts will be activated indirectly and unintentionally. However, when unwanted thoughts are relatively isolated from other associative networks, it is less likely that unwanted thoughts will become activated indirectly (see Case B in Figure 10.2).

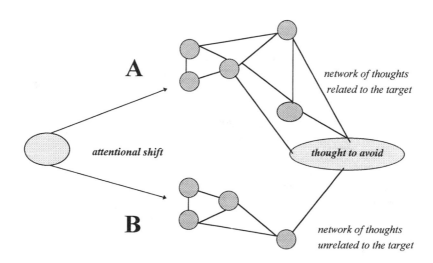

FIGURE 10.2. A graphic representation of two mental architectures that would lead to different outcomes during suppression. In Case A, attention is focused on thoughts that are indirectly associated with the unwanted thought. This increases the probability that activation will unintentionally spread to the very thought one is trying to suppress. In Case B, attention is focused on thoughts that are relatively unassociated with the unwanted thought. This substantially decreases the probability that the unwanted thoughts will become activated.

We propose that the architecture depicted in Case B characterizes the representational networks of dismissing–avoidant adults. If so, dismissing adults should be able to keep the attachment system relatively inactive by focusing on thoughts that are not associatively linked to attachment-related concerns. Thus, the way memory is structured plays a critical role in keeping the attachment system deactivated. Furthermore, because successful detachment results largely from the way memory is organized, suppression should be a fairly easy task for dismissing adults. Simply by focusing attention on something unrelated to attachment-related thoughts and feelings, they should be able to disengage their unwanted emotions. The *structure* of memory is doing most of the "work."

In their studies of repression, Hansen and Hansen (1988) proposed a mechanism similar to the one we are delineating here. Hansen and Hansen argue that one reason why repressive individuals recall fewer emotional memories is because these memories are relatively inaccessible for them.[2] This inaccessibility is thought to derive from the sparse number of associative connections between emotional memories and memories for other life experiences. As evidence for this argument, Hansen and Hansen conducted an experiment in which they asked subjects to retrieve memories that evoked feelings of anger, sadness, fear, and embarrassment. Generally, memories for emotionally significant events involve a rich mixture of dominant and nondominant emotional states (e.g., the recall of a sad memory often elicits the dominant emotion of sadness *and* the nondominant emotions of anger and anxiety). However, in this study, nondominant emotions were not experienced as strongly by repressive individuals as by other individuals. This finding suggests that repressors' memories for emotional events are not tightly connected to other emotional representations.

Other research on repressive individuals has led to similar conclusions. For instance, Davis (1987, 1990; Davis & Schwartz, 1987) found that repressive individuals recall fewer early childhood memories and take longer to retrieve the memories they do recall. These findings are consistent with the hypothesis that emotional memories are relatively dissociated from other memories in the minds of repressive individuals. Davis argues that these emotional memories are available but not easily accessible because of the paucity of associative interconnections. Once emotional memories are recalled by repressive individuals, however, these individuals are able to retrieve them later just as easily as nonrepressive individuals (see Davis, 1990).

As argued above, the structure of memory in dismissing adults is likely to be similar to that described by Hansen and Hansen (1988) for repressive adults. Thus, if memories that have the potential to activate the attachment system are not highly accessible in the memory structures of dismissing individuals, then the suppression of such memories should be fairly easy. It should be more difficult to make an inaccessible representation hyperaccessible than to make a relatively accessible thought hyperaccessible. Although no research has explicitly examined the organization of memory for dismissing–avoidant individuals, Mikulincer and his colleagues (Mikulincer & Orbach, 1995) have done some research on avoidant adults more generally that lends credibility to our hypothesis. Mikulincer and Orbach (1995) asked participants to recall early childhood memories specific to certain emotions (e.g., happiness, sadness, anger). They found that avoidant adults took longer to retrieve early childhood memories of negative experiences. Furthermore, similar to the Hansen and Hansen (1988) findings, the emotional memories recalled by avoidant individuals were not characterized by a diffuse array of nondominant emotions. Instead, these memories were specific to the particular emotion the avoidants had been asked to reflect upon. Unfortunately, this study did not examine *dismissing*-avoidance in particular and did not explore the distinction between attachment-related and nonattachment-related memories. Nevertheless, the findings lend credence to the hypothesis that the general representational networks of dismissing–avoidant adults are less likely to share connections with networks that might trigger emotional responses. It would be beneficial for future research to focus on dismissing-avoidance specifically and attempt to determine the ways in which memories for attachment-related experiences are organized for dismissing adults.

Attentional and Encoding Processes

If the structural organization of memory is a critical component in keeping the attachment system deactivated, it is important to understand the cognitive processes that give rise to that structural organization. Research strongly suggests that an individual's processing goals play a key role in the way information is consolidated in memory (Craik & Lockhart, 1972). For example, when people focus on specific features of a stimulus (e.g., semantic features), they are more likely to organize their memory of that stimulus around the feature that was attended to (Tulving & Thomson, 1973; Wyer & Srull, 1986). Similarly, when people process a stimulus in a way that involves reference to the self (Kuiper & Rogers, 1979), recall for that stimulus is enhanced. Such effects probably occur because the evaluation of self-relevant stimuli requires more elaborative processing (e.g., one needs to determine whether or not the information is threatening or favorable) and because information about the self has multiple links in memory, thereby providing more retrieval cues and pathways (Linville, 1982).

In order for attentional processes to support a defensively organized memory system, attention must be focused away from aspects of experience that may activate attachment-related thoughts and emotions. Dismissing–avoidant adults, therefore, will be less likely to incorporate attachment-related experiences into their self-concepts and less likely to elaborate on thoughts and feelings that partially activate attachment distress. By excluding attachment-related concerns from one's attentional focus, it becomes easier to maintain the relative deactivation of the attachment system.

Again, research on repressive personality styles illustrates how these attentional processes may operate to support a dissociated memory system. Hansen, Hansen, and Shantz (1992) conducted an experiment to determine whether the inaccessibility of the emotional memories for repressive individuals was due to the way the memories were encoded or the way they were retrieved. They presented subjects with facial expressions of emotion and asked them to rate the intensity of several different emotions that could have been associated with each expression. Repressors and nonrepressors rated the dominant emotional expressions equivalently. That is, facial expressions of sadness were rated as equally sad by both groups. However, repressors were less likely to rate these expressions as characteristic of nondominant emotional states (such as anxiety and anger). Thus, repressors do not focus on nondominant emotions when initially attending to an event. By limiting their attention to generalized, nonspecific features, they reduce the likelihood that specific emotional features will be incorporated into memory. Hence, the probability that specific emotional features will be recalled later is decreased.

Social and Interpersonal Processes

We argued earlier that when individuals are motivated to avoid attachment-related emotions, they will be less likely to attend to and elaborate upon events that may activate the attachment system. Over time, this process should lead to relatively dissociated memory systems for experiences related to attachment, emotions, and relationships. In addition to affecting the way memory becomes structured, defensive avoidance should affect the way an individual's caregiving, sexual, and attachment behavior becomes structured. Social interactions should reflect, and shape, the defensive organization of dismissing-avoidance.

Generally, behaviors involving intimate contact and caring are thought to facilitate attachment formation (Hazan & Zeifman, 1994). To prevent feelings of dependence and attachment, dismissing–avoidants may not allow themselves to engage in intimate behaviors with their romantic partners. We examined this hypothesis by administering Kunce and Shaver's (1994) caregiving scales, scales assessing sexual intimacy (Hazan, Zeifman, & Middleton, 1994), and Griffin and Bartholomew's (1994) RSQ measure of dismissing-avoidance to a sample of 100 dating students. The Kunce and Shaver scales assess four dimensions of romantic caregiving: cooperation versus control, proximity versus distance, compulsive caregiving, and sensitivity versus insensitivity. If dismissing–avoidant adults avoid caring for and supporting their partners as a way to maintain emotional distance, there should be negative correlations between dismissing-avoidance and scales tapping sensitive caring, cooperative caring, and proximity. Consistent with this hypothesis, dismissing-avoidance was negatively correlated with two of these caregiving dimensions (see Table 10.2). Specifically, dismissing participants reported being overly controlling and critical when helping their partners and reported pulling away when their partners needed support or comfort.

If dismissing adults avoid behaviors that facilitate attachment formation, dismissing-avoidance should be negatively correlated with preferences for sexual and physical intimacy—forms of behavior that may facilitate emotional bonding. Consistent with this prediction, dismissing-avoidance was negatively correlated with preferences for engaging in intimate behaviors such as holding hands, mutual gazing, cuddling, and kissing (see Table 10.2). There was also a tendency for dismissing-avoidance to be associated with the expression of less affection during sexual activities. Interestingly, dismissing–avoidant adults engaged in sexual activities with their partners just as frequently as did other participants. Thus, dismissing adults do not avoid sexual activity per se, but they do avoid the kind of intimacy that might facilitate emotional bonding, such as cuddling and expressing affection.

Finally, if dismissing–avoidant adults are avoiding experiences that might facilitate attachment formation or make them vulnerable to rejection, they should be less likely to use their romantic partners as attachment figures. According to Hazan and her colleagues (Hazan, Hutt,

TABLE 10.2. Correlations between Dismissing-Avoidance and Caregiving Styles and Sexual Behavior

	Dismissing-avoidance
Caregiving styles	
Cooperation versus control	−.33
Proximity versus distance	−.29
Compulsive caregiving	.05
Sensitivity versus insensitivity	.15
Physical intimacy	
Holding hands	−.44
Mutual gazing	−.29
Cuddling	−.34
Kissing	−.34
Feeling comfortable and safe when held	−.43
Discuss love for one another after sex	−.15
Have sex to express love and affection	−.17
Tell partner how much I love him/her during sex	−.23
My partner and I have sex frequently	.10

$n = 100$, $SE = .10$

Note. Dismissing-avoidance was measured with Griffin and Bartholomew's (1994) Relationship Styles Questionnaire (RSQ).

Sturgeon, & Bricker, 1991), the attachment figure serves as (1) a target for *proximity maintenance*, (2) a *safe haven* to turn to in times of distress, and (3) a *secure base* from which to explore the world. Thus, if dismissing adults are relatively unattached to their partners, we should find that their partners do not serve these functions for them. We examined this hypothesis in a sample of 217 dating undergraduates by administering a revised version of Hazan's WHOTO measure (Fraley & Davis, 1997; Hazan et al., 1991) and Griffin and Bartholomew's (1994) RSQ measure of dismissing-avoidance. Hazan's measure identifies the person to whom an individual is attached by asking various questions about who serves as a target for proximity-maintenance, safe haven, and secure base. Our revised version of the WHOTO is scored in way that allows us to determine the *extent* to which a particular target (in this case, a romantic partner) is used as an attachment figure (see Fraley & Davis, 1997, for a complete description of the measure). For instance, an individual who uses his or her partner as a secure base receives a higher score than an individual who uses his or her partner only as a target for proximity maintenance.

Consistent with the hypothesis that dismissing adults are less likely to establish attachment relationships with their partners, dismissing-avoidance was correlated negatively with the extent to which the romantic partner fulfilled the three attachment-related functions ($r = -.29$). Furthermore, there was a positive, although weak, correlation between dismissing-avoidance and using the *self* as a secure base ($r = .14$). Along similar lines, Fraley and Davis (1997) examined a sample of single adults and found that dismissing-avoidance was negatively correlated with using one's best friend as a secure base. Therefore, several lines of evidence indicate that dismissing–avoidant adults are less likely to form an attachment to their peers. Instead, it appears that there is a slight tendency for dismissing adults to rely on themselves as a secure base rather than relying on someone else.

To summarize, we believe that the defensive organization of attachment, caregiving, and sexual behavior serves to create and maintain the defensive memory structures that are hypothesized to characterize the minds of dismissing adults. By avoiding situations in which feelings of attachment or rejection may arise, it is less likely that dismissing adults will encode a wide variety of attachment-related experiences, ruminate and elaborate upon such experiences, and structure their values and goals around such experiences.

Derailing Attachment-Related Defenses

We have argued that dismissing defenses are fairly powerful because of their self-maintaining nature. Specifically, we argued that the desire to avoid attachment-related experiences leads to an underrepresentation of attachment-related memory structures. In turn, the paucity of attachment-related representations reduces the likelihood that dismissing–avoidant individuals will seek out and elaborate upon novel attachment-related experiences. Despite the powerful nature of this self-perpetuating organization, we suspect that there are certain circumstances in which it will break down. In particular, the system should be ineffective when dismissing adults are made to focus unwillingly on attachment-related events.

The Adult Attachment Interview (AAI) is a structured interview that requires people to reflect on their early attachment experiences and discuss their current views and interpretations of those experiences (George, Kaplan, & Main, 1985). Even if an individual would prefer not to think about these issues, the interview requires him or her to do so. Dozier and Kobak (1992) employed the AAI to examine the association between dismissing attachment and psychophysiology.[3] They found a positive correlation between dismissing attachment and physiological responses to questions that required interviewees to focus on early experiences of attachment and rejection. Their findings indicate that attachment-related experiences can lead to substantial arousal when a dismissing person is made to focus on thoughts that he or she would prefer to avoid.

Although defenses can break down when a person is made to focus on unwanted thoughts, we suspect that there are rarely moments in the context of natural interaction when dismissing individuals face such pressures. For example, in situations of separation or loss, dismissing adults can choose to ignore their partner or restrict their access to places, photos, or memories that serve as unpleasant reminders of that person. In such situations, dismissing individuals may experience some unavoidable anxiety and despair, but the degree of distress should be substantially less than that experienced by someone who is actively ruminating over a loss.

Summary and Suggestions for Future Research

In summary, we have suggested that dismissing adults are able to remain detached because of the defensive manner in which the systems mediating their memory, attentional processes, and social behavior are organized. We argued that the desire to avoid attachment-related emotions leads to a failure to attend to or elaborate upon attachment-related experiences. Furthermore, this goal prevents the dismissing individual from engaging in behaviors that might facilitate attachment formation, such as intimate physical contact, responsive caregiving, and emotional reliance on others. In conjunction, these attentional and social processes allow a person to create and maintain a dissociative memory system for attachment-related concerns and experiences.

Several aspects of the reasoning presented here require empirical scrutiny in the future. For example, if memories for attachment-related events are inaccessible and relatively dissociated for dismissing adults, then recall of these memories should result in longer retrieval latencies and fewer total recalled memories. Moreover, when these memories are recalled or made accessible, they should, for a short time at least, be just as accessible as nonattachment-related memories (cf. Davis, 1990).

Another testable prediction of the model concerns the autonomous nature of defense. Relative levels of detachment should be observed even when a dismissing individual lacks conscious control over his or her thoughts. Because the organization of long-term memory is *independent* of momentary changes in conscious goals and strategies, detachment should be effective even when the dismissing individual lacks the ability to consciously or explicitly control his or her thoughts.

Future research also needs to examine the conditions under which defenses do and do not work. As noted earlier, the Dozier and Kobak (1992) study indicates that dismissing strategies fail when an individual is forced to focus on disturbing topics. It is also possible that other factors interact with dismissing-avoidance to affect the success of defensive strategies. For example, the degree of attachment to a parent or romantic partner (Fraley & Davis, 1997; Hazan et al., 1991) should be a critical factor in how dismissing adults react to separation or loss. It may be that dismissing adults *do* become substantially distressed when they are emotionally invested in someone. In fact, such investments may help to explain why Dozier and Kobak observed physiological indications of distress in dismissing adults. These adults may have felt attached to their early caregivers or parents (the focus of the interview questions) even if they wanted to feel independent from them. However, in the case of romantic relationships (the focus of our studies), they may never allow themselves to become attached to their partners, in which case, defenses may be effective.

THE DEVELOPMENT OF
DISMISSING-AVOIDANCE

Up to this point, our discussion has focused mostly on the defensive organization of dismissing-avoidance in adulthood. To fully understand the role of defenses in adult attachment, it is necessary to address the factors that lead an individual to organize his or her thoughts and behaviors around the goal of intimacy avoidance. In this section, we propose a hypothesis about the development of this cognitive organization and dismissing-avoidance more generally.

Because the conceptualization of dismissing-avoidance has occurred only recently (Bartholomew, 1990), there have not been any longitudinal studies examining the etiology of this pattern of attachment. However, because the behavior of both dismissing–avoidant adults and avoidant infants appears to be organized around the same goal (i.e., avoidance of intimacy with and reliance upon others), it seems reasonable to assume that both patterns of avoidance share a common origin. Most of the research on insecure-avoidance in infancy has suggested that this attachment pattern can be traced to a history of experiences with a rejecting or insensitive caregiver (Isabella & Belsky, 1991; Kiser, Bates, Maslin, & Bayles, 1986; Lamb, Gaensbauer, Malkin, & Schultz, 1985; Main, 1990; Main & Weston, 1982). For example, Ainsworth and her colleagues (Ainsworth et al., 1978) found that maternal rejection, lack of maternal emotional expression, and unpleasant experiences related to close bodily contact, all assessed during home observations during the infant's first year of life, were predictors of insecure–avoidant attachment at 12 months of age.

According to attachment theory (Ainsworth et al., 1978; Bowlby, 1969/1982), the quality of the infant–caregiver relationship plays a critical role in shaping the expectations that the infant develops about the responsiveness of others and the worthiness of the self. When infants are exposed to warm, responsive, and sensitive caregiving, they are theorized to develop positive expectations about the availability and responsiveness of others and positive views of themselves as capable and worthy. When infants are exposed to rejection or emotional unresponsiveness, they are theorized to develop the expectation that others will not be available or responsive if needed. These expectations, or *working models*, are theorized to form the basis for the child's future interactions, influencing the way he or she interprets, initiates, and responds to social interactions with peers and adults (Pastor, 1981; Waters, Wippman, & Sroufe, 1979). When the child comes to expect that others will not be responsive to his or her needs, these expectations may promote the child's use of avoidant strategies, the development of compulsive self-reliance, and the expectation that others are unpredictable or unreliable.

Several studies have linked self-reliance (a component of adult dismissing-avoidance) to attachment classification at 12 months of age. For example, Berlin, Cassidy, and Belsky (1995) administered a loneliness questionnaire to 64 children ranging from 5 to 7 years of age. These authors found that children who were classified as insecure–avoidant at 12 months of age were less likely to report being lonely in early childhood. This suggests that there is a link between early childhood rejection (to the extent that it influences attachment classification) and the development of a model of the self as not needing others. Secondly, Cassidy (1988) asked 52 six-year-olds to tell a story in response to pictures depicting emotionally charged conflicts between a child and its mother. The stories told by avoidant children tended to minimize distress on the part of the child and to dismiss the parents as sources of comfort or support. These children also created stories in which the conflict was resolved by the child alone, without parental assistance. In other words, the avoidant children had developed a sense of self-reliance and an expectation that others could not, or need not, be counted on for support.

In addition to rejecting their infant's bids for closeness, the caregivers of avoidant infants actively discourage emotional expression (Bartholomew, 1990; Main, 1990; Main & Weston, 1982). According to Grossmann, Grossmann, and Schwan (1986), mothers of infants classified as insecure–avoidant in the strange situation were more likely to withdraw from their infants when the infants expressed negative affect. However, these mothers freely interacted with their infants when the infants were content. This interpersonal dynamic may encourage an infant to shut off his or her emotions as a way to maintain a caregiver's approval. Interestingly, Grossmann et al. (1986) also claimed that avoidant infants are less likely to communicate with their mothers when upset, suggesting that they learn how to regulate their emotional displays by deactivating or blocking their emotions. Over time, this habitual shutting-off process may have an effect on the way cognition and memory become organized.

According to several authors (Belsky, Steinberg, & Draper, 1991; Case, 1996; Cassidy & Kobak, 1988; Main & Weston, 1982), the avoidant pattern of attachment allows a child to maintain contact with an attachment figure under conditions in which the figure cannot be counted on for support. Under such conditions, avoidance may be an adaptive strategy. Main and Weston (1982) argued that the optimal strategy for maintaining proximity to a rejecting attachment figure is to conceal attachment-related distress, particularly in situations where the expression of attachment anxiety (such as crying, screaming, or clinging) is punished or differentially ignored. This is particularly likely to occur when the caregiver and infant inhabit a stressful environment. According to Belsky et al. (1991), contextual stress affects the caregiver's ability to provide responsive and warm support for the infant, which in turn affects the child's interpersonal development. These conditions are thought to influence the somatic development of the child and lead to early reproductive maturity and low-investment or short-term mating strategies during adolescence. According to Belsky et al. (1991), these mating strategies can be viewed as adaptive from an ultimate perspective, because they promote the net survival of offspring in an unstable or unpredictable environment.

Interestingly, there is some indication that the sexual strategies of dismissing–avoidant adults are similar to those that would be expected if, as children, they had been exposed to the kind of early caregiving environment discussed by Belsky et al. (1991). For example, Clark (1996) found an association between dismissing-avoidance and unrestricted sexuality (Simpson & Gangestad, 1992). Dismissing adults were more likely to believe that sex without love is acceptable and that multiple partners are preferable. Furthermore, the data reported here (see Table 10.2) indicate that the sexual strategies of dismissing–avoidants downplay the importance of intimacy and closeness, qualities strongly characteristic of a high-investment mating strategy.

In sum, factors that promote insecure-avoidance in infancy (such as parental rejection and stressful rearing environments) may also promote self-reliance, a central theme in the self-concept of dismissing–avoidant adults. Early manifestations of independence may allow a child to construct (at least implicitly) knowledge structures in which the self and goals are relatively dissociated from representations of attachment-related experiences. These autonomous attachment-related networks should, in turn, be less likely to become activated by other experiences, thereby allowing an individual to keep the attachment system in a relative state of deactivation. Additionally, the early discouragement of emotional expression may lead a child to try to shut off emotional states. With time, these attempts may become overlearned and allow the individual to deactivate the attachment system when attention is focused away from attachment-related issues. Collectively, the result of these developmental processes is proposed to be an emotional, cognitive, and behavioral organization that inhibits the formation of close, intimate attachments. An informal model of the proposed processes underlying the development of dismissing-avoidance is presented in Figure 10.3.

SIMILARITIES AND DIFFERENCES BETWEEN DISMISSING-AVOIDANCE AND THE REPRESSIVE PERSONALITY STYLE

In many ways, the dynamics of dismissing-avoidance are similar to those underlying the repressive personality style (Weinberger, Schwartz, & Davidson, 1979; Weinberger, 1990). For example, the attentional and memory processes of repressors (Hansen & Hansen, 1988; Hansen, Hansen, & Shantz, 1992) also appear to characterize those of dismissing adults. However, we believe that these defenses serve different goals in each case. We will briefly discuss ways in which the constructs of dismissing-avoidance and the repressive personality style differ.

Repressive individuals report low anxiety on self-report measures (i.e., the Manifest Anxiety Scale) but tend to score high on measures of social desirability (i.e., the Marlowe–Crowne Social Desirability Scale or Eysenck's Lie Scale). This suggests that their low levels of self-reported anxiety reflect defensiveness rather than a true absence of anxiety (Weinberger, 1990). Accordingly, Weinberger and his colleagues have shown that repressive individuals exhibit physiological arousal even when they deny experiencing distress (Asendorpf & Scherer, 1983; Weinberger et al., 1979).

Dismissing adults report low levels of anxiety about relationships. That is, they claim not to worry about abandonment. However, as we

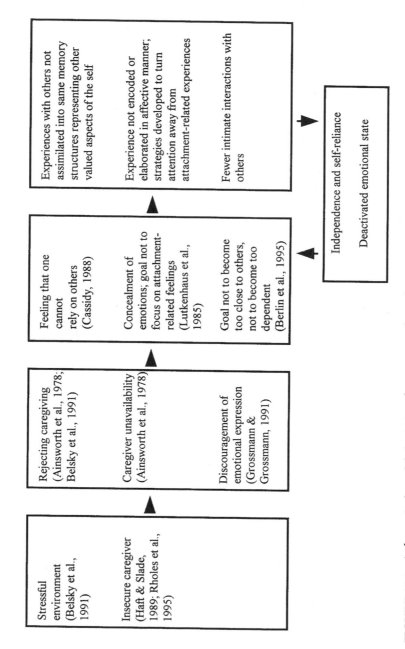

FIGURE 10.3. A theoretical model depicting the processes hypothesized to give rise to the defensive organization of the attachment system and, more specifically, to dismissing-avoidance.

argued earlier, these low levels of anxiety appear to be accurate reflections, rather than distortions, of latent emotional states. Because of the way the systems mediating attention, memory, and behavior have become organized for dismissing adults, these adults are actually able to deactivate their emotions when need be. Therefore, dismissing-avoidance should not correspond closely to the repressive personality style.

In Table 10.3 we present correlations between the attachment dimensions, the Manifest Anxiety Scale, and the Marlowe–Crowne Social Desirability scale. As can be seen, the Manifest Anxiety Scale is correlated moderately with Bartholomew's Anxiety dimension. However, the repressive pattern of low anxiety and high social desirability appears to correspond more strongly with security than with dismissing-avoidance.

These data indicate that the repressive personality style does not correspond to the construct of dismissing-avoidance. We suggest that these constructs differ because repressors are primarily concerned with being socially appropriate, whereas dismissing individuals are concerned with avoiding rejection by someone upon whom they could become emotionally dependent. Repressive adolescents are described by their classmates as being more likely to follow rules and more likely to adhere to socially appropriate standards (Weinberger, 1990). Moreover, repressors are thought to come from "very socially appropriate, *highly connected families*" (Weinberger, 1990, p. 375, emphasis added). In contrast, the evidence presented in the previous section suggests that dismissing adults do not come from "highly connected families." Instead, it appears that the families of dismissing individuals implicitly or explicitly encourage independence and self-reliance instead of connection. Furthermore, dismissing adults are likely to be rated as *hostile* by their peers (Kobak & Sceery, 1988)—a quality that may accompany extreme self-reliance, but not social appropriateness. We believe that the socially appropriate way to present oneself would be characterized by security and warmth, not hostility,

TABLE 10.3. Correlations between Attachment Styles and the Components of the Repressive Personality Style

Attachment style	Repressor components	
	Manifest anxiety	Social desirability
Secure	−.42	.23
Fearful	.37	−.15
Preoccupied	.29	−.22
Dismissing	.07	.21

$n = 117, SE = .09$

Note. Attachment styles were measured with Griffin and Bartholomew's (1994) Relationship Styles Questionnaire (RSQ). The components of repression were measured with the Marlowe–Crowne Social Desirability Scale and the Manifest Anxiety Scale. The repressive pattern (low anxiety, high social desirability) does not strongly characterize dismissing-avoidance. If anything, the pattern more closely resembles secure attachment.

introversion, coldness, and compulsive independence (Bartholomew & Horowitz, 1991; Kobak & Sceery, 1988).

In summary, although the mechanisms of defense may be similar for repressors and dismissing adults, the functions that these mechanisms serve are different. In the case of repressive adults, they maintain socially acceptable emotional facades. In the case of dismissing-avoidance, they help to deactivate the attachment system by preventing emotional attachment.

SUMMARY AND FINAL COMMENTS

When Bowlby (1980, Chapter 4) was attempting to outline his information processing theory of defense in the late 1970s, he was constrained by the cognitive and personality theories available at the time. For example, it was widely held that repression was a process that required a special vigilance mechanism or filtering device (Erdelyi, 1974, 1985, 1993). Inspired by evidence purported to demonstrate that information was screened, evaluated, and censored by an unconscious monitoring system (Dixon, 1971; Norman, 1976), Bowlby hypothesized that repression is a critical component to successful defense.

Since the late 1970s, the fields of personality and cognitive science have greatly advanced. For example, current theories of repression neither postulate nor require a special filtering device to select and censor threatening information (e.g., Hansen & Hansen, 1988). Moreover, many writers in cognitive psychology have called into question early research on perceptual vigilance and autonomous filtering systems (Baddeley, 1990; Bower, 1990; Holmes, 1990; Loftus & Ketcham, 1994; Schacter, 1996). If Bowlby were alive today, he might well revise his ideas about defense to make them more consistent with what we currently know about the brain and cognition.

In this chapter we, like Bowlby, have tried to delineate the mechanisms underlying defense within a framework provided by our contemporaries in the cognitive sciences. We have hypothesized that the adult pattern of dismissing-avoidance is rooted in early childhood experiences with rejecting, unpredictable, or inexpressive caregivers. These experiences have been shown to be associated with the development of self-reliance and repeated attempts to conceal attachment-related distress—critical facets in the conceptualization of adult dismissing-avoidance (Bartholomew, 1990). We believe that these experiences set the stage for the habitual redirection of attention away from attachment-related issues during stressful episodes and thus facilitate the construction of relatively isolated representations of attachment-related experiences in memory. Because of this organization of memory, dismissing–avoidant adults are able to deactivate cognitive and emotional components of their attachment systems. In conjunction, these processes and structures operate to create and maintain a self-perpetuating and resilient defensive psychology.

ACKNOWLEDGMENTS

We would like to thank Jim Cassandro, Catherine Clark, Steve Rholes, Jeff Simpson, and Caroline Tancredy for their helpful comments and suggestions on previous drafts of this chapter.

NOTES

1. As can be seen in Figure 10.1, the theoretical patterns of dismissing-avoidance and preoccupation are psychological opposites of one another. Because of space limitations we will not discuss preoccupation per se; however, it should be noted that the processes and mechanisms we discuss with respect to dismissing-avoidance apply to preoccupation inversely.

2. Repressive individuals are those who score low on self-report measures of anxiety but also score high on measures of social desirability.

3. Unfortunately, it is not yet clear how dismissingness scored from the AAI compares to dismissingness scored from self-reports. For the purposes of the present chapter, we assume that both measures are tapping the same latent psychological organization.

REFERENCES

Ainsworth, M. D. S., Blehar, M. C., Waters, E., & Wall, S. (1978). *Patterns of attachment.* Hillsdale, NJ: Erlbaum.

Asendorpf, J. B., & Scherer, K. R. (1983). The discrepant repressor: Differentiation between low anxiety, high anxiety, and repression of anxiety by autonomic–facial–verbal patterns of behavior. *Journal of Personality and Social Psychology, 45,* 1334–1346.

Baddeley, A. (1990). *Human memory.* Boston, MA: Allyn & Bacon.

Bartholomew, K. (1990). Avoidance of intimacy: An attachment perspective. *Journal of Social and Personal Relationships, 7,* 147–178.

Bartholomew, K., & Horowitz, L. M. (1991). Attachment styles among young adults: A test of a four-category model. *Journal of Personality and Social Psychology, 61,* 226–244.

Belsky, J., Steinberg, L., & Draper, P. (1991). Childhood experience, interpersonal development, and reproductive strategy: An evolutionary theory of socialization. *Child Development, 62,* 647–670.

Berlin, L. J., Cassidy, J., & Belsky, J. (1995). Loneliness in young children and infant–mother attachment: A longitudinal study. *Merrill–Palmer Quarterly, 41,* 91–103.

Bower, G. H. (1990). Awareness, the unconscious, and repression: An experimental psychologist's perspective. In J. L. Singer (Ed.), *Repression and dissociation:*

Implications for personality theory, psychopathology, and health (pp. 209–231). Chicago: University of Chicago Press.

Bowlby, J. (1980). *Attachment and loss: Vol. 3. Loss: Sadness and depression.* New York: Basic Books.

Bowlby, J. (1982). *Attachment and loss: Vol. 1. Attachment.* New York: Basic Books. (Original work published 1969)

Case, R. (1996). The role of psychological defense in the representation and regulation of close personal relationships across the life span. In G. G. Noam & K. W. Fischer (Eds.), *Development and vulnerability in close relationships* (pp. 59–88). Mahwah, NJ: Erlbaum.

Cassidy, J. (1988). Child–mother attachment and the self in six-year-olds. *Child Development, 59,* 121–134.

Cassidy, J., & Kobak, R. R. (1988). Avoidance and its relation to other defensive processes. In J. Belsky & T. Nezworski (Eds.), *Clinical implications of attachment theory* (pp. 300–323). Hillsdale, NJ: Erlbaum.

Clark, C. L. (1996). *Strategic behaviors in romantic relationship initiation.* Unpublished manuscript. University of California, Davis.

Craik, F. I. M., & Lockhart, R. S. (1972). Levels of processing: A framework for memory research. *Journal of Verbal Learning and Verbal Behavior, 11,* 671–684.

Cramer, P. (1987). The development of defense mechanisms. *Journal of Personality, 55,* 597–614.

Davis, P. J. (1987). Repression and the inaccessibility of affective memories. *Journal of Personality and Social Psychology, 53,* 585–593.

Davis, P. J. (1990). Repression and the inaccessibility of affective memories. In J. L. Singer (Ed.), *Repression and dissociation: Implications for personality theory, psychopathology, and health* (pp. 387–403). Chicago: University of Chicago Press.

Davis, J. P., & Schwartz, G. E. (1987). Repression and the inaccessibility of affective memories. *Journal of Personality and Social Psychology, 52,* 155–163.

DePaulo, B. M., Lanier, K., & Davis, T. (1983). Detecting the deceit of the motivated liar. *Journal of Personality and Social Psychology, 45,* 1096–1103.

Dixon, N. F. (1971). *Subliminal perception: The nature of a controversy.* London: McGraw-Hill.

Dozier, M., & Kobak, R. R. (1992). Psychophysiology in attachment interviews: Converging evidence for deactivating strategies. *Child Development, 63,* 1473–1480.

Ekman, P., & Friesen, W. V. (1975). *Unmasking the face.* Englewood Cliffs, NJ: Prentice-Hall.

Erdelyi, M. H. (1974). A new look at the New Look: Perceptual defense and vigilance. *Psychological Review, 81,* 1–25.

Erdelyi, M. H. (1985). *Psychoanalysis: Freud's cognitive psychology.* New York: Freeman.

Erdelyi, M. H. (1993). Repression: The mechanism and the defense. In D. M. Wegner & J. W. Pennebaker (Eds.), *Handbook of mental control* (pp. 126–148). Englewood Cliffs, NJ: Prentice Hall.

Fraley, R. C., & Davis, K. E. (1997). Attachment formation and transfer in young adults' close friendships and romantic relationships. *Personal Relationships, 4,* 131–144.

Fraley, R. C., Davis, K. E., & Shaver, P. R. (1995). *Attachment behavior and relationship dissolution.* Unpublished manuscript, University of California, Davis.

Fraley, R. C., & Shaver, P. R. (1997a). *Airport separations: A naturalistic study of adult attachment dynamics in separating couples.* Manuscript submitted for publication.

Fraley, R. C., & Shaver, P. R. (1997b). Adult attachment and the suppression of unwanted thoughts. *Journal of Personality and Social Psychology, 73.*

Freud, A., & Burlingham, D. (1974). *Infants without families and reports on the Hampstead Nurseries 1939–1945.* London: Hogarth.

George, C., Kaplan, N., & Main, M. (1985). *The Adult Attachment Interview.* Unpublished manuscript, Department of Psychology, University of California, Berkeley.

Greenwald, A. G., & Banaji, M. R. (1995). Implicit social cognition: Attitudes, self-esteem, and stereotypes. *Psychological Review, 102,* 4–27.

Griffin, D. W., & Bartholomew, K. (1994). The metaphysics of measurement: The case of adult attachment. In K. Bartholomew & D. Perlman (Eds.), *Advances in personal relationships* (Vol. 5, pp. 17–52). London: Jessica Kingsley.

Gross, J. J., & Levenson, R. W. (1993). Emotional suppression: Physiology, self-report, and expressive behavior. *Journal of Personality and Social Psychology, 64,* 970–986.

Grossmann, K. E., & Grossmann, K. (1991). Attachment quality as an organizer of emotional and behavioral responses in a longitudinal perspective. In C. M. Parkes, J. Stevenson-Hinde, & P. Marris (Eds.), *Attachment across the life cycle* (pp. 124–171). New York: Cambridge University Press.

Grossmann, K. E., Grossmann, K., & Schwan, A. (1986). Capturing the wider view of attachment: A reanalysis of Ainsworth's Strange Situation. In C. E. Izard & P. B. Read (Eds.), *Measuring emotions in infants and children* (Vol. 2). Cambridge, England: Cambridge University Press.

Haft, W. L., & Slade, A. (1989). Affect attunement and maternal attachment: A pilot study. *Infant Mental Health Journal, 10,* 157–172.

Hansen, C. H., Hansen, R. D., & Shantz, D. W. (1992). Repression at encoding: Discrete appraisals of emotional stimuli. *Journal of Personality and Social Psychology, 63,* 1026–1035.

Hansen, R. D., & Hansen, C. H. (1988). Repression of emotionally tagged memories: The architecture of less complex emotions. *Journal of Personality and Social Psychology, 55,* 811–818.

Harrigan, J. A., Harrigan, K. M., Sale, B. A., & Rosenthal, R. (1996). Detecting anxiety and defensiveness from visual and auditory cues. *Journal of Personality, 64,* 675–709.

Hazan, C., Hutt, M. J., Sturgeon, J., & Bricker, T. (1991, April). *The process of relinquishing parents as attachment figures.* Paper presented at the biennial meeting of the Society for Research in Child Development, Seattle, WA.

Hazan, C., & Shaver, P. R. (1987). Romantic love conceptualized as an attachment process. *Journal of Personality and Social Psychology, 59,* 511–524.

Hazan, C., & Zeifman, D. (1994). Sex and the psychological tether. In K. Bartholomew & D. Perlman (Eds.), *Advances in personal relationships* (Vol. 5, pp. 151–180). London: Jessica Kingsley.

Hazan, C., Zeifman, D., & Middleton, K. (1994, July). *Adult romantic attachment, affection, and sex.* Paper presented at the 7th International Conference on Personal Relationships, Groningen, The Netherlands.

Heinicke, C., & Westheimer, I. (1966). *Brief separations.* New York: International Universities Press.

Holmes, D. S. (1990). The evidence for repression: An examination of sixty years of research. In J. L. Singer (Ed.), *Repression and dissociation: Implications for personality theory, psychopathology, and health* (pp. 85–102). Chicago: University of Chicago Press.

Isabella, R. A., & Belsky, J. (1991). Interactional synchrony and the origins of infant–mother attachment: A replication study. *Child Development, 62,* 373–384.

Kelly, A. E., & Kahn, J. H. (1994). Effects of suppression on personal intrusive thoughts. *Journal of Personality and Social Psychology, 66,* 998–1006.

Kiser, L. J., Bates, J. E., Maslin, C., & Bayles, K. (1986). Mother–infant play at six months as a predictor of attachment security at thirteen months. *Journal of the American Academy of Child Psychiatry, 25,* 68–75.

Kobak, R. R., & Sceery, A. (1988). Attachment in late adolescence: Working models, affect regulation, and representations of self and others. *Child Development, 59,* 135–146.

Koriat, A., Melkman, R., Averill, J. R., & Lazarus, R. S. (1972). The self-control of emotional reactions to a stressful film. *Journal of Personality, 40,* 601–619.

Kuiper, N. A., & Rogers, T. B. (1979). Encoding of personal information: Self-other differences. *Journal of Personality and Social Psychology, 37,* 499–514.

Kunce, L. J., & Shaver, P. R. (1994). An attachment-theoretical approach to caregiving in romantic relationships. In K. Bartholomew & D. Perlman (Eds.), *Advances in personal relationships* (Vol. 5, pp. 205–237). London: Jessica Kingsley.

Lamb, M. E., Gaensbauer, T. J., Malkin, C. M., & Schultz, L. A. (1985). The effects of child maltreatment on security of infant–adult attachment. *Infant Behavior and Development, 8,* 35–45.

Linville, P. W. (1982). Affective consequences of complexity regarding the self and others. In M. S. Clark & S. T. Fiske (Eds.), *Affect and cognition* (pp. 79–109). Hillsdale, NJ: Erlbaum.

Loftus, E., & Ketcham, K. (1994). *The myth of repressed memory: False memories and allegations of sexual abuse.* New York: St. Martin's Press.

Lutkenhaus, P., Grossmann, K. E., & Grossmann, K. (1985). Infant–mother attachment at 12 months and style of interaction with a stranger at the age of 3 years. *Child Development, 56,* 1538–1542.

Main, M. (1990). Parental aversion to infant-initiated contact is correlated with the parent's own rejection during childhood. In K. E. Barnard & T. B. Brazleton (Eds.), *Touch: The foundation of experience* (pp. 461–495). Madison, CT: International Universities Press.

Main, M., & Weston, D. R. (1982). Avoidance of the attachment figure in infancy: Descriptions and interpretations. In C. M. Parkes & J. Stevenson-Hinde (Eds.), *The place of attachment in human behavior* (pp. 31–59). New York: Basic Books.

Mikulincer, M., & Orbach, I. (1995). Attachment styles and repressive defensiveness: The accessibility and architecture of affective memories. *Journal of Personality and Social Psychology, 68,* 917–925.

Norman, D. A. (1976). *Memory and attention: Introduction to human information processing* (2nd ed.). New York: Wiley.

Pastor, D. L. (1981). The quality of mother–infant attachment and its relationship to toddlers' sociability with peers. *Developmental Psychology, 17,* 821–829.

Reiser, M. (1990). *Memory in mind and brain.* New York: Basic Books.

Rholes, W. S., Simpson, J. A., Blakely, B. S., Lanigan, L., & Allen, E. A. (1995). *Adult attachment styles, the desire to have children, and working models of parenthood.* Unpublished manuscript, Texas A & M University.

Robertson, J. (Producer). (1952). *A two-year-old goes to the hospital* [Film]. London: Tavistock Child Development Research Unit.

Schacter, D. L. (1996). *Searching for memory.* New York: Basic Books.

Simpson, J. A., & Gangestad, S. W. (1992). Sociosexuality and romantic partner choice. *Journal of Personality, 60,* 31–51.

Spangler, G., & Grossmann, K. E. (1993). Biobehavioral organization in securely and insecurely attached infants. *Child Development, 64,* 1439–1450.

Sroufe, L. A., & Waters, E. (1977). Heart rate as a convergent measure in clinical and developmental research. *Merrill–Palmer Quarterly, 23,* 3–27.

Tulving, E., & Thomson, D. M. (1973). Encoding specificity and retrieval processes in episodic memory. *Psychological Review, 80,* 352–373.

Waters, E., Matas, L., & Sroufe, L. A. (1975). Infants' reactions to an approaching stranger: Description, validation, and functional significance of wariness. *Child Development, 46,* 348–356.

Waters, E., Wippman, J., & Sroufe, L. A. (1979). Attachment, positive affect, and competence in the peer group: Two studies in construct validation. *Child Development, 50,* 821–829.

Wegner, D. M. (1989). *White bears and other unwanted thoughts: Suppression, obsession, and the psychology of mental control.* New York: Guilford Press.

Wegner, D. M. (1994). Ironic processes of mental control. *Psychological Review, 101,* 34–52.

Wegner, D. M., & Erber, R. (1992). The hyperaccessibility of suppressed thoughts. *Journal of Personality and Social Psychology, 63,* 903–912.

Wegner, D. M., & Gold, D. B. (1995). Fanning old flames: Emotional and cognitive effects of suppressing thoughts of a past relationship. *Journal of Personality and Social Psychology, 68,* 782–792.

Wegner, D. M., Schneider, D. J., Carter, S., III, & White, L. (1987). Paradoxical effects of thought suppression. *Journal of Personality and Social Psychology, 58,* 409–418.

Weinberger, D. A. (1990). The construct validity of the repressive coping style. In J. L. Singer (Ed.), *Repression and dissociation: Implications for personality theory, psychopathology, and health* (pp. 337–386). Chicago: University of Chicago Press.

Weinberger, D. A., Schwartz, G. E., & Davidson, R. J. (1979). Low-anxious, high-anxious, and repressive coping styles: Psychometric patterns and behavioral and physiological responses to stress. *Journal of Abnormal Psychology, 88,* 369–380.

Wyer, R. S., Jr., & Srull, T. K. (1986) Human cognition in its social context. *Psychological Review, 93,* 322–359.

11

Childhood Revisited

*The Intimate Relationships
of Individuals from Divorced
and Conflict-Ridden Families*

KATE HENRY
JOHN G. HOLMES

Attachment theorists assume that early "family of origin" experiences affect one's functioning in romantic relationships. More specifically, they postulate that familial experiences engender internal *working models* that continue to shape interpersonal response patterns in adulthood (Bowlby, 1977). For example, individuals with dismissing orientations—with positive self and negative other models—have been hypothesized to have had parents who discouraged the expression of negative affect (Bartholomew, 1990).

However, there is little "objective" empirical support for their position. While there are notable exceptions (e.g., Sroufe, Egeland, & Kreutzer, 1990), the association between early experiences and later attachment representations has been explored largely through retrospective accounts, for example, via clinical interviews (e.g., Main & Goldwyn, in press). This approach is problematic, as reports are likely to be biased significantly by current attitudes about relationships (Ross, 1989), making it difficult to determine whether one is obtaining a realistic portrayal of childhood experience. Accordingly, we felt it important to take advantage of less *subjective* markers of disruptions in family life, for example parental divorce.

The purpose of the present chapter is to discuss our investigation of the working models of adult children from divorced families (Divorce Individuals). We begin by describing the rationale behind our interest in this population. We also present a theory that accounts for discrepant findings in the divorce literature. Finally, we describe the way in which we tested our predictions. The implications of our results for attachment theory are discussed.

LONG-TERM EFFECTS OF DIVORCE

Our interest in Divorce Individuals represents a shift from the primacy of parent–child relationships in attachment theorizing. Specifically, we raise the possibility that working models can be shaped via observation of parents' marital relationships. We view the marital bond as an important source of influence on the development of attachment representations, a possible template for views of self and other in later romantic involvements. For example, we suspect that witnessing the erosion of a couple's love and trust tarnishes children's working models of adult attachment bonds. This is not to say that divorce may not affect the attachment system more directly, for example, by contaminating the relationship between parents and their children. On the contrary, children's relationships with their noncustodial parents seem particularly vulnerable to being compromised. Instead, it is our contention that both aspects of the divorce experience place Divorce Individuals at risk of developing negative general models of relationships.

There is some preliminary evidence to support our predictions. Relative to individuals from intact families (Intact Individuals), Divorce Individuals are generally more pessimistic about the future of potential involvements. For example, they envision themselves (1) being less trusting of hypothetical spouses (Brennan, 1994; Franklin, Janoff-Bulman, & Roberts, 1990) and (2) having less successful marriages (Franklin et al., 1990; Henry & Holmes, 1994) and dating relationships (Brennan, 1994).

However, the divorce literature is unclear as to whether their working models actually influence interpersonal adjustment. For example, while they have a higher divorce rate relative to their intact counterparts (Amato & Keith, 1991), this may not reflect relationship dysfunction per se, but instead, more accepting or permissive attitudes regarding divorce (e.g., Glenn & Kramer, 1987; Greenberg & Nay, 1982). That is, relative to Intact Individuals, they may be more likely to see divorce as a viable solution to interpersonal difficulties. Equally unenlightening are studies that look more specifically at relationship quality. For example, while Wallerstein and Blakeslee (1989) found Divorce Individuals to be extremely anxious about relationships—to be preoccupied with fears of abandonment and betrayal—the methodological weaknesses in their design made it difficult for researchers to be confident about the validity of their results. Particularly damaging was their failure to compare Divorce Individuals' responses to those of appropriate control groups.

In spite of the study's flaws, Wallerstein's findings continue to receive considerable attention in the popular press. Indeed, we are reluctant to dismiss her results, given their intuitive appeal. In light of their histories, it would be surprising if Divorce Individuals did *not* struggle with trust and commitment. The empirical fact remains, however, that we cannot be certain if their difficulties differentiate them from other groups. In fact, when more rigorous methodologies are used, Divorce Individuals appear similar to their intact counterparts. More specifically, they are just as happy, committed, trusting, and optimistic about the future of their relationships (Brennan & Shaver; 1993; Glenn & Kramer, 1987; Guttman, 1989; Henry & Holmes, 1994).

The literature thus presents us with a seemingly contradictory pattern of results. Which set of findings are we to believe? Are the negative general models of Divorce Individuals detrimental to interpersonal functioning (Wallerstein & Blakeslee, 1989), or have they found ways to effectively insulate themselves from their potential influence?

A SPECIFIC VULNERABILITY PERSPECTIVE

We argue that the answer lies between these extreme positions—that while pessimistic models undoubtedly intrude, they are not pervasive in their effects on interpersonal functioning. More specifically, we suggest that general negative expectations coexist with more positive schemas regarding current partners—schemas that have been shaped by experiences within the present relationship. In fact, we argue that it is these specific models that most frequently guide interpersonal perceptions (Collins & Read, 1994).

At the same time, we suspect that there exist areas of vulnerability—Achilles heels—that enable general models to usurp the influence of these dominant representations. These models are likely activated by events that recapitulate the most salient psychological features of the divorce experience—for example, "being left." Consider that, as children, Divorce Individuals observe one partner desert another. Moreover, they themselves are " left" by their noncustodial parents—in most cases, their fathers. As a result, they may magnify the perceived threat of abandonment in their own relationships—exaggerate the probability that their partners will leave *them*.

Divorce Individuals' hypothesized abandonment concerns suggest a preoccupied orientation toward relationships (Bartholomew, 1990; Shaver & Hazan, 1988), an orientation characterized by negative self and positive other models. Indeed, we expect to find this pattern more frequently among Divorce Individuals. We develop the rationale for this prediction more fully as the chapter unfolds; briefly, however, we view preoccupation as the legacy of the divorce experience. It is our contention that the event spawns marked concerns regarding one's worthiness in the eyes of partners.

But to what extent are Divorce Individuals' fears realized? Do they, in fact, recapitulate their parents' relationships? Are they more likely to be left? We conducted a longitudinal study to begin to answer these questions. Specifically, the study was designed to (1) uncover the content of Divorce Individuals' attachment representations, (2) identify the situations that precipitate their activation, and (3) document their effects on relationship functioning.

THE EFFECTS OF MARITAL CONFLICT

An important issue in designing the project concerned the selection of appropriate control groups. We wished to compare Divorce Individuals with individuals from intact families. But, given the heterogeneity of this population, we felt it important to distinguish between those who had (1) happily married parents, and (2) parents who had conflictual relationships (Conflict Individuals).

There are two main reasons for the latter groups' inclusion. First, the relative merits of separation versus exposure to continuing conflict have been the subject of much recent speculation. For example, in February 1995, *Time* magazine featured an article on the growing trend to strengthen marriage and prevent divorce for the sake of the children (Gleick, 1995). In July of the same year, the *Toronto Globe and Mail* (Philp, 1995) advised parents that their children would be better off if the family remained together, even if their marital relationship remained troubled or conflictual. In contrast, theorists have argued that prolonged exposure to conflict may be more detrimental than divorce to later functioning in relationships (e.g., Booth, Brinkerhoff, & White, 1984; Emery, 1982; Enos & Handal, 1986)—in other words, that it is conflict, not breakup, that predicts long-term adjustment. At the present time, there is very little evidence to support either position. As far as we know, the present study is the first to examine this issue empirically—to investigate whether being left or witnessing conflict is the seminal psychological experience.

Second, the conflict group is interesting in and of itself. Like their Divorce counterparts, Conflict Individuals enable us to test the hypothesized link between working models and familial experience. We would expect them to have developed negative attachment representations. However, rather than being preoccupied, like other researchers (e.g., Bartholomew, 1990; Belsky, Steinberg, & Draper, 1991) we predict a predominantly fearful orientation toward relationships. Why might this be the case? Why would they become avoidant, fearful of closeness and intimacy?

Consider that, to Conflict Individuals, conflict may seem an inevitable part of adult relationships. After all, they are exposed to frequent and intense fighting throughout their childhood. Given that most children are disturbed by parental strife, so disturbed in fact that they often attempt to intervene (e.g., by getting in the middle of their parents' fights or misbehaving to distract parents from their negative interactions), it would not be surprising if they developed defense mechanisms that enabled them to avoid experiencing further anxiety and emotional pain—more specifically, attachment representations that steered them away from romantic involvements.

THEORETICAL IMPLICATIONS

Given the likely similarities between the groups' early experiences (e.g., parental conflict, decreased availability on the part of maritally distressed caregivers), our anticipation of differences in Conflict Individuals' working models sets us apart from predictions that might be offered by object relations theorists (see Baldwin, 1992). While Bowlby (1977) stressed that model shifts may take place during childhood and adolescence, these theorists have argued that it is children's initial interactions with caregivers—more specifically, those that occur before they reach age 2—that mold representations of attachment. If this were the case, later developments in the parents' relationship (e.g., divorce vs. continued strife) would be largely irrelevant as far as working models were concerned. That is, they would do little to alter the content engendered during the critical period. Our inclusion of the "high parental conflict" group enables us to challenge this commonly held assumption, and provide some empirical support for Bowlby's notion that working models remain malleable at later stages of development.

To summarize, we predict fearfulness in Conflict Individuals: that is, negative models of both self and other. However, the extent of the influence of these representations remains to be seen. We expect Conflict Individuals to be vulnerable to conflict, for example, to exaggerate its association with dysfunction. Moreover, like Divorce Individuals, we anticipate that they will fear recapitulating their parents' relationship. But, it is unclear whether Conflict Individuals' models will pervasively shape their interpersonal response patterns. For example, will they be the lenses of relationship perception, or will Conflict Individuals, too, develop more positive schemas that usurp the influence of these negative general models?

METHOD

Selection Criteria

While Conflict Individuals' inclusion in our study was important for theoretical reasons, they were more difficult to identify relative to the divorce group, as they lacked an objective outcome variable to mark familial disruption (i.e., parents' marital status). As a result, recruitment was based on retrospective accounts of participants' parents' relationship.

Given the problems with this approach, we did our best to minimize memory biases. For example, we used behavioral criteria to avoid evaluative judgments regarding the nature of parental interactions. More specifically, we had participants rate the frequency and intensity of parental conflict during childhood. This Conflict Severity Index (CSI) had excellent internal consistency and test–retest reliability over a period of 4 weeks (alphas = .94 and .95, respectively), indicating that participants' recollections were extremely stable over time. Moreover, we had participants complete the index in an independent context in order to ensure that their accounts of their present relationships did not skew their recall of their parents' marital quality. Our measure was embedded in a booklet of questionnaires that was used by other researchers for the purpose of participant selection. This booklet was completed approximately 1 month prior to being recruited for our research project.

In addition, we adopted extremely conservative selection criteria to discriminate between individuals from high and low conflict families. Individuals were defined as Conflict Individuals if their scores on each item of the CSI exceeded the midpoint of the 7-point Likert scale—that is, if they indicated that their parents fought more frequently and intensely than most couples. Researchers have found it difficult to get participants to admit that their parents' relationship was more troubled than that of the average couple. Thus, we can be relatively confident that our group of Conflict Individuals were, indeed, exposed to considerable interparental strife as children. Individuals were defined as Intact Individuals if their scores on each item fell below the midpoint of the scale. The reader will note that, in using these criteria, we ensured that there would be no overlap between the intact groups. Conflict Individuals had to score 50% higher than Intacts on the CSI. Moreover, the difference in their group means was highly significant (*Ms* for Intact Individuals and Conflict Individuals = 3.12 and 10.72, respectively; $p < .001$).

Some may regard our CSI as a poor marker of familial disruption. In fact, it may be argued that our selection criteria would result in heterogeneous groups. For example, the CSI may include Conflict Individuals whose parents fought intensely, yet were happy with one another, and Intacts whose parents fought rarely, yet had strained relationships. However, there were very strong correlations between the CSI and measures that required participants to rate the quality of their parents' relationship (rs = .90 and .86)—the more conflictual the relationship, the more likely Conflict Individuals were to describe their parents as being dissatisfied with one another.

Sample

The sample for our longitudinal study consisted of 101 Divorce Individuals (62 females , 40 males), 65 Conflict Individuals (47 females, 18 males), and 98 Intact Individuals (62 females and 36 males). All of our participants were enrolled in an introductory psychology course at the University of Waterloo (mean age = 19.7 years). We felt it important to examine the relationships of individuals in late adolescence/early adulthood as this is the period where Divorce Individuals' anxieties about relationships have been reported to emerge (Wallerstein & Blakeslee, 1989). In order to participate, individuals had to be involved in a serious dating relationship. On average, participants had been seeing their partners for 19.7 months, and 3.8% of our sample were engaged, while 3.8% were living together. All other participants were dating exclusively, but living apart.

Procedure

At Time 1, participants were given a comprehensive booklet of questionnaires containing measures that assessed their general models of relationships—for example, their models of self and other and general relationship beliefs—as well as schemas that were specific to their relationships with current partners. Relationship-specific scales included traditional indices of relationship functioning—for example, satisfaction, trust, commitment, and conflict style—and measures that we developed to assess specific areas of vulnerability. Six months later, participants completed an abridged version of the original questionnaire.

On both occasions, participants were administered measures that assessed their attachment orientations. First, they were given a 21-item dimensional scale that required them to indicate their feelings toward romantic partners in general. In developing this measure, we included items used by a variety of other researchers (e.g., Brennan & Shaver, 1993; Carnelley, Pietromonaco, & Jaffe, 1994; Collins & Read, 1990; Simpson, Rholes, & Phillips, 1996), as well as additional statements that tapped the anxiety dimension.

Factor analyses revealed that our measure assessed the constructs that have been identified as important markers of attachment orientations (see Griffin & Bartholomew, 1994). The first factor assessed the anxiety dimension—the extent to which individuals worried about romantic partners' feelings for them. Individuals scoring highly on this 8-item subscale endorsed statements such as "I often worry partners will not want to stay with me," and "I sometimes worry that others do not value me as much as I value them." The second factor assessed the avoidant dimension—the extent to which individuals shunned interpersonal closeness in relationships. Individuals scoring highly on this 12-item subscale endorsed statements such as "I find it difficult to allow myself to depend on others," and "Often, love partners want me to be more intimate than I feel comfortable being." These factors were extremely reliable (Cronbach alphas = .88 and .81, respectively); indeed, our Anxiety dimension was more internally consistent than measures used in previous research (e.g., Collins & Read, 1990; Simpson et al., 1996).

In addition to our dimensional measure, participants completed Bartholomew and Horowitz's (1991) Relationship Questionnaire (RSQ). They were required to rate the extent to which four prototypical descriptions captured their interpersonal style in relationships. One of the reasons for including the RSQ was to examine the relationship between Bartholomew's self and other axes, and our attachment dimensions.[1] In a recent article Simpson et al. (1996) accumulated evidence that suggested that these axes were largely synonymous with their anxiety and avoidant subscales. We obtained patterns of correlations that supported this interpretation. Like Simpson et al.'s, our anxiety subscale appeared to be a measure of individuals' models of self—the extent to which they possessed negative views of themselves in relationships (rs = −.65 and −.13 with Bartholomew's self and other axes, respectively). We keyed items such that higher scores on this dimension indicated more negative self-representations. In contrast, the avoidance subscale reflected participants' orientation toward significant others (rs = −.22 and −.66 with Bartholomew's self and other axes, respectively), higher scores indicated more negative other models.

Given that our subscales assessed the same constructs as the RSQ, we elected to focus, primarily, on the results yielded by our Anxiety and Avoidant dimensions. While the RSQ has been widely used in attachment research, its single-item format makes it much less reliable than our measure: The internal consistency of its self and other axes was only .40 and .27, respectively. By using our scale we were better able to detect theoretically meaningful associations between working models and indices of relationship functioning.

The improvements in internal consistency also enabled us to create more reliable attachment categories. Most researchers utilizing self-report measures have allowed individuals to categorize themselves: They have participants read the four paragraphs on the RSQ and decide which one best captures their orientation toward relationships. However, according to Bartholomew, individuals' attachment styles are determined by the valence and extremity of their working models. It thus seemed reasonable to use scores on our self (anxiety) and other (avoidant) subscales to assign participants to attachment categories. Individuals with low scores on both of our axes (i.e., who had positive models of both self and other) were classified as secure in their orientation toward relationships, whereas those who were high on both axes were assigned to the fearful category. Participants who were low in anxiety but high in avoidance (i.e., who had positive self and negative other models) were categorized as dismissive; whereas those who were high in anxiety but low in avoidance (i.e., who had negative self and positive other models) were considered to be preoccupied in orientation. An important issue in developing our classification system concerned the way in which we would determine the valence of participants' representations. For example, how anxious did individuals have to be before they were coded as being high in anxiety (i.e., as having negative models of self)? We felt that it was inappropriate to use the median to dichotomize our continuous variables, as an examination of the distribution of the RSQ suggested that there was an unequal number of "highs" and "lows" in our sample. The percentage of individuals who were secure, preoccupied, dismissing and fearful were 46%, 12%, 15%, and 26% respectively. Similar percentages have been obtained by other researchers, including those who use clinical interviews to categorize individuals' attachment orientations. Collapsing across categories, we found that 61% of our participants characterized themselves as having positive models of self (i.e., as being either secure or dismissing in orientation), and 58% as having positive models of other (i.e., as being either secure or preoccupied in orientation). Thus, the 60th percentile seemed an appropriate cut-off point for our own self and other axes.

While researchers have seldom used a multi-item scale for the purpose of categorization,[2] our approach offers several advantages over the RSQ. First, as others have argued, it is difficult to capture the valences of attachment representations with single items (i.e., paragraphs). Indeed, the results of our correlational analyses suggested that the RSQ may not map cleanly onto Bartholomew's theoretical model. For example, there was no relationship between the RSQ's preoccupied dimension and our other axis. On the contrary, instead of having positive representations of romantic partners, RSQ preoccupieds' scores on the avoidant dimension varied considerably.

Second, it is not clear whether the RSQ successfully categorizes dismissing–avoidants. According to Main, Kaplan, and Cassidy (1985), these individuals are well defended where relationships are concerned. This implies that assessment devices may need to be less transparent to capture their interpersonal style in relationships. The use of a multi-item scale—where variables of interest are unknown to participants—may more reliably detect the presence of this attachment orientation.

Third, an examination of the distribution of attachment styles using our categorization system revealed higher percentages of individuals in all three "insecure" categories. We would argue that our results make more sense than the RSQ's, given the selection criteria for inclusion in our study. This was far from a random sample. On the contrary, participants were recruited on the basis of family of origin experiences thought to predispose them to insecurity.

In light of the benefits of utilizing our measure, we will focus, primarily, on the results yielded by our multi-item scale. Categorical results based on responses to the RSQ will be discussed only when they deviate significantly from those obtained using our classification system. Specifics of other measures will be discussed in the Results section.

RESULTS

As predicted, we found significant differences between the working models of Intact Individuals and both groups of interest, as well as unique patterns of vulnerability in relationships. However, our analyses also revealed important gender differences across our family of origin categories. We will begin by examining the females' results: Specifically, the ways in which women from divorced and conflict-ridden families differed from their intact counterparts. This discussion is followed by a brief summary of the findings for males. While lower sample sizes prevented us from being confident about their results, the most interesting contrasts will be highlighted.

Daughters of Divorce (Divorce Daughters)

Family of Origin Experiences

Our predictions regarding Divorce Individuals were based on the assumption that their phenomenological experiences in their families of origin would differ from those of Intact Individuals. We expected Divorce Individuals to have been exposed to more dysfunctional models of marital relationships. In addition, we predicted that they would have had compromised bonds with their parents. Interestingly, we found these hypothesized differences to exist in the years prior to the divorce. For example, relative to daughters from intact families (Intact Daughters), Divorce Daughters' parents were reported to have less satisfactory relationships, and to fight more frequently and intensely with one another. Divorce Daughters also recalled being extremely disturbed by the severity of parental conflict in the home.

In addition, Divorce Daughters described having poorer relationships with their parents than Intact Daughters ($M = 5.42$ vs. $M = 6.03$ for mothers; $M = 4.06$ vs. $M = 5.86$ for fathers). Their relationship with their fathers seemed especially vulnerable to being compromised. Not only was it significantly poorer than Divorce Daughters' relationships with their mothers, but it deteriorated significantly following the initial separation ($M = 3.69$). Interestingly, these effects were most pronounced when it was the father who left the matrimonial home. The reader will note that this was the case for the majority of Divorce Daughters in our sample—74% of them remained with their mothers after the dissolution of the marital relationship.

Their perceptions regarding the reasons for the divorce may help to account for the divergence in the quality of their relationships with parents. Most of the women in our sample blamed their fathers for the marital break-up. Moreover, they reported being dissatisfied with the amount of post-divorce contact that they had with him. These factors may have engendered in Divorce Daughters negative feelings that made relationship-enhancing interactions with their fathers difficult after the breakup. The implications of these results for their interpersonal functioning are discussed later in the chapter.

Implications for Working Models

The differences in Divorce Daughters' family of origin experiences were associated with divergent orientations toward relationships. Table 11.1 displays the percentages of Divorce and Intact Daughters in each attachment category, as well as their means on dimensional indices of working models. Most critically, relative to Intact Daughters, Divorce Daughters

TABLE 11.1. Percentages and Means of Divorce and Intact Daughters' Attachment Orientations

Measure	Divorce Daughters	Intact Daughters
Attachment categories (percentages[a])		
Secure	32.8%	53.2%
Preoccupied	34.4%	19.4%
Fearful	21.3%	14.5%
Dismissing	11.5%	12.9%
Attachment dimensions (means[b])		
Model of self (RSQ)	4.12[*]	4.59
Model of other (RSQ)	4.09	4.12
General models (means)		
Global self-esteem	3.17	3.32

[a]Percentages reported represent the percentage of individuals within each sample that fall into each attachment category. Note that the chi-square value for the 2×4 table was statistically significant ($p < .01$).

[b]On the RSQ, higher scores reflect more positive working models.

[*]$p < .05$. Asterisks denote significant differences in group means on a particular variable (e.g., model of self).

were much less likely to be categorized as secure. Further, as predicted, Divorce Daughters' insecurity was manifested in specific ways. They were much more likely to be preoccupied—to hold negative views of themselves in relationships, yet to think positively about significant others.[3]

To a certain extent, Divorce Daughters also clustered within the fearful category. This clustering was unexpected; however, it underlined the impact of divorce on Divorce Daughters' self-representations. Whereas their orientations toward significant others varied considerably, their self models were significantly affected by the divorce experience. Interestingly, Divorce Daughters felt good about themselves in other domains. For example, they were just as confident as Intacts about their social skills, academic abilities, physical appearance, and general self-worth. It was only their image of themselves in relationships that was "damaged." They doubted their worthiness in the eyes of partners.

We also explored general beliefs that were more interpersonal or dyadic in nature. Consistent with previous research, we found Divorce Daughters to be more pessimistic about relationships in general—to view them as less enduring and less likely to remain fulfilling. Particularly significant were Divorce Daughters' responses on our measure of conflict efficacy. They were more likely to report feeling helpless about interpersonal difficulties. It was as though they believed that, given their inadequacies, there was little that they could do to resolve certain issues with romantic partners.

Interpersonal Functioning

Although Divorce Daughters' working models appeared qualitatively different from those of their intact counterparts, it was important to determine whether they actually influenced interpersonal functioning. For example, did they color relationship perception? Were we to have limited ourselves to assessing traditional markers of relationship functioning (e.g., satisfaction), we might have concluded that the answer was "no"—that Divorce Daughters had somehow protected themselves from their attachment representations. Relative to Intacts, they were just as satisfied, committed, trusting, and in love with their partners. Moreover, much to our surprise, they were just as optimistic about the future of their ongoing relationships when asked to rate the probability that a variety of positive and negative events would occur (e.g., their love continuing to grow, their partners and themselves discovering areas in which their needs conflicted in a serious way, and so on; adapted from Holmes & Murray, 1996). The fact that Divorce Daughters felt positively about their current attachments supported our predictions regarding the existence of more specific relational schemas. Presumably, their experience in their own relationships engendered a network of expectations and beliefs that usurped the influence of working models derived from the divorce experience.

Should we then feel secure about Divorce Daughters' relationships? On the contrary, an examination of their responses to theory-driven scales suggested that their negative general representations continued to be important, albeit in specific ways. As predicted, Divorce Daughters had areas of interpersonal vulnerability that indicated that their pessimistic models had an insidious impact on their perceptions of their relationships.

Specific Vulnerabilities

Vulnerabilities were assessed by asking participants to rate the extent to which they became anxious in specific interpersonal situations—for example, during conflictual interactions and discussions about the future. As far as we know, we are the first to assess vulnerabilities in this manner. Accordingly, we will present our results for the total sample before describing Divorce Daughters' concerns more specifically. For the sample as a whole, we found quite divergent patterns of vulnerability for those with negative models of self versus other. As Table 11.2 illustrates, those high in anxiety were more likely to worry about being abandoned and about interpersonal strife. In addition, they craved considerable reassurance that they were valued by their lovers. Those high on the avoidance dimension did not share these concerns. Instead, their vulnerabilities were related to ambivalence about closeness and intimacy (a more detailed discussion of these vulnerabilities appears later in the chapter).[4]

Given Divorce Daughters' negative models of self, it was not surprising that they struggled with vulnerabilities associated with the anxiety dimension. Moreover, as predicted, their most pressing concerns were related to the most salient psychological features of the divorce experience (see Table 11.3). Divorce Daughters were significantly more likely to

TABLE 11.2. Pearson Correlations between Specific Vulnerabilities and Anxiety (Self) and Avoidance (Other) Subscales for the Total Sample

Vulnerability	Anxiety dimension	Avoidance dimension[a]
Abandonment concerns	.60[***]	.19[*]
Worries about partner becoming emotionally distanced	.46[***]	−.045
Need for reassurance about partners' feelings	.50[***]	−.24[*]
Worries about conflict	.36[**]	.085
Closeness concerns		
Concerns about partners' "intimacy" demands	−.005	.38[***]
Approach–avoidance conflicts	.22[*]	.43[***]

[a]Note that, for each vulnerability, the magnitude of its correlation with the anxiety dimension was compared with its correlation with the avoidant dimension. In all cases, correlations were statistically different from one another ($p < .01$).
[*]$p < .05$; [**]$p < .01$; [***]$p < .001$.

TABLE 11.3. Means of Divorce and Intact Daughters' Specific Vulnerabilities in Relationships

Vulnerability	Divorce Daughters	Intact Daughters
Abandonment concerns		
Worries about being left for better alternative partners	3.32**	2.84
Worries about driving partners from the relationship	2.59*	2.19
Conflict concerns		
Disturbed by conflictual interactions	3.84**	3.03
Severity of conflict		
Conflict Severity Index	3.10****	2.15
Destructive Conflict Styles	3.26****	2.64

*$p < .10$; **$p < .05$; ****$p < .001$. Asterisks denote significant differences in group means on a particular variable.

worry about abandonment. They were concerned about partners one day leaving them for more attractive third parties. They also worried that their lovers would eventually discover in them intolerable qualities that drove them from the relationship, reflecting marked concerns that they were not "good enough" to continue to attract current partners.

Possible Origins of Divorce Daughters' Insecurities

While there are likely many contributing factors, we speculate that the quality of Divorce Daughters' relationships with their fathers played a critical role in shaping these self-views. As Collins and Read (1990) have found, individuals' models of opposite-sex parents can be important predictors of aspects of their heterosexual relationships. Consider the impact of fathers' departure from the matrimonial home: Many Divorce Daughters recalled feeling as though their fathers had abandoned *them* as opposed to their marriages. This is not unusual. Often, children's difficulty understanding the reasons for the divorce causes them to personalize experiences, even to blame themselves for familial events. In fact, in our clinical work with children of divorce, we have frequently heard comments like the following: "If I had only been better . . . cleaned my room when I was supposed to . . . been prettier, got better marks . . . maybe he wouldn't have left . . . maybe my parents would have stopped fighting . . . maybe they would have kept loving each other."

It is possible, then, that their fathers' departure marked the beginning of the development of negative self-representations. It is as though this event engendered in Divorce Daughters a belief that they were not "worth staying with." One can imagine such beliefs becoming ingrained in their attachment networks when their relationships with their fathers deteriorated further—as our data indicated was the case for the majority of

Divorce Daughters in our sample—and then generalizing to relationships with other significant male attachment figures (i.e., romantic partners).

In addition, Divorce Daughters' understanding of the divorce may have cultivated their abandonment concerns. The fact that most held their fathers responsible for the breakup may have affected their perceptions of control in relationships. From their perspective, *men* ended involvements—*men* left. Why would their partner behave differently?

Conflict Anxiety

A second area of vulnerability for Divorce Daughters was related to conflict. As a group, they reported being more anxious than Intact Daughters when they and their partners fought. As noted earlier in the chapter, conflict was a salient part of Divorce Daughters' family life. They described intense predivorce fighting between their parents. Moreover, it marked the beginning of the dissolution of their parents' marital bond. We speculate that Divorce Daughters' own conflicts remind them of the fragility of relationships, and prime their fears that their partners may one day elect to abandon them.

The reader will note that Divorce Daughters' conflict anxieties are likely to manifest themselves quite frequently. Relative to Intacts, they had much more conflictual relationships with their partners. Conflict was assessed by having participants rate the frequency and intensity of negative interactions in their relationships. In addition, they completed a 36-item scale (adapted from Holmes & Murray, 1996) that measured the degree to which they fell into destructive interaction patterns in their relationships—for example, reciprocal cycles of criticism and blame (e.g., "If my partner criticizes me, I often cannot help but criticize him/her in return"), and demand/withdraw patterns (e.g., "When my partner and I are dealing with a difficult issue, I often end up demanding or pressing him/her to talk, while my partner tends to withdraw or refuse to discuss the problem further"; see Heavey & Christensen, 1993).

Given their conflictual interactions with partners, it is remarkable that Divorce Daughters were able to maintain such positive feelings about their relationships. They were fighting, disturbed by the amount of conflict in their relationships, and worried about abandonment, yet their vulnerabilities failed to influence their feelings of security in their romantic involvements. How was this possible?

The Defensive Hypothesis

Unfortunately, the lack of controlled empirical work examining Divorce Daughters' relationship process (e.g., in the laboratory or via diary studies) forces us to speculate about the mechanisms that would yield our obtained pattern of results. One possibility is that Divorce Daughters compartmentalize their pessimistic attachment representations, they mobilize defenses that render them less accessible to conscious awareness. Their ability to minimize the influence of negative models on ongoing relationships would be adaptive, enabling them to risk closeness and intimacy. It would be difficult for Divorce Daughters to become involved, romantically, were their fears to be ever present. However, we were pessimistic about their ability to suppress their concerns over time. We suspected that, in certain situations, Divorce Daughters' tarnished self models would become extremely accessible, resulting in schema-driven interpersonal perception. That is, we expected specific features of their relationship experiences to activate divorce-related concerns (e.g., Baldwin, 1992). For example, when partners withdrew emotionally or spent time with attractive others, we envisioned Divorce Daughters magnifying even further the perceived threat of abandonment in their relationships. Presumably, they would begin to worry about partners leaving them, and perhaps engage in maladaptive "relationship maintenance activity" to avert this interpersonal disaster.

Longitudinal Results

We suspected that their negative models would eventually become intrusive enough to erode their attachment bonds. We have preliminary evidence to support this prediction. Divorce Daughters had a dramatically higher breakup rate than Intact Daughters at Time 2, despite their earlier reports of satisfaction with their relationships (41% of Divorce Daughters' vs. only 18% of Intact Daughters' relationships broke up; $p < .01$). Moreover, Divorce Daughters' breakups appeared to be related to their areas of vulnerability.

Divorce and Intact Daughters whose relationships dissolved were compared with those whose relationships continued in order to determine the best predictors of relationship status. As might reasonably be expected, Intact Daughters' breakups were associated with lower levels of satisfaction and love at Time 1. In addition, Intact Daughters who broke up viewed their partners more negatively than those who continued to date one another. Thus, in line with most research findings, their breakups were predicted by variables that suggested that they were not happy in those particular dating relationships.

In contrast, Divorce Daughters' breakups appeared vulnerability related. Preoccupation predicted relationship dissolution: Divorce Daughters who broke up were significantly more likely to be preoccupied in orientation than Divorce Daughters who remained with their partners. This finding is particularly striking given that this attachment style did not predict breakup for Intacts. On the contrary, it was the secure individuals whose relationships were most likely to end. It was not the case then that individuals who had negative self but positive other models had less stable attachments. Rather, they had to have lived through the divorce experience in order to be vulnerable to breakup. Why might this be the case?

We suspect that Divorce Daughters' family of origin experiences magnify and focus the concerns that are typically associated with a preoccupied orientation. For example, while most preoccupieds fear abandonment, Divorce Daughters have experienced it first-hand. They were left by one of the most significant male attachment figures in their lives. Thus, the threat may seem more real to them than it does to preoccupied Intact Daughters; they may be particularly "ready" to interpret partners' behavior as a sign of rejection.

Consistent with this hypothesis, worries about abandonment predicted breakup for Divorce, but not Intact Daughters. Moreover, they reported having more difficulty in situations where partners appeared to be withdrawing emotionally from the relationship. For example, Divorce Daughters who broke up were more likely than those who stayed together to become anxious when their partners were moody or refused to talk. Divorce Daughters' breakups were also associated with lower scores on our conflict efficacy index. The less faith they had in their abilities to resolve relationship difficulties, the more likely their bonds were to dissolve.

How might this combination of variables have precipitated breakup? One possibility was that partners, tired of the manifestations of Divorce Daughters' insecurity, elected to end the relationship. However, an examination of the data revealed that Divorce Daughters were the ones who initiated their breakups. We would argue that they did so to protect themselves from reexperiencing the painful affect associated with being left. From Divorce Daughters' perspective, there were signs that their partners would abandon them in the future. Moreover, they believed that there was little that they could do to resolve the difficulties that might drive partners from the relationship. Better to leave first than to recapitulate one of the most painful aspects of their childhood experience.

Interestingly, these "leavers" also appeared to distance themselves emotionally from partners while they were dating. For example, they were more likely to say that, in the future, they might abandon their lovers for someone else. Moreover, they reported being less committed to their relationships than Divorce Daughters who remained with their partners, despite the fact that they were just as satisfied and in love. It was as though they kept their partners at arms' length to minimize the impact of their lovers' inevitable departure from the relationship.

But were their strategies necessary? Did they have to maintain psychological distance between themselves and their partners, and to leave to avoid recapitulation? Unfortunately, we did not assess Divorce Daughters' partners' feelings about their relationships. Consequently, we have no way of evaluating the validity of Divorce Daughters' perceptions. It is certainly possible that their partners were dissatisfied with them. As Shaver and Hazan (1988) have argued, preoccupieds are often experienced as emotionally draining. Partners may very well have left, given time. However, we suspect that Divorce Daughters' fears were ill founded.

Their predictions regarding the probability that partners would one day abandon them were based on their assumptions that they would be viewed as inadequate. They *assumed* that their partners would evaluate them less favorably than they would alternative lovers. However, in a recent study Holmes and Murray (1996) found that low self-esteem individuals (i.e., individuals with negative self models) were quite inaccurate in assessing partners' feelings for them. In contrast to their negative expectations, partners' evaluations were almost as positive as they were for high self-esteem individuals. Ironically, the partners of "lows" thought that they were, indeed, responsive, warm, affectionate, and understanding. These findings suggest that Divorce Daughters' abandonment concerns were based not in reality, but in fantasies engendered by their negative general models of themselves in relationships.

In all probability, such schemas lead Divorce Daughters to misinterpret innocuous behaviors on the part of partners. For example, they may frequently infer impending relationship distress where none exists. Consider the following excerpt from a transcript of one of Wallerstein and Blakeslee's (1989) clinical interviews: "I'm always afraid that if my boyfriend is 30 minutes late, he is with another woman. He works with a female employee. I start wondering whether sex would be better with her, whether he'll fall in love with her, whether they'll fall in love with each other" (p. 52). Sadly, such fears may incite Divorce Daughters to act in ways that rob them of long-lasting intimacy. Their anxiety about recapitulation prompts them to leave before their partners can demonstrate their continuing commitment to the relationship—before they can convey their feelings regarding Divorce Daughters' value as relationship partners.

We now examine the results of our Daughters of Conflict (Conflict Daughters) to determine whether they, too, were affected adversely by their family of origin experiences.

Daughters of Conflict (Conflict Daughters)

Family of Origin Experiences

In many ways, Conflict Daughters' childhood and adolescence was similar to Divorce Daughters' predivorce experience. For example, their parents fought just as frequently and intensely as the parents of Divorce Daughters. Moreover, the parents were viewed by daughters as being extremely dissatisfied with one another. However, a closer examination of Divorce and Conflict Daughters' reports revealed subtle differences later in childhood that had the potential to affect their interpersonal functioning.

First, Divorce Daughters' experience with conflict shifted following the divorce. Their parents' arguments decreased in frequency, while Conflict Daughters continued to be exposed to disturbing interparental strife. Also significant was the difference in Conflict Daughters' parent-child relationships. Whereas Divorce Daughters had adequate relationships with their mothers to counter negative interpersonal experience, relative to Intacts, Conflict Daughters reported compromised attachments with both parents ($M = 4.62$ vs. $M = 6.03$ for mothers; $M = 4.46$ vs. $M = 5.86$ for fathers). Indeed, Conflict Daughters' quality ratings were equal in magnitude to Divorce Daughters' descriptions of their poorest relationship: their bond with their fathers.

Implications for Working Models

We expected Conflict Daughters' family of origin experiences to be associated with dysfunctional working models. But, consistent with Bowlby's (1977) theorizing, we thought that their orientations toward relationships would differ from those of Divorce Daughters. It was our contention that the events that set Conflict Daughters apart from their divorce counterparts later in childhood would be important in determining the content of their general working models.

As predicted, the manifestations of Conflict Daughters' insecurity were different from those of Divorce Daughters (see Table 11.4). Instead of being anxious in orientation (i.e., preoccupied), Conflict Daughters

TABLE 11.4. Percentages and Means of Conflict and Intact Daughters' Attachment Orientations

Measure	Conflict Daughters	Intact Daughters
Attachment categories (percentages[a])		
Secure	29.8%	53.2%
Fearful	29.8%	14.5%
Dismissing	27.7%	12.9%
Preoccupied	12.8%	19.4%
Attachment dimensions (means)		
Model of Self (RSQ)	4.11[*]	4.59
Model of Other (RSQ)	3.61[**]	4.12
General models (means)		
Global self-esteem	3.06[*]	3.32

[a]Note that the chi-square value for the 2 × 4 table was statistically significant ($p < .01$).
[*]$p < .05$; [**]$p < .01$. Asterisks denote significant differences in group means on a particular variable (e.g., model of self).

clustered within the two avoidant attachment categories. They were more likely than Intacts to be either fearful—to have negative models of both self and other—or dismissing, with negative models of others but positive views of themselves.[5]

Our dimensional analyses revealed that, when negative self models existed, they extended beyond the realm of relationships. In contrast to Divorce Daughters, Conflict Daughters felt more negatively about themselves generally, and were less confident about their social skills. The potential thus existed for their self models to affect more diverse areas of their lives. However, our categorical results suggested that their models of other were more important in conceptualizing their *interpersonal* dynamics. Fully 58% of the Conflict Daughter sample had negative other representations. In stark contrast, only 27% of Intact Daughters fell into negative other attachment categories.

We would argue that this sad portrait of Conflict Daughters' internal representations—the "variable self, negative other" pattern—makes sense given their family of origin experiences. It was possible for us to imagine factors buffering Conflict Daughters' self-evaluations, such as, familial emphasis on achievement versus interpersonal sources of esteem. However, it would have been difficult for Conflict Daughters to combat the evidence in their families regarding the nonresponsiveness of others. Their parents fought constantly. They were not happy with one another. Moreover, given the compromised nature of their parent–child relationships, Conflict Daughters could not count on caregivers to provide comfort and support. How could Conflict Daughters help but grow up to view significant others with skepticism and mistrust?

Interpersonal Functioning

Surprisingly, Conflict Daughters found ways to insulate their feelings about their ongoing relationships from their negative general models. Despite their histories, they developed positive specific schemas about their current involvements, schemas that enabled them to feel satisfied, committed, and optimistic about their futures. Indeed, so powerful were these schemas that Conflict Daughters were actually able to overcome general pessimism about others' dependability to trust their current dating partners to the same degree as Intacts.

Were we to have relied solely on these traditional indices, we might have concluded that Conflict Daughters had discovered a supportive attachment figure who restored their faith in close relationships. However, an examination of Conflict Daughters' vulnerabilities revealed differences in the quality of their attachments with partners—differences that suggested that they continued to be profoundly affected by their family of origin experiences.

Specific Vulnerabilities

Our correlational results suggested that individuals with negative other representations would worry not about withdrawal on the part of their partners, but instead about "approach" behaviors, that is, behaviors intended to increase the level of closeness in their relationships (see Table 11.2). Consistent with these findings, Conflict Daughters were more likely than Intacts to become anxious when their partners made "intimacy demands." They worried when their partners requested emotional support or an increased commitment to the relationship. Further, Conflict Daughters were more likely to struggle with approach–avoidance conflicts, to fluctuate between desiring and shying away from closeness and intimacy with their partners. For example, they endorsed items like the following: "I miss my partner intensely when we are apart; but want desperately to escape when we manage to make time for one another." "While I want attention and affection, I feel uncomfortable when I get it" (see Table 11.5).

Conflict Daughters' closeness concerns were associated with attitudes that enabled them to emotionally distance themselves from their partners. For example, Conflict Daughters were more likely to say that they would one day abandon their relationships for better alternatives. It was as though they needed a mental escape route, a way to reassure themselves that they were involved only casually with their current dating partners.

Conflict Anxiety

In addition to closeness, we anticipated that conflict would emerge as a significant area of concern. While our general correlation matrix associ-

TABLE 11.5. Means of Conflict and Intact Daughters' Specific Vulnerabilities in Relationships

Vulnerability	Conflict Daughters	Intact Daughters
Closeness concerns		
Worries about partners' intimacy demands	2.80**	2.32
Approach–avoidance conflicts	3.14**	2.58
Probability that self will abandon partner in the future	3.07*	2.59
Conflict concerns		
Disturbed by conflictual interactions	3.47	3.03
Severity of conflict		
Conflict Severity Index	2.81**	2.15
Destructive Conflict Styles	3.26**	2.64

*$p < .10$; **$p < .05$. Asterisks denote significant differences in group means on a particular variable.

ated conflict anxieties with self models, we expected Conflict Daughters to be the proverbial exception to the rule. We imagined them exaggerating conflict's association with dysfunction, and interpreting its occurrence in their own relationships as a sign that they were becoming like their parents. However, much to our surprise, Conflict Daughters were not bothered by conflictual interactions with their partners. They fought just as intensely and destructively as Divorce Daughters, but were significantly less anxious about it.

Conflict Daughters' frame of reference may help us understand their tolerance for greater levels of dissension in their relationships. Perhaps their own arguments pale in comparison to the severity of conflict witnessed between their parents throughout childhood and adolescence. Indeed, we speculate that Conflict Daughters' skewed norms, in part, account for their favorable evaluation of their relationships. As long as they continue to fight less frequently than their parents, they can feel good about the quality of their attachments with partners.

Longitudinal Results

Although Conflict Daughters were satisfied with their relationships, we viewed them as being at risk, ultimately vulnerable to the contaminating effects of their negative general models. Specifically, we expected them to have the highest breakup rate at Time 2. They fought more than is typical of most dating couples. Moreover, they were afraid of engaging in the kinds of intimacy-building behaviors that would counteract these negative interactions. We envisioned two possible breakup scenarios. As the demands for interdependence increased, we imagined Conflict Daughters bolting from their relationships. Equally plausible was the possibility that Conflict Daughters' partners would leave *them*. Unless they, too, were interpersonally avoidant, they would likely tire of being kept at arms' length. However, neither Conflict Daughters nor their partners abandoned their relationships. Contrary to our predictions, Conflict Daughters' breakup rate was no higher than that of Intact Daughters (25% vs. 18%, respectively; $p > .10$). Indeed, their relationships were significantly more likely than those of Divorce Daughters to be intact at Time 2 (25% vs. 44%, respectively; $p < .05$).

In arriving at an understanding of this startling pattern of results, we concluded that we had underplayed the importance of the most significant aspect of Conflict Daughters' childhood experience. We were studying a group whose parents fought constantly and were markedly dissatisfied with one another, but who *remained together* in spite of the dysfunctional aspects of their relationships. Perhaps, we should have anticipated that Conflict Daughters would follow suit.

Of course, *they* might not be cognizant of the similarities between their and their parents' relationships. As we argued earlier in the chapter, their norms may skew their evaluations of the quality of their attachments. Nevertheless, the pattern of results disturbed us, as it argued for the intergenerational transmission of relationship dysfunction. While we had anticipated a certain degree of behavioral mimicry—such as the repetition of negative interaction patterns and deficits in conflict resolution skills—we did not expect Conflict Daughters to remain, complacently, in attachments that approximated their parents' marital relationship.

The pattern of results *may* shift over time. Conflict may, eventually, drive Conflict Daughters from their relationships as they gain more direct experience with dating. Indeed, other researchers have found "sleeper effects" where this variable is concerned (e.g., Markman, 1981). Similarly, Conflict Daughters' ambivalence about closeness may ultimately create rifts with their partners. As we speculated earlier, the longer the relationship—the greater the demands for closeness and intimacy—the more likely partners may be to tire of Conflict Daughters' distancing strategies. At the 6-month mark, however, both daughters of divorce and conflict behaviorally recapitulated their parents' relationships: Divorce Daughters fought and broke up; Conflict Daughters fought and remained with their partners.

Were males as likely to repeat familial patterns? Unfortunately, as we noted earlier in the chapter, lower sample sizes made it more difficult for us to interpret their results. Indeed, in many places, we were forced to speculate about their interpersonal dynamics. However, although the data was more ambiguous than that for females, findings emerged that suggested that they, too, were affected by their family of origin experiences.

Sons of Divorce (Divorce Sons)

Family of Origin Experiences

The early experiences of sons from divorcing families were similar to those of their female counterparts. They witnessed frequent and intense fighting between their parents, and viewed them as being markedly dissatisfied with one another. Moreover, like daughters, they reported having poorer relationships with their fathers, relative to Intact Sons ($M = 4.45$ vs. $M = 5.98$). However, unlike Divorce Daughters, Divorce Sons had excellent relationships with their opposite-sex parents. Their mother–son bonds were comparable to those of Intacts ($M = 5.74$ vs. $M = 6.03$, ns). Did this important relationship function as a protective factor in the development of their attachment representations?

Implications for Working Models

According to our own categorical analyses, the representations of Divorce Sons were equivalent to those of Intact Sons (see Table 11.6). They were

TABLE 11.6. Percentages and Means of Divorce and Intact Sons' Attachment Orientations

Measure	Divorce Sons	Intact Sons
Attachment categories[a]		
Secure	35.0%	38.9%
Fearful	12.5%	11.1%
Dismissing	27.5%	30.6%
Preoccupied	25.0%	19.4%
Attachment dimensions (means)		
Model of Self (RSQ)	4.66	4.49
Model of Other (RSQ)	4.38[*]	3.85
General models (means)		
Global self-esteem	3.38	3.52

[a]Note that the chi-square value for the 2×4 table was not statistically significant ($p = .995$).
[*]$p < .05$. Asterisk denotes significant differences in group means on a particular variable.

just as likely to be secure. Moreover, they were neither more anxious, nor more avoidant of closeness and intimacy than their intact counterparts. In fact, on the RSQ, Divorce Sons looked more secure than Intacts. They had more positive models of other. Divorce Sons also held positive general beliefs about relationships. For example, they perceived couples to have just as much efficacy in dealing with conflict as Intact Sons, and were optimistic about their relational futures. How do we understand this pattern of results?

One possibility was that their mothers' responsiveness indeed protected them from the effects of more disruptive familial events. As was discussed earlier in the chapter, children's relationships with their opposite-sex parents may play a critical role in shaping relational models. In fact, it has been argued that they are more critical influences than are same-sex parent ties (Collins & Read, 1990). However, subsequent analyses suggested that Divorce Sons may have been defensive (i.e., self-deceiving) in their perceptions of their attachment styles. Their scores on relationship-specific subscales led us to suspect that they were not nearly as secure as they believed themselves to be.

Interpersonal Functioning

While Divorce Sons were just as satisfied, in love, and trusting of their partners, they were less likely than Intacts to envision their relationships enduring. Analyses were suggestive of lower degrees of commitment on the part of Divorce Sons, compared to Intact Sons ($M = 5.33$ vs. $M = 5.81$)[6] and optimism about their futures with current partners ($M = 5.05$ vs. $M = 5.58$, $p < .10$) . Divorce Sons' pessimism stemmed not from concerns about being abandoned by their lovers; instead, Divorce Sons imagined *themselves* terminating their involvements at some point in the future.

Proponents of the "maternal buffering" hypothesis just described might argue that these responses were consistent with secure general models. After all, the Divorce Sons in our sample were young, only beginning to date. Perhaps they chose not to commit prematurely. Perhaps they preferred to sample relationships to clarify their interpersonal needs (e.g., to determine what they valued in romantic partners, what they were willing to tolerate, and so on). We were skeptical of this interpretation, however, feeling instead that Divorce Sons' responses stemmed from underlying fears of closeness and commitment.

Specific Vulnerabilities

At first our skepticism was more intuitive than data driven. No clear patterns of vulnerability emerged at Time 1. On the one hand, relative to Intacts, Divorce Sons reported having more approach–avoidance conflicts—that is, more ambivalence about closeness and intimacy ($M = 3.33$ vs. $M = 2.77$, $p = .064$). But, on the other, they were reportedly comfortable in "intimacy-demanding" situations. However, when we analyzed our follow-up data, we found more compelling evidence to support our defensive hypothesis.

Longitudinal Results

Like Divorce Daughters, Divorce Sons had dramatically higher breakup rates relative to Intacts (44.4% vs. 24.1%, $p < .10$). Moreover, in *all* cases, they were the initiators, they left their partners. Did they leave for rational reasons? (For example, were they not satisfied—were their needs not being met?) On the contrary, neither Divorce Sons' level of satisfaction, love, or positivity about their partners predicted breakup. Divorce Sons' relationships were considerably more conflictual than those of Intacts ($M = 3.19$ vs. $M = 2.33$, $p = .018$). Perhaps it was their negative interactions that led them to infer that they were not with the "right" person. However conflict, too, failed to emerge as a significant predictor of breakup. Instead, it was Divorce Sons' *closeness concerns* that precipitated their exits from their relationships. Divorce Sons who broke up were more likely than those who remained together to become anxious when their partners made intimacy demands. They struggled more intensely with approach–avoidance conflicts. Moreover, they were more likely to maintain emotional distance between themselves and their partners. For example, they were less committed to their relationships, and more likely to say that they would one day leave.

This pattern seems consistent with the intrapersonal conflicts experienced by individuals who have avoidant orientations toward relationships. Indeed, while Divorce Sons were reportedly no different than Intact Sons on the avoidance subscale, avoidant orientation nevertheless emerged as a significant predictor of Divorce Sons' breakups. The more negative Divorce Sons' general view of others, the more likely they were to leave their partners at Time 2. Similarly, the more dismissing in orientation, the less stable their relationships over the 6-month period.

In light of our follow-up results, we argue that Divorce Sons' scores on our attachment subscales reflected not their actual models of self and other, but instead, defensive constructions that minimized their anxieties about closeness and intimacy. In one sense, these constructions were adaptive. Were Divorce Sons to have acknowledged their skepticism about others, they might never have risked intimate involvement. At the same time, we suspect that they encouraged behaviors that, in the long run, only perpetuate Divorce Sons' less conscious, negative relational models:

Imagine Divorce Sons and their partners interacting in ways that recapitulate the most painful aspects of the divorce experience—for example, fighting more often and more severely than do Intact Sons. How do they experience this event? Do they begin to worry explicitly about being hurt by their partners, or do their underlying closeness vulnerabilities result in their distancing further from the relationship? We suspect the latter to be the case. While Divorce Sons may experience negative emotional arousal during the interaction, we do not envision them having access to the reason for their distress. Instead, they may defensively withdraw further from their partners, interpreting the event as evidence that they are not with the "right" person. Eventually, Divorce Sons would leave, never challenging their assumptions about the dangers of closeness, never learning of their partners' potentially responsive nature.

Sons of Conflict (Conflict Sons)

Family of Origin Experiences

Conflict Sons' family of origin experiences were similar to those of the other "clinical" groups. Their parents had unsatisfactory, conflictual relationships, and their fathers had difficulty being responsive to them. Interestingly, however, Conflict Sons' relationships with their mothers were significantly better than those of Conflict Daughters. While statistically lower in quality than Intact Sons' mother–son attachments ($M = 5.26$ vs. $M = 6.03$), the relationships were "good enough" (potentially) to buffer Conflict Sons from more dysfunctional connections in the home.

Implications for Working Models

Consistent with this hypothesis, Conflict Sons reported being just as secure as Intacts; they were just as likely to have developed positive representations of self and other (see Table 11.7). Again, however, we were reluctant to trust these results, given the message from other relational indices. For example, Conflict Sons were considerably more negative about themselves in general, scoring lower than Intacts on a global measure of esteem. In addition, they had tarnished general beliefs about relationships. They were more pessimistic about their futures with hypothetical partners. They viewed relationships as unpredictable. Moreover, they perceived couples to have little efficacy in resolving interpersonal difficulties.

Interpersonal Functioning

The specific relational schemas of Conflict Sons were also markedly negative. They were more likely to be confused about their feelings where their partners were concerned. Conflict Sons were just as in love as Intact Sons but, despite this, were more likely to evaluate their partners in negative terms—for example, to say that they were critical, impatient, and unresponsive ($M = 4.58$ vs. $M = 3.36$, $p = .003$). Indeed, they were the only group to report being unhappy with their lovers. Further, Conflict Sons were significantly less trusting of their partners than Intact Sons ($M = 5.04$ vs. $M = 5.81$, $p = .014$), and less optimistic that their relationships would continue ($M = 4.63$ vs. $M = 5.58$, $p = .018$).

Specific Vulnerabilities

In addition, Conflict Sons emerged as the most vulnerable family of origin group. They exhibited all of the concerns that were found earlier to be associated with negative self-representations (see Table 11.8). They were

TABLE 11.7. Percentages and Means of Conflict and Intact Sons' Attachment Orientations

Measure	Conflict Sons	Intact Sons
Attachment categories[a]		
Secure	41.2%	38.9%
Fearful	11.8%	11.1%
Dismissing	23.5%	30.6%
Preoccupied	23.0%	19.4%
Attachment dimensions (means)		
Model of Self (RSQ)	4.14	4.49
Model of Other (RSQ)	4.09	3.85
General models (means)		
Global Self-Esteem	2.98***	3.52

[a]Note that the chi-square value for the 2 × 4 table was not statistically significant ($p = .995$).
*** $p < .001$. Asterisks denote significant differences in group means on a particular variable.

TABLE 11.8. Means of Conflict and Intact Sons' Specific Vulnerabilities in Relationships

Vulnerability	Conflict Sons	Intact Sons
Abandonment concerns		
Worries about being left for better alternative partners	3.38[*]	2.85
Worries about driving partners from the relationship	2.97[**]	2.21
Worries about partners interacting with attractive others	5.11[*]	4.22
Worries about partners distancing, emotionally, from the relationship	4.30[*]	3.77
Need for reassurance regarding partners' feelings for them	3.86	3.22
Conflict concerns		
Disturbed by conflictual interactions	4.22[***]	2.83
Severity of conflict		
Conflict Severity Index	3.28[**]	2.33
Destructive Conflict Styles	3.70[***]	2.76
Closeness concerns		
Approach–avoidance conflicts	3.74[***]	2.77
Probability that self will abandon partner in the future	3.10[*]	2.32

[*]$p < .10$; [**]$p < .05$; [***]$p < .01$. Asterisks denote significant differences in group means on a particular variable.

more likely to worry about abandonment, that their partners would one day leave them for someone "better." They also feared that their partners would discover in them flaws that drove them from the relationship. (The reader will note that Conflict Sons' means on these variables were equivalent to those of Divorce Daughters.) Conflict Sons found it stressful when their partners interacted with attractive others. Moreover, they were more likely to become anxious when they felt their partner withdrawing emotionally from the relationship. Not surprisingly, they required considerable reassurance that their partners continued to value them as mates.

In addition to abandonment concerns, Conflict Sons reacted adversely to conflict in their relationships. They fought more frequently and intensely than Intact Sons. Moreover, they were disturbed by the nature of these interactions. Conflict Sons also endorsed items that were consistent with closeness concerns. For example, they reported having stronger approach–avoidance conflicts in their relationships than Intact Sons. They were also more likely to say that they would one day abandon their partners.

In light of these findings, we would have expected the concerns of Conflict Sons to be reflected on our attachment subscales, in particular the anxiety (self) axis. Yet their scores were equivalent to Intact Sons on all but the global self-esteem measure. Why might this be the case?

It seems unlikely that they were being defensive in their responses, given their openness about their myriad of vulnerabilities. Equally unlikely are statistical explanations, such as lower sample sizes/ insufficient power. Their mean differences were moderate at best. Unfortunately, we have no viable explanation for the results on the attachment scales. Instead, we remain puzzled that their dysfunctional profiles and general low self-esteem were not reflected more dramatically in their working models of self and other in relationships.

Longitudinal Results

Attachment issues aside, Conflict Sons seemed the most fragile of our "clinical" groups. Low in self-esteem, dissatisfied with partners, incredibly vulnerable in relationships, we thought them prime candidates for breakup at Time 2. However, again, we were wrong! Their breakup rate was equivalent to that of Intact Sons (30.8% vs. 24.1%, *ns*)—considerably lower than that of their divorced counterparts (44%).

Thus, it appears that Conflict Sons, too, behaviorally recapitulated their parents' relationship, perhaps to a greater extent than Conflict Daughters. They continued to date despite anxiety-provoking interactions and acknowledged relationship dissatisfaction. They remained with people whom they found difficult to trust, and whom they regarded as unresponsive to their needs.

Why would Conflict Sons remain in such dissatisfactory relationships? We speculate that Conflict Sons' continued commitment to their partners was, in part, a function of their pessimism regarding the availability of better alternative involvements (Drigotas & Rusbult, 1992). They may have believed themselves incapable of attracting better partners. Not only was their self-esteem extremely low, but by virtue of their dysfunctional childhood models of attachment, they sadly expected little from romantic relationships.

GENERAL DISCUSSION

Our findings presented us with an intriguing paradox. Both adult children of divorce and of conflict held negative general beliefs about relationships. They emerged from their childhoods disillusioned, and all too cognizant of the pitfalls of intimacy. They expected not to live happily ever after but, instead, to be hurt in relationships. Yet their schemas for their current involvements failed to incorporate the pessimism engendered by their family of origin experiences. With the exception of Conflict Sons, they felt good about their ongoing relationships. They were satisfied and in love, trusting, even optimistic about their futures. There were, of course, *signs* of vulnerability—evidence of fault lines in their rosy constructions of their relationships. Their attachments were anxiety-provoking and fraught with destructive conflict. But, in summarizing their feelings about their partners, these signs were ignored, glossed over in favor of more positive evaluations of their relationships.

We argue that these positive perceptions were maintained via powerful defensive processes, such as compartmentalization and denial. In essence, Divorce and Conflict Individuals disavowed their dysfunctional beliefs, making them less accessible to conscious awareness. With their protective mechanisms in place, they were able to take the "leap of faith" that we suspect is necessary to risk intimate involvement. In a sense, they restored, artificially, the optimism about relationships that characterizes Intact Individuals (Murray, Holmes, & Griffin, 1996a), optimism that serves the desire for a sense of "felt security" in their relationships.

Their feelings of security were transient, however. Presumably, negative models continued to operate, exerting an insidious influence on interpersonal functioning. Their fears haunted Divorce and Conflict Individuals, leading them to magnify the perceived threat of negative outcomes in their relationships (e.g., abandonment, partner unresponsiveness, and partner intimacy demands). Moreover, we suspect that their fears were, in part, responsible for the conflictual nature of their involvements. Divorce and Conflict Individuals' insecurities likely elicited behavioral responses that precipitated conflict with partners. Divorce Daughters' abandonment concerns, for example, might have placed them at risk of falling into demand/withdraw cycles of interaction. In an effort to avoid being left, they may have been hypervigilant for evidence of partners' dissatisfaction, often attempting to engage them in relationship maintenance discussions. Instead of accepting partners' accounts of moodiness (e.g., "I'm tired" or "I had a bad day"), they may have continued to dig for model-confirming explanations (e.g., "I'm not happy with you" or "You did something to annoy me"). Further, their general models may have driven them to overcompensate for their fears. Divorce Individuals preempted their partners: They left before they were left. Conflict Individuals, ambivalent about closeness and worried about their partners' intimacy demands, elected to distance themselves emotionally, robbing partners of the opportunity to shun *them*.

Thus, while *perhaps* adaptive in some respects, negative general models predisposed these groups to repeat dysfunctional familial patterns. Indeed, we were stunned by the extent to which both groups mimicked the nature of parental interactions: They fought more frequently and intensely with their partners, and recapitulated their parents' relationship outcomes.

Implications for Relationship Research

As a field, we have tended to rely on traditional indices of relationship quality to predict breakup, such as concurrent indices of satisfaction, trust, and, more recently, optimism (e.g., Murray et al., 1996a). However, these measures had little predictive power for the clinical groups in our sample. Divorce Sons and Daughters were happy at Time 1, yet their relationships ended. Conflict Sons' relationships remained intact, despite negative feelings about their involvements. It seems, then, that assessments of more specific vulnerabilities may be called for in relationship research.

More specific assessment devices—developed from theoretical models regarding the weaknesses likely to develop in particular populations—may enable us to more accurately identify the factors that place couples at risk for relationship dysfunction. Our understanding of the phenomenological experiences of children of divorce and conflict guided us in generating hypotheses regarding their areas of vulnerability. For example, Divorce Individuals' childhood experience with abandonment was predicted to spawn marked concerns about being left by romantic partners. These hypotheses led to the development of measures that mimicked the most traumatic aspects of their early experience (e.g., conflict, being left, being rejected in interactions with caregivers, and so on), enabling us to identify unique, powerful predictors of Divorce and Conflict Individuals' relationship outcomes.

The Malleability of Working Models

Adult children of divorce and conflict are, clearly, at risk in their involvements. But are they doomed to recapitulate their parents' experience? Must they always be haunted by their interpersonal fears? From our perspective, this is an empirical question. One could make a case either way. For example, their models may be amenable to change; after all, they were based on "old" data, and formed via experiences in their families of origin. Perhaps more recent events could alter their content. For example, if Divorce Daughters were to remain with faithful, responsive partners, they might begin to think differently about themselves—to question their feelings of inadequacy as mates (e.g., Murray, Holmes, & Griffin, 1996b). Similarly, if Divorce Sons and Conflict Daughters risked interpersonal closeness, they might learn to differentiate their partners from significant others in their families of origin.

However, we were skeptical. We could imagine them continuing to be self-defeating in their interaction patterns: Divorce Daughters leaving because of systematically underestimating the positivity of partners' feeling for them, and engaging in behaviors that led partners to respond in schema-confirming ways. It is conceivable, for example, that Divorce Daughters' partners would tire of their doubts, perhaps even feel hurt by apparent manifestations of distrust. They may elect to abandon the relationship in search of alternative partners who had more faith in their commitment.

Conflict Sons' models may also resist alteration. Their relationships were dissatisfactory, anxiety-provoking, and highly conflictual, making it unlikely that they would have schema-disconfirming experiences. Indeed, we envisioned them caught in a vicious cycle. The longer they stayed with their partners, the stronger their belief system about the poverty of close relationships. The stronger their belief system, the weaker their faith that better alternatives existed. The fewer perceived alternatives, the longer they would remain in their current involvements, and so on.

This is not to say that our clinical groups would be resistant to treatment interventions that targeted their negative attachment representations. On the contrary, they may benefit significantly from insight-oriented approaches that elucidate the reasons for their insecurities in relationships (Dozier & Tyrrell, Chapter 9, this volume). With the help of a therapist, they might be able to identify and alter self-defeating behavior patterns. For example, Divorce Daughters may learn that, ironically, it is their insecurities—their worries about their inadequacy in the eyes of partners—that make them less attractive as mates. Couple therapy may also be useful. Partners may benefit from insight into their mates' intrapersonal dynamics; for instance, it may reduce their likelihood of partners personalizing Divorce and Conflict Individuals' insecurities (e.g., "It is not that he or she does not trust me, rather, the divorce/conflict experience made these particular situations difficult for him or her"). Together, they could then work toward reducing the frequency of destructive interaction patterns in their relationship.

However, they may need to present for therapy before they can begin to break out of these negative interaction patterns. Sadly, Divorce Sons may never seek help for their interpersonal difficulties. Relative to other groups, they seem least aware of their vulnerabilities in relationships. They defensively deny intimacy concerns and blame their partners for the dissolution of their bonds. Their defensiveness may reduce the likelihood that they would identify intrapersonal issues that interfered with their ability to sustain satisfactory relationships. Instead of seeking help, and, ultimately, comprehending the role that their own issues play in their romantic experiences, they seem likely to continue to attribute their unstable history to a failure to meet the "right" partner.

Clinical Implications

Our findings highlight the usefulness of placing clients' interpersonal difficulties in a broader developmental context. With the possible exception of Divorce Sons, these groups are likely overrepresented in clinic referrals for both individual and couple therapy. Consistent with this hypothesis, Wallerstein and Blakeslee (1989) reported that over 50% of her sample were counseled for interpersonal difficulties. An understanding of these individuals' vulnerabilities will likely facilitate the therapeutic process.

Our results also have implications for earlier intervention programs—programs that target children of divorce (e.g., Kalter et al.,

1985)—as they highlight potential gender differences in their adjustment to separation. Girls' self models seem particularly vulnerable to being compromised by the divorce experience. We argued that their pheno-menological experience of their fathers' departure from the home helped to account for our diverging pattern of results. Daughters watch their fathers leave. They feel abandoned, and perhaps worry that they are somehow to blame for his exit (they were not smart enough or pretty enough). Moreover, they regard him as being responsible for the divorce. We suspect that these perceptions become prototypical of the ways in which they regard other male attachment figures. That is, they learn that men leave them—that men end their relationships because of Divorce Daughters' inadequacy.

Boys, too, experience abandonment by their male caregivers. They, too, blame their fathers for the divorce. But they struggle with different issues by virtue of their same-sex status. In contrast to females, sons learn that they have a certain power in relationships. They, perhaps, worry that they, too, are leavers—that they may be the cause of others' pain and suffering. However, these fears would soon be alleviated, as they found ways to differentiate themselves from their fathers during childhood and adolescence. Sadly, they end up recapitulating their fathers' behavior: They exhibit less commitment and initiate their breakups, perhaps hurting their partners in the process. Their defenses seem to protect them from this realization. As far as Divorce Sons are concerned, their partners are to blame for the dissolution of the relationship.

These findings suggest that both prevention and crisis interventions for children of divorce should target the father–daughter relationship. Girls who maintain positive attachments with their male caregivers, who have more balanced views regarding the reasons for the divorce, and who are given strong messages regarding their own blamelessness for their fathers' departure may develop more positive self-schemas. Future re-search should explore the implications of paternal custody to determine whether similar cross-gender effects emerge when mothers leave the matrimonial home. We suspect that in father-run households it is sons who are vulnerable to developing preoccupied orientations toward rela-tionships.

Finally, it may be important for clinicians to develop and implement intervention programs for children of conflict. We worry most about this group. While they are just as likely as Divorce Individuals to struggle romantically, they may be at risk of developing more general psychopa-thology. They had lower self-esteem, and were less confident in social situations. Moreover, their family of origin experiences—specifically, their compromised relationships with *both* parents—suggested that they had fewer social supports, relative to Divorce Individuals, to buffer the effects of negative interpersonal events. As adults, they may be vulnerable to depression, especially if they remain in dissatisfactory, conflictual relationships. Future research will need to evaluate the accuracy of our pessimistic predictions where they are concerned. Like other commentators, we remain to be convinced that "it is better to stay together for the sake of the children." Theirs seems the sadder of the two familial legacies.

ACKNOWLEDGMENTS

This research was supported by a Doctoral Fellowship to Kate Henry from the Social Sciences and Humanities Research Council of Canada (SSHRC) and by SSHRC research grants to John Holmes. Portions of this research were presented at the International Society for the Study of Personal Relationships convention in Banff, Alberta, in August 1996, and the American Psychological Association convention in Toronto, Ontario, in August 1996.

NOTES

1. Bartholomew's self and other axes were created using the quantitative rating scales on the RSQ. Participants were required to rate, on 7-point Likert scales, the extent to which each of the four paragraphs characterized their style in relationships. The self axis was created by subtracting the sum of participants' ratings to the negative self categories from the sum of their ratings to the positive self categories: self model = (secure + dismissing) – (preoccupied + fearful). The other axis was created by subtracting the sum of ratings to the negative-other categories from the sum of ratings to the positive-other categories: other model = (secure + preoccupied) – (dismissing + fearful).

2. In several studies (e.g., Simpson et al., 1996), researchers have statistically mimicked typological systems by examining interaction terms for the two dimensions.

3. Some might argue that preoccupied individuals' models of other are not isomorphic with the positive "other" views held by secures, that is, while hopeful, preoccupieds are more guarded and uncertain of their romantic partners. These qualities may very well characterize individuals with preoccupied orientations toward relationships. However, we remain to be convinced that they suggest differences in their other models. While preoccupieds may worry about their partners' commitment to the relationship—while they may fear abandonment—it is our contention that their uncertainty stems not from beliefs that others are less dependable, but instead from their negative models of self. From preoccupieds' perspective, there is something about themselves that might lead partners to hurt or leave them. They believe their partners would *not* behave similarly with lovers who were not so "fundamentally flawed."

4. As was discussed in the Method section of the chapter, we obtained much weaker correlations with the RSQ's self and other axes (e.g., for abandonment concerns, $r = .32$ vs. $r = .6$ with our scale; for conflict anxieties, $r = .17$ vs. $r = .36$; for closeness concerns, $r = .24$ vs. $r = .43$). Many of these vulnerabilities would have gone undetected or been dismissed as uninteresting were we to have relied solely on the RSQ to assess participants' attachment orientations.

5. As predicted, Conflict Daughters' "dismissingness" was not detected by

the RSQ. On the contrary, according to Bartholomew's categorization system, Intact Daughters were more likely to be dismissing (50% of Intact Daughters vs. only 33% of Conflict Daughters clustered within this attachment category).

6. Lower sample sizes resulted in many marginal effects for males. When $p > .10$, we used the results from our female sample to judge the relative importance of the differences among means. Generally, differences that exceeded .5 on our indices were considered meaningful enough to report.

REFERENCES

Amato, P. R., & Keith, B. (1991). Parental divorce and adult well-being: A meta-analysis. *Journal of Marriage and the Family, 53,* 43–58.

Baldwin, M. W. (1992). Relational schemas and the processing of social information. *Psychological Bulletin, 112*(3), 461–484.

Bartholomew, K. (1990). Avoidance of intimacy: An attachment perspective. *Journal of Social and Personal Relationships, 7,* 147–178.

Bartholomew, K., & Horowitz, L. M. (1991). Attachment styles among young adults: A test of a four-category model. *Journal of Personality and Social Psychology, 61,* 225–234.

Belsky, J., Steinberg, L., & Draper, P. (1991). Childhood experience, interpersonal development and reproductive strategy: An evolutionary theory of socialization. *Child Development, 62*(4), 647–670.

Booth, A., Brinkerhoff, D. B., & White, L. K. (1984). The impact of parental divorce on courtship. *Journal of Marriage and the Family, 46,* 85–94.

Bowlby, J. (1977). The making and breaking of affectional bonds. *British Journal of Psychiatry, 130,* 201–210.

Brennan, K. (1994). *Expectations of future relationships, marriage, and divorce: An investigation of children from divorced and intact families.* Unpublished manuscript, University of Texas at Austin.

Brennan, K., & Shaver, P. R. (1993). Attachment styles and parental divorce. *Journal of Divorce and Remarriage, 23,* 161–175.

Carnelley, K. B., Pietromonaco, P., & Jaffe, K. (1994). Depression, working models of others, and relationship functioning. *Journal of Personality and Social Psychology, 66*(1), 127–140.

Collins, N. L., & Read, S. J. (1990). Adult attachment, working models, and relationship quality in dating couples. *Journal of Personality and Social Psychology, 58,* 644–663.

Collins, N. L., & Read, S. J. (1994). Cognitive representations of attachment: The structure and function of working models. *Advances in Personal Relationships, 5,* 53–90.

Drigotas, S. M., & Rusbult, C. E. (1992). Should I stay or should I go? A dependence model of breakups. *Journal of Personality and Social Psychology, 62*(1), 62–87.

Emery, R. E. (1982). Interparental conflict and the children of discord and divorce. *Psychological Bulletin, 92,* 310–330.

Enos, D. M., & Handal, P. J. (1986). The relation of parent marital status and perceived family conflict to adjustment in white adolescents. *Journal of Consulting and Clinical Psychology, 54,* 820–824.

Franklin, K. M., Janoff-Bulman, R., & Roberts, J. E. (1990). Long-term impact of parental divorce on optimism and trust: Changes in general assumptions or narrow beliefs? *Journal of Personality and Social Psychology, 50*(4), 743–755.

Gleick, E. (1995, February 27). For better, for worse: The growing movement to strengthen marriage and prevent divorce. *Time,* pp. 48–56.

Glenn, N. D., & Kramer, K. B. (1987). The marriages and divorces of the children of divorce. *Journal of Marriage and the Family, 49,* 811–825.

Greenberg, E. F., & Nay, R. W. (1982). The intergenerational transmission of marital instability reconsidered. *Journal of Marriage and the Family, 44,* 335–347.

Griffin, D., & Bartholomew, K. (1994). Models of the self and other: Fundamental dimensions underlying measures of adult attachment. *Journal of Personality and Social Psychology, 67*(3) 430–445.

Guttman, J. (1989). Intimacy in young adult males' relationships as a function of divorced and non-divorced family of origin structure [Special issue: Children of divorce: Developmental and clinical issues]. *Journal of Divorce, 12,* 253–261.

Heavey, L., Layne, C., & Christensen, A. (1993). Gender and conflict structure in marital interaction: A replication and extension. *Journal of Consulting and Clinical Psychology, 61*(1), 16–27.

Henry, K., & Holmes, J. G. (1994). *The disjunction between the general and specific relational schemas of adult children of divorce.* Unpublished data, University of Waterloo.

Holmes, J. G., & Murray, S. (1996). *Positive illusions in close relationships: Is love blind, or prescient?* Paper presented at the annual meeting of the American Psychological Association, Toronto.

Kalter, N., et al. (1985). *Time-limited developmental facilitation groups for children of divorce.* Author.

Main, M., & Goldwyn, R. (in press). Interview-based adult attachment classifications: Related to infant–mother and infant–father attachment. *Developmental Psychology.*

Main, M., Kaplan, N., & Cassidy, J. (1985). Security in infancy, childhood, and adulthood: A move to the level of representation. In I. Bretherton & E. Waters (Eds.), Growing points in attachment theory and research. *Monographs of the Society for Research in Child Development, 50,* 66–104.

Markman, H. J. (1981). Prediction of marital distress: A 5-year follow-up. *Journal of Consulting and Clinical Psychology, 49,* 760–762.

Murray, S. L., Holmes, J. B. & Griffin, D. W. (1996a). The benefits of positive illusions: Idealization and the construction of satisfaction in close relationships. *Journal of Personality and Social Psychology, 70,* 79–98.

Murray, S. L., Holmes, J. B., & Griffin, D. W. (1996b). The self-fulfilling nature of positive illusions in romantic relationships: Love is not blind, but prescient. *Journal of Personality and Social Psychology, 71,* 1155–1180.

Philp, M. (1995, July 15). Studies roll back rosy view of divorce. Latest advice: Stay together for the kids. *Globe and Mail* (Toronto), pp. A1, A6.

Ross, M. (1989). Relation of implicit theories to the construction of personal histories. *Psychological Review, 96,* 341–357.

Shaver, P. R., & Hazan, C. (1988). A biased overview of the study of love. *Journal of Social and Personal Relationships, 5,* 473–501.

Simpson, J. A., Rholes, W. S., & Phillips, D. (1996). The impact of conflict on close relationships: An attachment perspective. *Journal of Psychology and Social Psychology, 71*(5), 899–914.

Sroufe, L. A., Egeland, B., & Kreutzer, T. (1990). The fate of early experience following developmental change: Longitudinal approaches to individual adaptation in childhood. *Child Development, 61*, 1363–1373.

Wallerstein, J. S., & Blakeslee, S. (1989). *Second chances.* New York: Ticknor & Fields.

12

The Associations between Adult Attachment and Couple Violence

The Role of Communication Patterns and Relationship Satisfaction

NIGEL ROBERTS
PATRICIA NOLLER

It seems a contradiction that marriage, the primary source of support and love for many, can simultaneously represent an environment in which people are more likely to be physically assaulted than in society in general (Gelles, 1990). How can an atmosphere of love and warmth also foster a situation in which people are at risk of physical attack? It has been suggested that attachment theory can offer some insight into the apparent paradox of the association between violence, on the one hand, and love and intimacy on the other (Mayseless, 1991). However, to date, little empirical research has been conducted on the possible relation between adult attachment and couple violence.

In this chapter we present theory and research on the association between adult attachment and couple violence in married and cohabiting relationships. Moreover, we attempt to identify the ways in which adult attachment may influence whether people use violence against their partners. Primarily, it is suggested that the association between attachment and couple violence can be explained by the dysfunctional communication patterns that are linked with insecure attachment, and that create an environment in which couple violence is more likely to occur. We also examine other ways in which communication may influence the relation between attachment and violence, as well as investigating the role of relationship satisfaction and partners' use of violence in the link between attachment and violence. Because of our emphasis on the couple rather than the individual, and our focus on relationship issues such as couple communication patterns and relationship satisfaction, we are adopting a systems approach to the study of couple violence.

THE SYSTEMIC APPROACH
TO COUPLE VIOLENCE

Over the last 20 years, couple violence has been studied from a wide range of different sociological and psychological perspectives, most notably from the feminist (e.g., Yllo, 1983), social-learning (e.g., O'Leary, 1988), and family systems approaches (e.g., Giles-Sims, 1983). Nevertheless, there exists considerable debate about the causes of couple violence and about the appropriate theoretical and methodological perspective from which the issue should be studied; political controversy over this highly emotive subject has slowed progress in understanding the etiology of couple violence, particularly from a systems perspective (Gelles, 1990; Rosenbaum, 1988).

General Systems theorists focus on the dyad as the unit of analysis when studying couple violence, examining those features of the couple that make them more prone to using violence. The central proposition of a systems approach to couple violence is that violence is the product of a dysfunctional family or marital system, rather than of individual pathology (Gelles, 1985). Violence is viewed not as an outcome, but as part of an ongoing process (Gelles & Maynard, 1987). That is, rather than assuming a simple linear cause-and-effect process, systems theory portrays the elements in a model as interrelated and, through the action of feedback processes, mutually causal in nature. For instance, a self-concept as a "violent person" may increase the risk of actually performing a violent act, which in turn, will reinforce the "violent person" self-concept, further increasing the likelihood of future violence (Straus, 1973).

One limitation of many studies investigating the role of communication patterns in the etiology of couple violence is that they have ignored female-to-male violence (e.g., Burman, Margolin, & John, 1993; Lloyd, 1990). Consequently, not only have researchers neglected an important aspect of couple violence, but the comparison groups in these studies may have been inappropriate, with female-to-male violence being present in some of the "nonviolent" relationships as well as some of the violent relationships.

Systemic approaches to the study of interpersonal violence have been heavily criticized by feminist researchers. Central to the feminist position is the belief that the systemic approach relieves the perpetrator of responsibility for his violence, by viewing violence as a product of the family system (e.g., Avis, 1992; Bograd, 1992; Hansen, 1992). This view is limited in two respects. First, no matter what factors contribute to the maintenance of violence in a relationship, any violent act is always the individual choice of the perpetrator (Gottman et al., 1995).

Second, research that has not used women's shelters or hospital samples strongly suggests that, in the majority of violent relationships, both partners are violent (Henton, Cate, Koval, Lloyd, & Christopher, 1983; O'Leary, Barling, Arias, & Rosenbaum, 1989; Stets & Henderson, 1991; Straus & Gelles, 1990). Research suggests, therefore, that violence begets violence, with many couples feeding off each other's use of violence. These findings clearly indicate that the roots of couple violence lie within the relationship (Henton et al., 1983), as well as within the individual and the culture.

ORDINARY COUPLE VIOLENCE VERSUS TERRORISTIC VIOLENCE

It is important to emphasize, however, that not all violent relationships are mutually violent in nature, and that this fact may be partially explained by the proposal that there are different types of "batterers" (Gondolf, 1988; Holtzworth-Munroe & Stuart, 1994; Johnson, 1993). In particular, Johnson (1993) builds a case for the existence of two qualitatively and quantitatively different forms of couple violence: "patriarchal terrorism" and "ordinary couple violence." The former involves men who perpetrate more severe and more frequent violence against their partners, and who report little remorse for doing so (Gondolf, 1988). They are also more violent outside of the relationship (Gondolf, 1988; Gottman et al., 1995). In contrast, the second and more common group of batterers identified, also labeled "typical batterers" or "family-only batterers," perpetrate fewer and less severe acts of violence, restrict violence to their couple relationships, and report remorse for their violence (Gondolf, 1988; Holtzworth-Munroe & Stuart, 1994).

Johnson (1993) claims that research where subjects have been recruited using random sampling procedures (e.g., Straus & Gelles, 1990), media advertisements (e.g., Margolin, 1988), marriage counseling services (Vivian, Malone, & O'Leary, 1989, cited in O'Leary & Vivian, 1990) and student samples (e.g., Bookwala, Frieze, Smith, & Ryan, 1992) present a picture of couple violence where men and women are equally violent, with most violence being of a "minor" nature (pushing, shoving, and slapping) and occurring relatively infrequently. Johnson (1993) suggests that the women studied by most feminist researchers, recruited mainly from women's shelters, emergency rooms, and criminal courts, are the recipients of "psychopathic" or "terroristic" violence, whereas subjects recruited through community samples are more likely to represent those who experience "ordinary couple violence" in their relationships.

ATTACHMENT AND COUPLE VIOLENCE

The potential contribution of attachment theory to increasing our understanding of the etiology of couple violence has been noted by a number of researchers and theorists. Mayseless (1991) suggests that one of the most useful contributions of attachment theory is its ability to explain the apparent contradiction between violence and intimacy. That is, attachment theory, by focusing on the regulation of intimacy in close relationships, can help our understanding of how violence can be related to love and intimacy.

Attachment has been measured using a variety of techniques. However, there is some support for the proposition that adult attachment can be adequately represented in terms of two underlying dimensions (Feeney, Noller, & Hanrahan, 1994; Simpson, 1990). These dimensions reflect the degree to which an individual feels uncomfortable in close romantic relationships (labeled Discomfort with Closeness) and the degree to which he or she fears abandonment from romantic partners (Anxiety over Abandonment). High Discomfort with Closeness involves a belief that attachment figures are untrustworthy and cannot be relied upon to provide assistance in times of need. In contrast, high Anxiety over Abandonment involves a belief that one is "unlovable" and unworthy of help from attachment figures in times of need. Another common way of viewing attachment has been by way of four discrete categories; preoccupied, fearful–avoidant, dismissing–avoidant, and secure (Bartholomew & Horowitz, 1991). However, these four categories are easily conceptualized in terms of the two underlying dimensions of attachment. Fearful and dismissing individuals report more Discomfort with Closeness, whereas preoccupied and fearful individuals report higher levels of Anxiety over Abandonment (Feeney, 1995).

The relevance of attachment in the etiology of couple violence is indicated by a number of findings. First, many recipients of violence in dating relationships interpret their abuse as a sign of love (Henton et al., 1983). Second, the first occurrence of violence tends to coincide with periods of transition from one level of intimacy to another. In dating relationships, violence is most likely to occur for the first time following the couple becoming seriously involved (Henton et al., 1983). Similarly, Rounsaville (1978) found that 40% of all first occurrences of couple violence in his married sample occurred immediately following marriage or pregnancy.

Third, a large number of violent people are not violent outside of the marital relationship, with violence directed only toward those with whom they are most intimate (Gondolf, 1988; Straus & Gelles, 1990). This finding is particularly true for females. Ben-David (1993) suggests that theorists need to account for this difference between women's use of violence in the private and public domains. If attachment insecurities are seen to underlie women's use of violence, it is easy to explain why women are far less likely to be violent in the public domain, where attachment insecurities do not arise, relative to the private domain.

An association between attachment and couple violence has been noted in a number of early qualitative investigations of the causes of couple violence. Mattinson and Sinclair (1979) described the violent couples in their sample as characterized by an intense fear of separation, and as using violence to control the proximity of their partner. Coleman (1980) also described the violent men in his sample as desiring close proximity with their spouses, although he saw them as having a simultaneous fear of intimacy.

More recently, Retzinger (1991a, 1991b) has proposed a model of marital conflict in which threatened bonds result in the emotional reaction of shame which, if unacknowledged by the partner, leads to rage and violence. Her model is relevant to the current study in two ways. First, it is concerned with the relations among attachment, couple communication patterns, and couple violence. Second, it is clearly systemic in nature, in that both partners play a role in the escalation of negative emotion and any ensuing violence. On the other hand, Retzinger does not incorporate individual differences in the form of attachment style into her model. Nevertheless, her work has provided evidence for a relation between threatened bonds (attachment) and couple violence.

Dutton and Browning (1988) present more direct evidence that couple violence is related to the regulation of intimacy and the maintenance of proximity within the relationship. They found that violent men reported heightened anger and more aggression than nonviolent men in response to viewing videotaped conflict interactions of a woman displaying behaviors that distanced her from her partner. These scenes were also reported to be the most relevant to the relationships of violent men, but not of nonviolent comparisons.

Finally, Dutton, Saunders, Starzomski, and Bartholomew (1994) found that men in treatment for domestic violence reported being more fearful and preoccupied than a control group of men recruited from the community. Although the community group also contained some violent men, this finding suggests that attachment is related to men's use of couple violence. Furthermore, Dutton et al. (1994) found anxious attachment to be related to what they called a "personality constellation of abusiveness in intimate relationships" (p. 1379), identified by previous research (Dutton, 1994). In addition, both fearful and preoccupied attachment (but not dismissing attachment) were positively associated with men's use of psychological abuse.

Thus, there is some support in the literature for an association between attachment (particularly fear of abandonment) and couple violence. On the other hand, little quantitative work has been published that demonstrates clear links between attachment and couples' use of physical violence. Furthermore, Pistole and Tarrant (1993) recently found that, in a sample of 62 convicted male batterers, the four attachment styles were represented in proportions similar to those obtained in previous research using nonviolent men, and these researchers were thus unable to provide evidence of a link between attachment and couple violence. Indeed, they concluded that the effects of threats to attachment on couple violence is equivalent across attachment styles.

Pistole and Tarrant's (1993) study is limited in a number of respects, including the absence of any nonviolent comparison group and an exclusive focus on an identified and possibly extreme group of violent individuals. In other words, Pistole and Tarrant (1993) may have been studying the role of attachment in what Johnson (1993) refers to as "patriarchal terrorism," rather than "ordinary couple violence." A further reason that Pistole and Tarrant were unable to obtain evidence for an association between insecure attachment and couple violence may lie in the individual differences approach that these researchers adopted.

It may be important to look at both partners' attachment, as well as the interaction of partners' attachment in predicting whether couples are violent. Research has suggested that a secure partner may provide a buffering effect for the behavior of insecure individuals (e.g., Cohn, Silver, Cowan, Cowan, & Pearson, 1992). Alternatively, the pairing of two insecure individuals may prove a highly volatile combination, especially if one partner is scared of abandonment whereas the other fears intimacy. This combination of attachments is seen as especially dangerous because of the conflicting needs for intimacy involved. In particular, a person who is anxious over abandonment may find the emotional distance of a partner who is uncomfortable with closeness extremely anxiety provoking, and violence may result to protest that distance. As noted by Feeney (1994), examining the interaction between partners' attachment styles shifts the focus from the individual to the dyad, and thus represents a more systemic view of the attachment process.

Couple Violence, Attachment, and Communication Patterns

One important way in which insecure attachment may lead to an increased risk of couple violence is through the development of dysfunctional communication patterns. It is possible that insecure attachment leads to dysfunctional patterns of couple communication, and that these patterns of communication increase the likelihood of couple violence occurring. That is, insecure attachment may drive the dysfunctional patterns of interaction that lead to violence or, speaking more technically, communication patterns may mediate the relation between attachment and violence. There is considerable evidence for such a relation existing; research has demonstrated clear associations both between attachment and dysfunctional communication, and between dysfunctional communication and couple violence.

Adult attachment is inextricably linked with how individuals express their emotions and the level of intimacy in their romantic relationships. Both the degree to which people are uncomfortable with closeness and the extent to which they worry about being abandoned have important implications for the ways in which they interact with romantic partners.

First, Discomfort with Closeness is primarily associated with a lack of emotional involvement in relationships and a strong tendency to deny negative affect. The behavior of individuals who are uncomfortable with closeness is directed toward avoiding intimate contact and the negative affect associated with rejection. They report being emotionally inexpressive and lacking warmth (Bartholomew & Horowitz, 1991), and they report more relief following the breakup of a relationship (Feeney & Noller, 1992). Furthermore, they see their relationships as involving poorer communication, less closeness, less disclosure, and less acknowledgment of others' disclosures (Collins & Read, 1990; Feeney, Noller, & Callan, 1994; Kobak & Hazan, 1991).

In contrast, the behavior of individuals who are anxious over abandonment is directed toward maintaining close proximity to their attachment figure, and any negative affect which may be a threat to that proximity is dealt with in an obsessive manner. Anxiety over Abandonment is associated with hypervigilant attention to negative affect (Collins & Read, 1994; Feeney, Noller, & Callan, 1994; Kobak & Sceery, 1988). Furthermore, Anxiety over Abandonment is associated with high levels of disclosure in self-disclosure tasks, albeit disclosure that is lacking in flexibility and topical reciprocity (Mikulincer & Nachshon, 1991).

There is good reason to expect attachment to affect the way that individuals deal with relationship conflict, in particular. Levels of marital conflict are related to attachment, with conflict levels consistently being related to Anxiety over Abandonment (Collins & Read, 1990; Feeney, Noller, & Callan, 1994; Levy & Davis, 1988) and less consistently to Discomfort with Closeness (Levy & Davis, 1988). Attachment is concerned with the availability of attachment figures, and conflict can be seen as a threat to a partner's availability (Pistole, 1989). It is further suggested, somewhat paradoxically, that conflict may offer the opportunity for increased intimacy between partners through the sharing of their beliefs and feelings, and the airing of their grievances (Straus, 1979; Vuchinich, 1987). Therefore, conflict may represent a highly anxiety-provoking situation for individuals who are anxious over abandonment *and* for those who are uncomfortable with closeness.

If conflict does represent a highly threatening situation for those who are anxious over abandonment, then those individuals have three options. First, they can "integrate" with their "abandoning" partners by simply submitting to their partners' wishes. Second, they can attempt to prevent a partner's "abandonment" by dominating partners through the use of hostility and exaggerated displays of anger and coercion. Finally, they can avoid the possible abandonment by withdrawing from the conflict, essentially fleeing from the unpleasantness that conflict brings with it, and denying its very existence.

To some extent, the same three options may be open to those who are uncomfortable with closeness, if conflict is associated with expressions of intimacy. These individuals can simply "end" the conflict as quickly as possible, by either "submitting" to their partners or attempting to dominate their partners through the use of hostility and coercion. Alternatively, they could withdraw from the conflict altogether and so avoid its associated unpleasantness. Furthermore, given their fear of intimacy, it is difficult to see how these individuals could easily engage in any of the skills commonly associated with conflict resolution in close relationships, such as self-disclosure, negotiation, active listening, or the open discussion of intimate feelings and beliefs.

Attachment and Communication Skills during Conflict

Individuals with insecure attachment have poorer problem-solving skills than those who are securely attached (Kobak & Hazan, 1991), at least during conflict with attachment figures. Couples in which both partners are secure are more assertive (Feeney, 1990). The fearful–avoidant attachment style is associated with interpersonal problems involving passivity and nonassertion (Bartholomew & Horowitz, 1991). Previous research supports a linkage between a lack of assertion (submission) and Anxiety over Abandonment, in particular. Individuals who are anxious over abandonment have been found to be more "obliging" of their partner during conflict than those who are uncomfortable with closeness (Pistole, 1989). On the other hand, Levy and Davis (1988) failed to obtain any relations between obliging approaches to conflict and adult attachment.

However, more generally, both Discomfort with Closeness and Anxiety over abandonment are related to a lack of communication skills during relationship conflict. Discomfort with Closeness and Anxiety over Abandonment are inversely related to people's self-reported use of mutually constructive communication during conflict (Fitzpatrick, Fey, Segrin, & Schiff, 1993). Further, people who are anxious over abandonment and those who are uncomfortable with closeness are less likely to use integrating and compromising approaches to conflict than are securely attached individuals (Levy & Davis, 1988; Pistole, 1989).

Attachment and Withdrawal from Conflict

Marriages where both partners are secure have been shown to involve less withdrawal (Feeney, 1990; Senchak & Leonard, 1992) than marriages in which the wife is insecure (Senchak & Leonard, 1992). Furthermore, secure husbands are more involved in marital interaction than are insecurely attached husbands (Cohn et al., 1992). Wives' Anxiety over Abandonment has been linked, both concurrently and longitudinally, to asymmetrical destructive patterns that involve one partner making demands while the other withdraws (Feeney, Noller, & Callan, 1994; Fitzpatrick et al., 1993). Furthermore, wives' Anxiety over Abandonment is positively correlated with the frequency with which wives use avoidance strategies in response to marital conflict (Feeney, 1990).

Research has failed to reveal consistent associations between Discomfort with Closeness and withdrawal from conflict. A number of researchers have not found specific links between Discomfort with Closeness and the avoidance of conflict (Feeney, 1990; Levy & Davis, 1988; Pistole, 1989). However, Fitzpatrick et al. (1993) found a significant association between Discomfort with Closeness (Avoidance) and people's tendency to withdraw from conflict, as well as their tendency to engage in cycles of interaction with their partners in which one partner makes demands while the other withdraws.

Attachment and Hostility during Conflict

Verbal aggression is used less by secure couples than couples in which either both partners are insecure or the wife is insecure (Senchak & Leonard, 1992). In addition, Kobak and Hazan (1991) found that the insecurity of both husbands and wives is related to wives' dysfunctional displays of anger during conflict resolution. Although individuals who are uncomfortable with closeness are rated as generally more hostile by their peers (Kobak & Sceery, 1988), specific links between Discomfort with Closeness and people's displays of hostility and their use of coercion during conflict with romantic partners have not been identified by researchers. In contrast, theory and research both point toward strong links between Anxiety over Abandonment and the use of dominating approaches to conflict resolution.

Theoretically, displays of anxiety and anger are natural processes used to protest the inaccessibility of an attachment figure (Bowlby, 1988). High levels of Anxiety over Abandonment are associated with high emotional expressivity (Bartholomew & Horowitz, 1991), and involve an obsession with distress and conflict (Feeney, Noller, & Callan, 1994; Kobak & Sceery, 1988). Research supports an association between Anxiety over Abandonment and the use of dominating and coercive tactics during conflict (Bartholomew & Horowitz, 1991; Feeney, Noller, & Callan, 1994; Levy & Davis, 1988).

Communication Patterns and Couple Violence

To some extent these findings regarding the differences in conflict interaction between secure and insecure couples are paralleled by findings regarding the differences between violent and nonviolent couples. There is evidence that violent couples, compared to nonviolent couples, lack communication skills, tend to withdraw from conflict, and show heightened levels of anger and hostility.

Communication Skills and Couple Violence

A number of studies have revealed that violent couples appear to lack communication skills. Margolin (1988) found that wives in violent relationships showed less self-disclosure and more communication apprehension than other wives. Using both self-report and observational techniques, strong links have been established between poor problem-solving skills and a lack of assertion (Infante, Chandler, & Rudd, 1989; Lloyd, 1990; Margolin, 1988; Margolin, Burman, & John, 1989; Rosenbaum & O'Leary, 1981; Telch & Lindquist, 1984).

It is important to note, however, that the lack of assertion displayed by people involved in violent marriages may be specific to the relationship with the partner (Margolin, 1988). Therefore, findings regarding the communication skills of couples in terms of how they resolve conflict (whether observational or self-report) cannot be simply interpreted as violent couples lacking communication skills (Holtzworth-Munroe, 1992). Rather, the lack of communication skills that violent couples display during conflict resolution reflects some type of interference in their ability to use the skills that they display outside of the marital relationship, suggesting that the communication of violent couples is better viewed as a relationship issue than as an individual skills-deficit issue (Whitchurch & Pace, 1993).

Withdrawal from Conflict and Couple Violence

A number of researchers have identified an association between couple violence and withdrawal from conflict. Using both self-report and observational methods, couple violence is positively linked to high levels of withdrawal from conflict, both concurrently (Lloyd, 1990; Margolin, Burman, & John, 1989) and longitudinally (Smith, Vivian, & O'Leary, 1991).

Furthermore, the sequencing of withdrawal in the conflict of violent couples is also important. Couples in violent relationships tend to reciprocate one another's withdrawal, and violent husbands tend to respond to wives' verbal aggression with increased withdrawal (Margolin, John, & O'Brien, 1989). Finally, couples in which the man is violent are more likely to report a pattern of one partner making demands while the other withdraws (Babcock, Waltz, Jacobson, & Gottman, 1993).

Heightened Hostility and Couple Violence

Verbal aggression is an important predictor of couple violence, both concurrently and longitudinally (Infante et al., 1989; Murphy & O'Leary, 1989; O'Leary & Vivian, 1990). Observational studies show that violent couples display more hostile negative affect (such as anger and contempt) and hostile behaviors during their conflict (Burman et al., 1993; Margolin, Burman, & John, 1989; Margolin, John, & Gleberman, 1988; Vivian & O'Leary, 1987). Men in violent relationships report feeling higher levels of anger than other men during couple conflict (Margolin et al., 1988), and violent couples report getting more angry and more verbally aggressive toward their partner in their conflict interactions, compared with nonviolent couples (Lloyd, 1990).

Interactions between Attachment and Communication

Alternatively, it is possible that a combination of insecure attachment and dysfunctional couple communication predicts whether couples are violent. Rather than insecure attachment driving the communication patterns that predict violence, it may be the case that insecure attachment only predicts the presence of violence in a relationship, if particular interaction patterns characterize the relationship. In other words, attachment security may interact with couple communication to create an environment in which violence is more likely to occur. For example, individuals who are anxious over abandonment may perceive their partners' withdrawal from conflict as highly threatening (relative to those who are securely attached), because withdrawal is interpreted as an act of emotional abandonment. Violence may then be used as a means of preventing the distancing behavior of partners. Alternatively, a person using withdrawal to escape a distressing conflict interaction may be pursued by the partner (i.e., the demand–withdraw pattern of interaction). In this case, a person who is insecurely attached may be so distressed by this "pursuit" that he or she uses violence as a means of halting the partner's pursuit. However, in both cases, it is the interaction between individuals' attachment and couple communication patterns that predicts the occurrence of violence.

Similarly, interactions between attachment security and expressions of hostility and anger are easily envisaged. Although some use of hostility and anger by a partner may be accepted by most people, if it is directed toward someone who is insecurely attached, the situation is potentially explosive. Similarly, the frustrations born out of a lack of good communication skills may be more deeply felt by those for whom complete emotional intimacy is so important. Thus, Anxiety over Abandonment could also interact with communication skills to predict violence in a relationship.

Summary

In summary, three relatively clear findings emerge from the literature regarding the interaction patterns of violent couples. Couples in violent relationships suffer from communication deficits that are at least heightened during marital interaction, and they tend to withdraw from conflict and to express heightened levels of hostility and anger during conflict interaction. Furthermore, these findings regarding the communication of violent couples parallel findings relating adult attachment to couple communication. It is suggested that this pattern of findings indicates that insecure attachment may fuel the couple communication patterns that are associated with couple violence, with communication processes mediating the association between attachment and couple violence. However, a further possibility is that attachment and communication patterns interact to predict the presence of violence within a couple relationship.

Relationship Satisfaction and Partner Violence

Research into couple violence has revealed two important covariates of couple violence. First, previous research has demonstrated that relationship satisfaction is reliably related to couple violence (Bookwala, Frieze, & Grote, 1994; Julian & McKenry, 1993; O'Leary et al., 1989; Smith et al., 1991). Indeed, O'Leary (1988) suggests that relationship dissatisfaction is a necessary precursor to violence. Second, research that has not used women's shelter or hospital samples strongly suggests that in the majority of relationships, couple violence is mutual in nature (Henton et al., 1983; O'Leary et al., 1989; Straus & Gelles, 1990). Thus, one of the most important predictors of whether individuals hit their partner may be whether the partner hits them.

It seems important for researchers to at least investigate whether the specific variables of interest add to the prediction of individuals' use of couple violence provided by measures of relationship satisfaction and partners' use of violence (Rosenbaum, 1988). However, in the present study, how these important covariates interrelate with the variables of interest (attachment and couple violence) is also investigated more fully.

We investigated whether relationship satisfaction mediates the association between adult attachment and the use of couple violence. Given the plethora of research demonstrating associations between adult attachment and relationship satisfaction (e.g., Feeney, Noller, & Callan, 1994; Simpson, 1990) and between relationship satisfaction and couple violence (Bookwala et al., 1994; Julian & McKenry, 1993; O'Leary et al., 1989), it is possible that relationship satisfaction is the process through which attachment influences couple violence. We considered it important to investigate this issue, in order to determine whether any mediating role communication patterns may play in the association between attachment and couple violence is simply due to the covariate of relationship satisfaction, which is reliably associated with couple communication, attachment, and couple violence.

Second, it was postulated that attachment could moderate the relation between partners' use of violence. A slap by a partner is likely to prompt a fairly extreme response by many people, including a retaliatory act of violence. Nevertheless, the manner in which the initial act of violence is interpreted by the victim is likely to shape his or her response. It is considered likely that a person's attachment will affect his or her interpretation of a partner's use of violence, and thereby mold any response to that violence. In particular, a person who is anxious over abandonment may view a partner's use of violence as a sign of rejection—requiring a protest over that rejection, possibly in the form of violence. People who are anxious over abandonment may then be more likely to respond to the violence of a partner with violence of their own, than would people who are not anxious over abandonment.

METHOD

Participants and Procedure

All subjects were either married or had been living with their partner in a de facto relationship for at least 12 months. Subjects were recruited through counseling and community centers, and through the first-year psychology pool at the University of Queensland. By recruiting from these two sources we hoped that a broader range of people would be included in the study than if recruitment had occurred solely through the more accessible student sample. Furthermore, it was expected that recruiting from agencies involved in helping those experiencing relationship difficulties would ensure a greater proportion of subjects who experience violence and marital dissatisfaction. In all, 181 questionnaires were returned in which both partners completed the surveys; of these, 89 were returned by first-year psychology students and their partners.

Demographic information for the two samples is provided in Table 12.1. Couples from the community sample tended to be older, to have been in a relationship for a longer period and to have had more children

TABLE 12.1. Comparison of Demographic Variables for the Student and Community Samples

	Sample source	
	Student	Community
Categorical variables		
Number in de facto relationships	25* (28.7%)	15 (16%)
Number in marriages	62* (71.3%)	79 (84%)
Number of males completing or having completed a university degree	52* (59.8%)	38 (40.4%)
Number of females completing or having completed a university degree	49* (56.3%)	30 (31.9%)
Number of males previously married	17 (19.5%)	19 (20.2%)
Number of females previously married	9* (10.3%)	23 (24.5%)
Continuous variables		
Mean age of males	33.7*	37.5
	(SD = 9.8)	(SD = 9.8)
Mean age of females	31.2*	35.7
	(SD = 8.7)	(9.0)
Mean years married or cohabiting	7.0*	10.6
	(SD = 6.9)	(SD = 8.8)
Mean number of children from present relationship	0.8*	1.4
	(SD = 1.1)	(SD = 1.3)
Mean number of males' children from previous relationships	0.2	0.5
	(SD = 0.6)	(SD = 1.3)
Mean number of females' children from previous relationships	0.2	0.4
	(SD = 0.6)	(SD = 0.8)

Note. Asterisks indicate the presence of a significant difference across the two samples at $p < .05$. For categorical variables percentages are given in parentheses.

than the couples from the student sample. Community couples were also less likely to be living in de facto relationships and more likely to be married. Both males and females from the community sample were less likely to be completing or to have already completed a university degree than the student sample.

Measures

Attachment Scales

The Relationship Styles Questionnaire (RSQ; Griffin & Bartholomew, 1994) is a 30-item self-report measure of adult attachment. The questionnaire contains items from the adult attachment literature, including Hazan and Shaver's (1987) measure, Collins and Read's (1990) measure, and Bartholomew and Horowitz's (1991) measure of adult attachment.

A factor analysis conducted on this 30-item measure of attachment style resulted in a two-factor solution. The two factors were labeled Discomfort with Closeness and Anxiety over Abandonment; together they explained 41.3% of the variance in the 30 items. The final two scales possess high levels of internal consistency as measured by Cronbach's alpha for both Anxiety over Abandonment (alpha = .86) and Discomfort with Closeness (alpha = .88) and bear strong resemblance to the two factors obtained by previous researchers (e.g., Feeney, Noller, & Callan, 1994; Simpson, 1990). The Anxiety over Abandonment scale is made up of 8 items that involve a fear of being alone and a preoccupation with complete emotional intimacy with others (e.g., "I worry about being abandoned"; "I find that others are reluctant to get as close as I would like"). In contrast, the Discomfort with Closeness scale consists of 12 items that reflect an apprehension over forming dependent relationships or establishing emotional intimacy with others (e.g., "I am nervous when anyone gets too close to me"; "I find it difficult to trust others completely").

Communication Patterns Questionnaire

The Communication Patterns Questionnaire (Christensen, 1988; Christensen & Sullaway, 1984) is a 35-item instrument designed to measure couples' usual patterns of interaction before, during, and after marital conflict. Noller and White (1990) conducted a study on the validity of the Communication Patterns Questionnaire. They found that most items of the questionnaire possess good discriminant validity, discriminating between spouses of high, moderate, and low marital satisfaction.

Noller and White (1990) obtained four factors, which they labeled Coercion, Mutuality, Postconflict Distress and Destructive Process. The Coercion scale included items involving the use of threats and physical and verbal aggression by both partners. The Mutuality scale included items that involved partners using mutually constructive problem-solving skills, such as negotiation and expression, instead of both withdrawing from or avoiding conflict issues. The Postconflict Distress scale consisted of items that assessed the degree to which couples experienced emotional stress following marital conflict. Finally, the Destructive Process scale contained items measuring the degree to which couples engage in a range of dysfunctional interactions, such as demand–withdraw and pressure–resist.

Because the Coercion scale includes items involving interpartner aggression, this scale was not included in any analyses in order to avoid spurious relations between communication and couple violence. Reliability coefficients for the Noller and White scales were satisfactory: Mutuality (alpha = .87), Postconflict Distress (alpha = .75), and Destructive Process (alpha = .84). In addition, interpartner agreement was calculated for all six of the scales: Mutuality (r = .66), Postconflict Distress (r = .43), and Destructive Process (r = .63). To further increase the reliability of these scales and to decrease the number of predictor variables, partners' scores on the same scales were summed for all further analyses.

Conflict Tactics Scales

The Conflict Tactics Scales are the most widely used measures of couple violence (Arias & Beach, 1987; Babcock, Waltz, Jacobson, & Gottman, 1993; Rosenbaum, 1988). The Conflict Tactics Scales have received considerable criticism from feminist researchers (e.g., Bograd, 1992; McHugh, 1992), but contain several valuable features that continue to make them useful for assessing the occurrence of *physical violence* in intimate relationships. The version of the Conflict Tactics Scales used in the present study is an 18-item measure consisting of three subscales: Reasoning, Verbal Aggression, and Physical Aggression. In the present study, where investigation was limited to the occurrence of physical violence in intimate relationships, only the Physical Aggression subscale was used. The Physical Aggression subscale requires the subject to indicate the number of times over the last 12 months that he or she has engaged in various acts of violence, ranging from throwing something at a partner to using a knife or gun against a partner (Items 11–18). However, because of the highly skewed nature of couple violence, scores on this scale were dichotomized for all analyses, as recommended by Straus (1990).[1]

The percentage of males and females who had used each of the violent tactics over the last 12 months is presented in Table 12.2. As can be seen from the table, the most common violent tactic used by people involves pushing, grabbing, and shoving partners. In the present sample, few couples report the presence in their relationships of more severe tactics, such as beating up a partner or using a knife or gun against a partner. These findings are consistent with previous research utilizing community and student samples (e.g., Bookwala et al., 1992; MacEwan & Barling, 1988), and reflect the violence in the current sample being char-

TABLE 12.2. Percentage Endorsement of Violent Conflict Tactics for Females and Males

Conflict tactic	Percentage endorsement	
	Females	Males
Threw something	28.7	19.9
Pushed, grabbed, or shoved	36.5	34.8
Slapped	24.9	16.0
Kicked, bit, or hit with fist	20.4	9.9
Hit or tried to hit with something	21.0	13.8
Beat up	2.8	7.2
Threatened with knife or gun	3.3	2.8
Threatened with knife or gun	1.7	2.2

Note. Percentages are based on reports of violence by either partner.

acterized more by "typical couple violence" than "patriarchal terrorism" (Johnson, 1993). Because individuals are more likely to underreport the violence in their relationships than to overreport it (Stets & Straus, 1990), any report of violence by either the perpetrator or victim is taken as an indication that violence has been perpetrated (Szinovacz & Egley, 1993).

The Dyadic Adjustment Scale

The Dyadic Adjustment Scale (Spanier, 1976) is a 32-item measure of relationship satisfaction with demonstrated reliability and validity. The overall scale has a high reliability as measured by Cronbach's coefficient alpha (alpha = .96).

RESULTS

Descriptive Statistics

As expected, couples recruited from the community sample were more likely than student couples to experience male-perpetrated violence in their relationships (48.9% vs. 29.9%). However, the difference between the percentage of couples from the two samples who reported experiencing female-perpetrated violence in their relationships (46.8% vs. 34.5%) failed to reach significance. Descriptive statistics (means and standard deviations) for the hypothesized predictors of couple violence are presented in Table 12.3, as a function of men's and women's use of violence. As can be seen from the table, violent relationships appear to be less happy, and partners appear to be less securely attached and to engage in more dysfunctional patterns of communication during conflict.

Relations between Attachment and Couple Violence

As outlined earlier, the effect of attachment on couple violence may be influenced by couple communication patterns. For example, someone with high Anxiety over Abandonment may be more likely to withdraw from conflict, and this withdrawal may increase the likelihood of violence occurring. Alternatively, people with high Anxiety over Abandonment may find the withdrawal of a partner highly threatening, and use violence as a means of preventing any withdrawal. These two possibilities place communication (withdrawal) as, first, a potential mediator of the relation between attachment (Anxiety over Abandonment) and couple violence, and, second, a potential moderator of the relation between attachment and couple violence

Baron and Kenny (1986) outline the differences between mediating and moderating variables, and the means by which to test for their

TABLE 12.3. Means and Standard Deviations of Predictor Variables across Violent and Nonviolent Subjects

Variable	Females		Males	
	Violent	Nonviolent	Violent	Nonviolent
Females' Relationship	94.5	110.6	94.5	110.3
Satisfaction (0–151)	(19.1)	(18.0)	(20.3)	(17.3)
Males' Relationship	95.7	110.6	95.5	110.4
Satisfaction (0–151)	(16.6)	(18.2)	(18.4)	(17.1)
Females' Anxiety over	20.1	17.5	19.7	17.9
Abandonment (8–40)	(6.5)	(6.6)	(6.2)	(6.9)
Males' Anxiety over	20.9	16.6	20.6	16.8
Abandonment (8–40)	(6.8)	(5.8)	(6.7)	(6.0)
Females' Discomfort with	32.7	31.7	34.0	30.8
Closeness (12–60)	(8.8)	(8.7)	(8.2)	(8.8)
Males' Discomfort with	33.7	31.9	34.1	31.7
Closeness (12–60)	(8.8)	(9.5)	(8.9)	(9.4)
Postconflict Distress (8–72)	42.5	32.4	42.5	32.6
	(11.1)	(12.8)	(11.2)	(12.8)
Mutuality (18–162)	97.3	118.3	99.3	116.6
	(23.5)	(24.6)	(25.0)	(25.0)
Destructive Process	73.6	49.4	74.4	49.4
(14–126)	(18.9)	(20.8)	(20.5)	(19.4)

Note. Possible range of scores are presented in parentheses after variable name. High scores always reflect a high level of the attribute being measured. Standard deviations are presented in parentheses below their respective means.

presence. They argue that a mediator variable represents the process through which the variable of interest influences the criterion variable, whereas a moderator variable alters the strength or direction of a relationship between two variables. The way in which mediation can be demonstrated with multiple predictor and mediating variables using hierarchical multiple regression analysis is outlined by Feeney (1994). Following demonstrated associations between the predictor and mediating variables (using bivariate correlation), a single hierarchical multiple regression can be performed by regressing the criterion variable on the predictor and mediating variables. At Step 1, the dependent variable is predicted from the predictor variables. At Step 2, the hypothesized mediating variables are entered into the regression equation. The presence of a mediating relationship is supported if the importance of the predictor variables decreases from Step 1 to Step 2, as reflected in a reduction in their standardized regression weights.

Is Attachment Related to Couple Violence?

The question of whether attachment is related to couple violence was assessed using hierarchical multiple regression analysis. Separate analyses were carried out for females and males, using subjects' own attachment (Step 1) and then their partners' attachment (Step 2) to predict whether or not subjects are violent toward their partners. Unless otherwise noted, all effects in the study are significant at the .05 level or better.

Evidence was found for a relation between own attachment and use of couple violence for both females and males. However, this relation was restricted to Anxiety over Abandonment ($\beta = .21$ and $\beta = .27$ for females and males, respectively). Partners' scores on the attachment scales significantly added to the prediction of females' but not males' violence. Again, this relation between attachment and couple violence was restricted to Anxiety over Abandonment ($\beta = .29$). Men's Anxiety over Abandonment was significantly related to whether they were the victims of couple violence, after controlling for females' attachment. In other words, both men and women were more likely to use violence against partners if they, themselves, feared abandonment, and women were also more likely to use violence against partners who were anxious over abandonment. In contrast, Discomfort with Closeness appeared to have little direct effect on whether or not violence was present in a relationship.

Do Couples' Attachment Styles Interact to Predict Violence?

A moderating relationship can be demonstrated using multiple regression analysis or logistic regression analysis.[2] In the present case, the question of whether partners' attachment styles interact to predict violence in their relationships was investigated using two logistic regression analyses, one each for males' and females' use of couple violence.

As a group, the two-way interactions between partners' attachment scores provided a significant increase in prediction of violence for females' violence, but only approached significance for males' violence ($p < .07$). However, for both females' violence and males' violence, the specific term for the interaction between the violent individual's Anxiety over Abandonment and his or her partner's Discomfort with Closeness reached significance ($pr = .12$, for both female and males).

Given that these interactions were the two that were most expected, it was considered appropriate to interpret them, despite the overall nonsignificant contribution of the four interaction terms for male violence. In order to interpret these two interactions, subjects were divided into groups according to whether they scored above the mean score on Discomfort with Closeness (high Discomfort with Closeness) or below the mean score (low Discomfort with Closeness). Violence was then regressed onto Anxiety over Abandonment, using logistic regression analysis, separately for couples in which the partner was either high or low in Discomfort with Closeness. Separate analyses were conducted for males and females.

For both females and males, the relation between their own Anxiety over Abandonment and their own use of violence was significant *only* if partners were uncomfortable with closeness ($prs = .28$ and $.31$, for females and males, respectively). These findings are consistent with the prediction that couples in which one person worries about being abandoned by romantic partners and the other is scared of intimacy are at greater risk of experiencing couple violence perpetrated by the anxious partner.

Does Communication Mediate between Attachment and Couple Violence?

Having demonstrated an association between attachment and couple violence, it is possible now to investigate whether communication mediates this association. To establish this mediating process, first we need to demonstrate an association between communication and couple violence. Then it is necessary to establish (in the present sample) relations between attachment and communication. Finally, we need to show that the relation between attachment and couple violence decreases, after controlling for communication patterns. This decrease can be demonstrated using hierarchical multiple regression analyses in which the criterion is regressed onto the hypothesized predictor variables at Step 1 and then the hypothesized mediators at Step 2. For perfect mediation it must be shown that any significant regression coefficients between the individual predictors and criterion variables at Step 1 are no longer significant at Step 2, when the hypothesized mediators are entered into the regression equation (Feeney, 1994).

The results of two multiple regression analyses confirmed that violence was related to couple communication. Together, the three scales were significantly related to whether or not subjects had perpetrated at least one act of violence against their partners over the last year, for both females and males. However, Destructive Process was the most important variable in predicting couple violence, for both female ($\beta = .36$) and male violence ($\beta = .48$), being the only scale to predict violence, independently of the other communication scales.

As shown in Table 12.4, insecure attachment and dysfunctional communication patterns were reliably related. Women's Discomfort with Closeness was the only attachment scale not to show significant associations with all three of the couple communication scales; it related only to Mutuality.

Finally, two hierarchical multiple regression analyses were performed, regressing couple violence on both partners' attachment (Step 1) and then the couple's communication patterns (Step 2), separately for female and male violence. Evidence consistent with a mediating process was obtained; the relation between attachment and couple violence failed to reach significance after controlling for communication patterns. In other words, communication patterns do account for the relation between attachment and couple violence. More specifically, the association be-

TABLE 12.4. Bivariate Correlations between Attachment Scales and Couple Communication, and between Attachment Scales and Relationship Satisfaction for Males and Females

Variable	Females		Males	
	Anxiety[a]	Discomfort[b]	Anxiety[a]	Discomfort[b]
	Communication			
Postconflict Distress	.31**	.10	.32**	.20**
Mutuality	−.23**	−.23**	−.27**	−.41**
Destructive Process	.34**	.12	.34**	.26**
	Relationship Satisfaction			
Female Relationship Satisfaction	−.26**	−.26**	−.33**	−.28**
Male Relationship Satisfaction	−.23**	−.20**	−.36**	−.31**

[a]Anxiety over abandonment.
[b]Discomfort with closeness.
**$p < .01$.

tween the Anxiety over Abandonment of both partners and female vio lence was mediated by couple communication patterns, as was the association between males' Anxiety over Abandonment and male violence.

These results are consistent with a situation in which one partner's fear of being abandoned leads to the development of destructive patterns of communication within a relationship, such as one partner making demands while the other withdraws, which in turn fosters an environment in which couple violence is more likely to occur.

Does Communication Moderate between Attachment and Couple Violence?

The question of whether couples' attachment styles and couples' communication patterns interact to predict violence in their relationships was investigated using four logistic regression analyses. Separate analyses were used for males' and females' use of couple violence, and for own and partner attachment. However, no evidence was found for communication patterns moderating the relation between attachment and couple violence.

Two Covariates of Couple Violence: Relationship Satisfaction and Partner Violence

As expected, relationship satisfaction and partner violence were significant predictors of the use of violence by both males and females. The association between partners' use of violence was particularly strong. (Relationship satisfaction did not provide independent prediction of men's or women's use of violence after statistically controlling for partner violence.) However, couple communication successfully added to the prediction of both men's and women's use of violence, after controlling for satisfaction and partner violence. Furthermore, the attachment measures added to the prediction of women's use of violence, after satisfaction and partner violence were statistically controlled, but not men's violence, suggesting that perhaps attachment processes are more important in the prediction of females' use of violence than men's use of violence.

However, even though communication continues to significantly predict violence after controlling for relationship satisfaction, it is important to examine whether relationship satisfaction also mediates the relation between attachment and violence. It is important to determine whether the mediating role that communication plays in the association between attachment and violence may simply be because of the variance communication processes share with relationship satisfaction.

Does Relationship Satisfaction Mediate between Attachment and Couple Violence?

We have already established an association between attachment and violence; therefore, three steps remain in order to demonstrate that relationship satisfaction mediates the association between adult attachment and couple violence. First, we need to demonstrate an association between relationship satisfaction and couple violence. Second, it is necessary to show that satisfaction and attachment are significantly related. Third, the association between attachment and couple violence must be shown to decrease once relationship satisfaction is statistically controlled.

The association between relationship satisfaction and couple violence was established using multiple regression analyses. Both females' and males' satisfaction was related to the use of violence by both women and men. As shown in Table 12.4, there is substantial evidence of an association between attachment and relationship satisfaction, with all eight correlations reaching significance. That is, high levels of relationship satisfaction experienced by both females and males are consistently related to low levels of attachment *insecurity*.

Finally, to ascertain whether the relation between attachment and couple violence decreases after controlling for relationship satisfaction, two hierarchical multiple regression analyses were performed, regressing couple violence on both partners' attachment scores (Step 1) and then their relationship satisfaction scores (Step 2), separately for female and male violence. Male Anxiety over Abandonment (the only attachment dimension to independently predict couple violence) continued to predict couple violence after controlling for relationship satisfaction. Although the standardized regression weights did show a drop in magnitude (from

β = .29 to β = .19, for female violence, and from β = .25 to β = .15, for male violence), these differences between the coefficients were not found to be significant using the method of comparing two regression coefficients outlined by Kleinbaum and Kupper (1978).

These results suggest therefore that the association between male Anxiety over Abandonment and couple violence is not mediated by relationship satisfaction. In other words, the findings are consistent with the presence of links between adult attachment and couple violence, independent of the process of relationship satisfaction. This finding is important because it strengthens the position that the process through which adult attachment predicts couple violence is couple communication patterns as opposed to relationship satisfaction.

Does Attachment Style Moderate the Association between Partners' Use of Couple Violence?

The question of whether individuals' attachment interacts with their partners' use of violence to predict their own use of violence was investigated using two logistic regression analyses. Separate analyses were used for males' and females' use of couple violence. Evidence for attachment moderating the association between partners' use of violence was only obtained for men. The overall effect, which was obtained for male violence, was due to a significant interaction between men's own Anxiety over Abandonment and females' use of violence in predicting males' use of violence (pr = .23).

The moderating effect of male Anxiety over Abandonment on the association between partners' use of couple violence was assessed using logistic regression analyses, separately for males who were low in Anxiety over Abandonment (below the mean) and those who were high in Anxiety over Abandonment (above the mean). In both cases, the association was significant; however, the association was stronger when males were high in Anxiety over Abandonment (pr = .53), than when they were low in Anxiety over Abandonment (pr = .39).

DISCUSSION

As predicted, couple violence was related to adult attachment. More specifically, individuals' Anxiety over Abandonment predicted whether or not they were violent toward their partners. Furthermore, male Anxiety over Abandonment predicted whether or not they were the victims of couple violence. The finding that Anxiety over Abandonment is more important than Discomfort with Closeness in predicting couple violence is consistent with previous research. Dutton and his colleagues have also found stronger links between fear over abandonment and abuse than between fear of intimacy and both emotional and physical abuse (Dutton & Browning, 1988; Dutton et al., 1994).

However, in adopting a more systemic approach to the investigation of couple violence by examining the interaction of partners' attachment in this study, we found that Discomfort with Closeness played an important role in the prediction of violence. Individuals' Anxiety over Abandonment was only associated with their use of violence if their partners were uncomfortable with closeness. This interaction between partners' attachment indicates that conflict over the optimal emotional climate of a relationship can create an environment in which couple violence is more likely to occur. In particular, a person's fear of abandonment may be exacerbated by a partner's fear of intimacy, and violence may consequently be used by the anxious partner as a means of controlling the emotional distance of the partner who is uncomfortable with closeness. It is important to note that, although this tactic may work in the short term to maintain the proximity of a partner, over time violence is likely to increase a person's discomfort with closeness. A self-perpetuating feedback loop may be established; violence may increase the victim's discomfort with intimacy, which in turn intensifies the abandonment insecurities of the partner, and thus increases the likelihood of future violence being perpetrated.

The findings of the present study concerning the association between attachment and couple violence contrast with those of Pistole and Tarrant (1993). These researchers concluded that individual differences in attachment are unimportant in the etiology of couple violence. However, our study differs from that of Pistole and Tarrant in a number of key ways. Firstly, Pistole and Tarrant used a sample of convicted male batterers, whereas in the current study subjects represented a more diverse range of people, being recruited from marriage counseling services, community centers, and a university. Second, because the association between violence and attachment was only of peripheral concern to these researchers, their study lacked some sophistication in that no nonviolent comparison group was used and that attachment was measured using a forced-choice measure rather than a continuous scale.

Couple violence is a complex phenomenon, and research over the last 20 years has clearly shown that the causes of couple violence are multiple in nature (Gelles & Maynard, 1987; Mayseless, 1991; Vivian & O'Leary, 1987). Therefore, with few exceptions, any single predictor is likely to account for only a relatively small proportion of the variance in couple violence. Consequently, in attempting to isolate the factors that contribute to the occurrence of couple violence, researchers need to be especially careful to maximize the sensitivity of the measurement devices they use. In investigating the role of attachment in predicting couple violence, it may be necessary to use more sensitive continuous measures of attachment, rather than categorical measures (Feeney, Noller, & Hanrahan,

1994). Researchers may also need to obtain reports of violence from both partners to obtain more accurate assessments of couples' use of violence (Szinovacz & Egley, 1993).

Communication

The hypothesis that communication patterns would *moderate* the association between attachment and violence was not supported. However, the hypothesis that communication patterns would *mediate* the relation between attachment and couple violence was supported. The association between Anxiety over Abandonment and violence could be explained by the dysfunctional communication patterns also associated with Anxiety over Abandonment.

The importance of the Destructive Process scale of the Communication Patterns Questionnaire in predicting whether or not couples are violent highlights the importance of the demand–withdraw pattern of interaction in the etiology of couple violence. This subscale is made up of items measuring the extent to which couples' conflict interactions are characterized by one partner criticizing, making demands, and applying pressure on the other partner, who withdraws from the interaction, defends him- or herself, or attempts to resist any pressure being applied (Noller & White, 1990). The importance of the demand–withdraw pattern of interaction supports previous research into the communication patterns of violent couples (Babcock et al., 1993; Lloyd, 1990; Margolin, John, & O'Brien, 1989).

The findings regarding the communication patterns of violent couples again point to the fact that couple violence has both relational and individual origins. The Communication Patterns Questionnaire was used because it specifically assesses the extent to which *dyads* engage in a range of complementary and supplementary patterns of interaction. Although at the dyadic level it is the dysfunctional communication patterns that make violence more likely to occur, these dysfunctional communication patterns may be, at least partially, due to the attachment styles people bring to their relationships.

Relationship Satisfaction and Partner Violence

As in previous research, both partner violence and relationship dissatisfaction were found to predict whether or not individuals were themselves violent. After controlling for partner violence and relationship satisfaction, communication continued to predict individuals' use of violence, and attachment continued to predict female but not male violence.

Furthermore, the association between Anxiety over Abandonment and couple violence could not be explained by the relationship dissatisfaction that was associated with both Anxiety over Abandonment and couple violence. In contrast to communication patterns, which were found to mediate the association between attachment and couple violence, relationship satisfaction could not account for the association between attachment and violence. These findings suggest that the role of couple communication patterns is more important that relationship satisfaction in explaining how Anxiety over Abandonment is associated with couple violence, and that the mediating role that communication was found to play is not due to the relationship dissatisfaction that is also associated with dysfunctional patterns of couple communication.

Finally, the hypothesis that the association between two partners' use of violence would be affected by adult attachment was also supported, although only for males. Men who were not anxious over abandonment were less likely to be violent toward violent partners than were men who were anxious over abandonment. These findings are important because they reveal that attachment influences one of the strongest findings in the couple violence literature, namely, the highly mutual nature of couple violence. Researchers who have employed random phone surveys, student samples, and marriage counseling samples have consistently found that one of the strongest predictors of whether someone is violent toward his or her romantic partner is whether the partner is violent toward him or her. The fact that attachment impacts upon this association, albeit only for men, is quite impressive, and again demonstrates how factors internal to the individual can influence the dyadic system.

Treatment Implications

Although controversial, couple therapy has been suggested as an important intervention strategy for treating couple violence (O'Leary & Smith, 1991; O'Leary & Vivian, 1990; Tolman & Bennet, 1990). Certainly, couple therapy is inappropriate in those cases where safety issues are prominent, or where the violence is characterized by what Johnson (1993) refers to as "patriarchal terrorism." However, in other cases involving "ordinary couple violence," conjoint counseling may be the treatment of choice. The present research supports that contention by demonstrating the importance of dyadic factors in predicting violence, such as couple communication patterns, relationship satisfaction, partners' violence, and the interaction of partners' attachment. Communication and conflict management training for couples certainly reduces the risk of their experiencing violence in their relationships, even at 5-year follow-ups (Markman, Renick, Floyd, Stanley, & Clements, 1993). In addition, research has shown that the problem-solving skills that people in violent relationships lack are spouse-specific in nature (Holtzworth-Munroe, 1992; Margolin, 1988), suggesting that it is the dyad rather than the individual that should be the focus of treatment. As O'Leary and Vivian (1990) point out, it is unlikely that gender-specific treatment strategies can adequately address the dysfunctional communication and relationship dissatisfaction that contribute to the occurrence of couple violence.

However, attachment insecurities may drive the dysfunctional communication patterns in which violent couples engage. Therefore, the results of the present study suggest that to help violent couples adopt new communication patterns, therapists and counselors need to address couples' attachment insecurities. Furthermore, practitioners may need to help couples investigate with each other their conflicting notions of the optimal emotional closeness for their relationship.

Time-out is an intervention strategy commonly used by practitioners to help people who are experiencing violence in their relationships (Edleson, 1984; Sonkin & Durphy, 1982; Veenstra & Scott, 1993). In such situations, time-out is taught for when an argument is believed to be getting out of control; people are instructed to remove themselves from the situation until they gain sufficient "internal control." When used properly, interactants return to discuss the issues when they are able to discuss them with more control and skill.

Time-out, though potentially useful, needs to be applied with some caution by practitioners. Furthermore, conjoint therapy may be necessary for the successful application of time-out because both partners must fully understand and agree to the process. If only one partner agrees to using time-out, then the process may correspond to little more than the demand–withdraw pattern of interaction, as one partner attempts to temporarily extricate him- or herself from the interaction, while the other partner attempts to pursue him or her. This situational is potentially dangerous because, as found in the present study, the demand–withdraw pattern of interaction may, in fact, contribute to the presence of violence in couple relationships. Furthermore, practitioners must be careful to distinguish time-out from withdrawal. It needs to be framed, not as a form of abandonment, but as a process designed to ensure both partners' physical safety, and to increase the likelihood of successful conflict resolution.

Limitations and Future Research

It is acknowledged that attachment accounts for only a relatively modest amount of variance in couple violence. However, as already noted, the causes of couple violence are multiple in nature (Gelles & Maynard, 1987; Mayseless, 1991; Vivian & O'Leary, 1987), and therefore, any one predictor is likely to account for a limited amount of variance in couple violence. For instance, even measures of patriarchy only account for some 10% of variance in couple violence (Straus, 1993).

More importantly, all the findings presented are correlational in nature, and therefore causation cannot be inferred from the current findings: It cannot be proved that it is not couple violence that is driving the dysfunctional communication patterns and insecure attachment, rather than visa versa. However, a number of important longitudinal studies have been conducted, and these do provide evidence that both couple communication and relationship satisfaction predict couples' later use of violence (Lloyd, 1989; O'Leary, Malone, & Tyree, 1989, cited in O'Leary & Vivian, 1990). Furthermore, helping couples learn better communication and conflict resolution skills reduces the risk of their experiencing violence in their relationships over a 5-year period (Markman et al., 1993).

Attachment, on the other hand, has yet to be linked longitudinally with couple violence. It is more difficult, therefore, to justify our position that attachment drives communication and violence in couple relationships. However, theoretically, attachment has its roots in childhood relationships with parents. Therefore, it is likely that attachment has primacy to any variable associated with a current adult relationship. Furthermore, in the present study, individuals were asked to indicate their approach to romantic relationships in general, not their attachment to their current partner. Finally, attachment has been found to predict later communication patterns and communication accuracy (Feeney, Noller, & Callan, 1994). Nevertheless, future research needs to be directed toward assessing the longitudinal effects of adult attachment on couples' use of violence, to more exactly ascertain the interrelations among attachment, communication, and couple violence. It would be particularly interesting to examine whether self-perpetuating feedback mechanisms are established between couple violence and adult attachment. For example, over time the violence of people who are anxious over abandonment may lead to their partners becoming more uncomfortable with closeness, which in turn increases the abandonment anxiety of the violent partner, thereby further increasing the likelihood that violence will occur.

The findings of this study are limited in being based purely on self-report measures. Future researchers may need to use observational techniques to clarify with greater certainty the interrelations among communication, attachment, and couple violence. The specific communication patterns that predict the development of couple violence longitudinally are yet to be identified, because little observational work has been applied to the study of the conflict interaction of violent couples. Although self-report measures provide invaluable initial insights into the communication of violent couples, their ability to fully assess the complexities of couple interaction is severely limited.

Conclusions

The findings from the present study show how insecure attachment influences whether both men and women are likely to use couple violence or be the victims of couple violence. They also show how attachment can foster an environment within the dyadic system characterized by dysfunctional communication patterns, which in turn increases the chance of violence being present in a relationship. These findings have important implications for the treatment of couple violence. In some cases couple therapy may be a vital component in the treatment of couple violence, although time-out, a common treatment strategy for couple violence, needs to be utilized with caution because of its potential to contribute to the patterns of interaction that already characterize the conflict of violent couples.

NOTES

1. Due to the highly skewed nature of couple violence data, Straus (1990) recommends the use of a dichotomous split of violent versus nonviolent subjects, and the use of logistic regression analysis to investigate its correlates. However, multiple regression can be used with a dichotomous dependent variable if a minimum of 100 cases are obtained, with no less than 25% of these belonging to the smaller category (Cleary & Angel, 1984; Tabachnick & Fidell, 1989). In general, therefore, linear regression techniques were used to analyze the results presented, because of the greater familiarity of most researchers with the use of linear regression techniques in demonstrating the presence of mediator variables.

2. In the present study, investigation of some moderator effects involved a dichotomous predictor and a dichotomous criterion; therefore, logistic regression analysis was used to examine all moderator effects. Unlike the analysis of interactions using multiple regression analysis, the analysis of interaction effects using logistic regression analysis does not require the use of hierarchical procedures in which interaction terms are entered after statistically controlling for main effects (Norusis, 1990). The criterion variable may simply be regressed on the interaction terms of interest. To ensure that an undue amount of variance in the interaction was not provided by any one of the two variables, they were first standardized, as is recommended for analysis of interactions using multiple regression analysis (Feeney, 1995; Jaccard, Turrisi, & Wan, 1990).

REFERENCES

Arias, I., & Beach, S. R. H. (1987). Validity of self-reports of marital violence. *Journal of Family Violence, 2*(2), 139–149.

Avis, J. (1992). Where are all the family therapists?: Abuse and violence within families and family therapy's response. *Journal of Marital and Family Therapy, 18,* 223–230.

Babcock, J. C., Waltz, J., Jacobson, N. S., & Gottman, J. M. (1993). Power and violence: The relation between communication patterns, power discrepancies, and domestic violence. *Journal of Consulting and Clinical Psychology, 61,* 40–50.

Baron, R. M., & Kenny, D. A. (1986). The moderator–mediator variable distinction in social psychological research: Conceptual, strategic, and statistical considerations. *Journal of Personality and Social Psychology, 51,* 1173–1182.

Bartholomew, K., & Horowitz, L. M. (1991). Attachment styles among young adults: A test of a four-category model. *Journal of Personality and Social Psychology, 61,* 226–244.

Ben-David, S. (1993). The two facets of female violence: The public and the domestic domains. *Journal of Family Violence, 8*(4), 345–359.

Bograd, M. (1992). Values in conflict: Challenges to family therapists' thinking. *Journal of Marital and Family Therapy, 18*(3), 245–256.

Bookwala, J., Frieze, I. H., & Grote, N. K. (1994). Love, aggression and satisfaction in dating relationships. *Journal of Social and Personal Relationships, 11,* 625–632.

Bookwala, J., Frieze, I. H., Smith, C., & Ryan, K. (1992). Predictors of dating violence: A multivariate analysis. *Violence and Victims, 7*(4), 297–311.

Bowlby, J. (1988). *A secure base.* New York: Basic Books.

Burman, B., Margolin, G., & John, R. S. (1993). America's angriest home videos: Behavioral contingencies observed in home reenactments of marital conflict. *Journal of Consulting and Clinical Psychology, 61,* 28–39.

Christensen, A. (1988). Dysfunctional interaction patterns in couples. In P. Noller & M. A. Fitzpatrick (Eds.), *Perspectives on marital interaction* (pp. 31–52). Clevedon, England: Multilingual Matters.

Christensen, S., & Sullaway, M. (1984). *Communication Patterns Questionnaire.* Unpublished manuscript, University of California, Los Angeles.

Cleary, P. D., & Angel, R. (1984). The analysis of relationships involving dichotomous dependent variables. *Journal of Health and Social Behavior, 25,* 334–348.

Cohn, D. A., Silver, D. H., Cowan, C. P., Cowan, P. A., & Pearson, J. (1992). Working models of childhood attachment and couple relationships. *Journal of Family Issues, 13*(4), 432–449.

Coleman, K. H. (1980). Conjugal violence: What 33 men report. *Journal of Marital and Family Therapy, 6,* 207–213.

Collins, N. S., & Read, S. J. (1990). Adult attachment, working models, and relationship quality in dating couples. *Journal of Personality and Social Psychology, 58,* 644–663.

Collins, N. S., & Read, S. J. (1994). Cognitive representations of attachment: The structure and function of working models. *Advances in Personal Relationships, 5,* 53–90.

Dutton, D. G. (1994). Behavioral and affective correlates of Borderline Personality Organization in wife assaulters. *International Journal of Criminal Justice and Behavior, 17*(3), 26–38.

Dutton, D. G., & Browning, J. J. (1988). Power struggles and intimacy anxieties as causative factors of wife assault. In G. Russell (Ed.), *Violence in intimate relationships* (pp. 163–175). Newbury Park, CA: Sage.

Dutton, D. G., Saunders, K., Starzomski, A., & Bartholomew, K. (1994). Intimacy-anger and insecure attachment as precursors of abuse in intimate relationships. *Journal of Applied Social Psychology, 24*(15), 1367–1386.

Edleson, J. L. (1984). Working with men who batter. *Social Work, 29,* 237–242.

Feeney, J. A. (1990). *The attachment perspective on adult romantic relationships.* Unpublished doctoral dissertation, University of Queensland, Brisbane, Australia.

Feeney, J. A. (1994). Attachment style, communication patterns, and satisfaction across the life cycle of marriage. *Personal Relationships, 1,* 333–348.

Feeney, J. A. (1995). Adult attachment and emotional control. *Personal Relationships, 2,* 143–159.

Feeney, J. A., & Noller, P. (1992). Attachment style and romantic love: Relationship dissolution. *Australian Journal of Psychology, 44,* 69–74.

Feeney, J. A., Noller, P., & Callan, V. J. (1994). Attachment style, communication and satisfaction in the early years of marriage. *Advances in Personal Relationships, 5,* 269–308.

Feeney, J. A., Noller, P., & Hanrahan, M. (1994). Assessing adult attachment. In M. B. Sperling & W. H. Berman (Eds.), *Attachment in adults: Clinical and developmental perspectives* (pp. 128–152). New York: Guilford Press.

Fitzpatrick, M. A., Fey, J., Segrin, C., & Schiff, J. L. (1993). Internal working models of relationships and marital communication patterns. *Journal of Language and Social Psychology, 12,* 103–131.

Gelles, R. J. (1985). Family violence. *Annual Review of Sociology, 11,* 347–367.

Gelles, R. J. (1990). Methodological issues in the study of family violence. In M. A. Straus & R. J. Gelles (Eds.), *Physical violence in American families: Risk factors and adaptations in 8,145 families* (pp. 17–28). New Brunswick, NJ: Transaction Press.

Gelles, R. J., & Maynard, P. E. (1987). A structural family systems approach to intervention in cases of family violence. *Family Relations, 36,* 270–275.

Giles-Sims, J. (1983). *Wife battering: A systems theory approach.* New York: Guilford Press.

Gondolf, E. W. (1988). Who are these guys?: Toward a behavioral typology of batterers. *Violence and Victims, 3,* 187–203.

Gottman, J. M., Jacobson, N. S., Rushe, R. H., Shortt, J. W., Babcock, J., La Taillade, J. J., & Waltz, J. (1995). The relationship between heart rate reactivity, emotionally aggressive behavior, and general violence in batterers. *Journal of Family Psychology, 9*(3), 227–248.

Griffin, D. W., & Bartholomew, K. (1994). The metaphysics of measurement: The case of adult attachment. *Advances in Personal Relationships, 5,* 17–52.

Hansen, M. (1992). Feminism and family therapy: A review of feminist critiques of approaches to family violence. In M. Hansen & M. Harway (Eds.), *Battering and family therapy: A feminist perspective* (pp. 69–81). Newbury Park, CA: Sage.

Hazan, C., & Shaver, P. (1987). Romantic love conceptualized as an attachment process. *Journal of Personality and Social Psychology, 52,* 511–524.

Henton, J., Cate, R., Koval, J., Lloyd, S., & Christopher, S. (1983). Romance and violence in dating relationships. *Journal of Family Issues, 4*(3), 467–482.

Holtzworth-Munroe, A. (1992). Social skill deficits in maritally violent men: Interpreting the data using a social information processing model. *Clinical Psychology Review, 12,* 605–617.

Holtzworth-Munroe, A., & Stuart, G. L. (1994). Typologies of male batterers: Three subtypes and the differences among them. *Psychological Bulletin, 116*(3), 476–497.

Infante, D. A., Chandler, T. A., & Rudd, J. E. (1989). Test of an argumentative skill deficiency model of interspousal violence. *Communication Monographs, 56,* 163–177.

Jaccard, J., Turrisi, R., & Wan, C. K. (1990). *Interaction effects in multiple regression.* Newbury Park, CA: Sage.

Johnson, M. P. (1993). *Violence against women in the American family: Are there two forms?* Paper presented at the Theory Construction and Research Methodology Workshop, National Council on Family Relations, Baltimore, MD.

Julian, T. W., & McKenry, P. C. (1993). Mediators of male violence toward female intimates. *Journal of Family Violence, 8*(1), 39–56.

Kleinbaum, D. G., & Kupper, L. L. (1978). *Applied regression analysis and other multivariable methods.* North Scituate, MA: Duxbury Press.

Kobak, R. R., & Hazan, C. (1991). Attachment in marriage: Effects of security and accuracy of working models. *Journal of Personality and Social Psychology, 60,* 861–869.

Kobak, R. R., & Sceery, A. (1988). Attachment in late adolescence: Working models, affect regulation, and representations of self and others. *Child Development, 59,* 135–146.

Levy, M. B., & Davis, K. D. (1988). Love styles and attachment styles compared: Their relations to each other and to various relationship characteristics. *Journal of Social and Personal Relationships, 5,* 439–471.

Lloyd, S. (1989). *The stability of physical aggression in marriage.* Paper presented at the annual conference of the National Council on Family Relations, New Orleans, LA.

Lloyd, S. (1990). Conflict types and strategies in violent marriages. *Journal of Family Violence, 5,* 269–284.

MacEwan, K. E., & Barling, J. (1988). Multiple stressors, violence in the family of origin, and marital aggression: A longitudinal investigation. *Journal of Family Violence, 3*(1), 73–87.

Margolin, G. (1988). Interpersonal and intrapersonal factors associated with marital violence. In G. T. Hotaling, D. Finkelhor, J. T. Kirkpatrick, & M. A. Straus (Eds.), *Family abuse and its consequences* (pp. 203–217). Newbury Park, CA: Sage.

Margolin, G., Burman, B., & John, R. S. (1989). Home observations of marital couples reenacting naturalistic conflicts. *Behavioral Assessment, 11,* 101–118.

Margolin, G., John, R. S., & Gleberman, L. (1988). Affective responses to conflictual discussion in violent and nonviolent couples. *Journal of Consulting and Clinical Psychology, 56,* 24–33.

Margolin, G., John, R. S., & O'Brien, M. (1989). Sequential affective patterns as a function of marital conflict style. *Journal of Social and Clinical Psychology, 56,* 24–33.

Markman, H. J., Renick, M. J., Floyd, F. J., Stanley, S. M., & Clements, M. (1993). Preventing marital distress through communication and conflict management training: A 4- and 5-year follow-up. *Journal of Consulting and Clinical Psychology, 61*(1), 70–77.

Mattinson, J., & Sinclair, I. (1979). *Mate and stalemate.* Oxford, England: Blackwell.

Mayseless, O. (1991). Adult attachment patterns and courtship violence. *Family Relations, 40,* 21–28.

McHugh, M. C. (1992). Studying battered women and batterers: Feminist perspectives on methodology. In M. Hansen & M. Harway (Eds.), *Battering and family therapy: A feminist perspective* (pp. 54–68). Newbury Park, CA: Sage.

Mikulincer, M., & Nachshon, O. (1991). Attachment styles and patterns of self-disclosure. *Journal of Personality and Social Psychology, 61,* 213–331.

Murphy, C., & O'Leary, K. D. (1989). Psychological aggression predicts physical aggression in early marriage. *Journal of Clinical and Consulting Psychology, 57,* 579–582.

Noller, P., & White, A. (1990). The validity of the Communication Patterns

Questionnaire. *Psychological Assessment: A Journal of Consulting and Clinical Psychology, 2,* 478–482.

Norusis, M. J. (1990). *SPSS advanced statistics user's guide.* Chicago: SPSS, Inc.

O'Leary, K. D. (1988). Physical aggression between spouses: A social learning theory perspective. In V. B. Van Hasselt, R. L. Morrison, A. S. Bellack, & M. Hersen (Eds.), *Handbook of family violence* (pp. 31–55). New York: Plenum Press.

O'Leary, K. D., Barling, J., Arias, I., & Rosenbaum, A. (1989). Prevalence and stability of physical aggression between spouses: A longitudinal analysis. *Journal of Consulting and Clinical Psychology, 57*(2), 263–268.

O'Leary, K. D., & Smith, D. A. (1991). Marital interactions. *Annual Review of Psychology, 42,* 191–212.

O'Leary, K. D., & Vivian, D. (1990). Physical aggression in marriage. In F. Fincham & T. Bradbury (Eds.), *Psychology of marriage* (pp. 323–348). New York: Guilford Press.

Pistole, M. (1989). Attachment in adult romantic relationships: Style of conflict resolution and relationship satisfaction. *Journal of Social and Personal Relationships, 6,* 505–510.

Pistole, M. C., & Tarrant, N. (1993). Attachment style and aggression in male batterers. *Family Therapy, 20*(3), 165–173.

Retzinger, S. M. (1991a). Shame, anger, and conflict: Case study of emotional violence. *Journal of Family Violence, 6*(1), 37–60.

Retzinger, S. M. (1991b). *Violent emotions: Shame and rage in marital quarrels.* Newbury Park, CA: Sage.

Rosenbaum, A. (1988). Methodological issues in marital violence research. *Journal of Family Violence, 3*(2), 91–104.

Rosenbaum, A., & O'Leary, D. (1981). Marital violence: Characteristics of abusive couples. *Journal of Consulting and Clinical Psychology, 49,* 63–71.

Rounsaville, B. J. (1978). Theories in marital violence: Evidence from a study of battered women. *Victimology: An International Journal, 3*(1), 11–31.

Senchak, M., & Leonard, K. E. (1992). Attachment styles and marital adjustment among newlywed couples. *Journal of Social and Personal Relationships, 9,* 51–64.

Simpson, J. (1990). Influence of attachment styles on romantic relationships. *Journal of Personality and Social Psychology, 59,* 971–980.

Smith, D. A., Vivian, D., & O'Leary, K. D. (1991). The misnomer proposition: A critical reappraisal of the longitudinal status of "negativity" in marital communication. *Behavioral Assessment, 13,* 7–24.

Sonkin, D. J., & Durphy, M. (1982). *Learning to live without violence: A handbook for men.* San Francisco: Volcano Press.

Spanier, G. B. (1976). Measuring dyadic adjustment: New scales for assessing the quality of marriage and similar dyads. *Journal of Marriage and the Family, 38,* 15–30.

Stets, J. E., & Henderson, D. A. (1991). Contextual factors surrounding conflict resolution while dating: Results from a national study. *Family Relations, 40,* 29–36.

Stets, J. E., & Straus, M. A. (1990). The marriage license as a hitting license: A comparison of assaults in dating, cohabiting, and married couples. In M. A. Straus & R. J. Gelles (Eds.), *Physical violence in American families: Risk factors and adaptations to violence in 8,145 families* (pp. 227–244). New Brunswick, NJ: Transaction Press.

Straus, M. A. (1973). A general systems theory approach to a theory of violence between family members. *Social Science Information, 12,* 105–125.

Straus, M. A. (1979). Measuring intrafamily conflict and violence: The conflict tactics (CT) scales. *Journal of Marriage and the Family, 41,* 75–86.

Straus, M. A. (1990). Measuring intrafamily conflict and violence: The Conflict Tactics (CT) Scale. In M. A. Straus & R. J. Gelles (Eds.), *Physical violence in American families: Risk factors and adaptations to violence in 8,145 families* (pp. 29–47). New Brunswick, NJ: Transaction Press.

Straus, M. A. (1993). *Discussion by Murray Straus on two papers.* Presented at the annual meeting of the National Council on Family Relations, Baltimore, MD.

Straus, M. A., & Gelles, R. J. (1990). How violent are American families?: Estimates from the National Family Violence Resurvey and other studies. In M. A. Straus & R. J. Gelles (Eds.), *Physical violence in American families: Risk factors and adaptations to violence in 8,145 families* (pp. 95–112). New Brunswick, NJ: Transaction Press.

Szinovacz, M., & Egley, S. C. (1993). *Aggregate and couple data on marital violence: Another look at the evidence.* Paper presented at the Theory Construction and Research Methodology Workshop, National Council on Family Relations, Baltimore, MD.

Tabachnick, B. G., & Fidell, L. S. (1989). *Using multivariate statistics.* New York: Harper & Row.

Telch, C. F., & Lindquist, C. U. (1984). Violent versus nonviolent couples: A comparison of patterns. *Psychotherapy, 21*(2), 242–248.

Tolman, R. M., & Bennet, L. W. (1990). A review of quantitative research on men who batter. *Journal of Interpersonal Violence, 5*(1), 87–118.

Veenstra, G. J., & Scott, C, G. (1993). A model for using time out as an intervention technique with families. *Journal of Family Violence, 8(1),* 71–87.

Vivian, D., & O'Leary, K. D. (1987). *Communication patterns in physically aggressive engaged couples.* Paper presented at the Third National Family Violence Research Conference, Durham, NH.

Vuchinich, S. (1987). Starting and stopping spontaneous family conflicts. *Journal of Marriage and the Family, 49,* 591–601.

Whitchurch, G. G., & Pace, J. L. (1993). Communication skills training and interspousal violence. *Journal of Applied Communication Research, 21*(1), 96–102.

Yllo, K. (1983). Using a feminist approach in quantitative research: A case study. In D. Finkelhor, R. J. Gelles, G. T. Hotaling, & M. A. Straus (Eds.), *The dark side of families: Current family violence research* (pp. 277–288). Beverly Hills, CA: Sage.

PART V

Conceptual and Empirical Extensions

13

Evolution, Pair-Bonding, and Reproductive Strategies

A Reconceptualization of Adult Attachment

LEE A. KIRKPATRICK

Since the publication of seminal work by Hazan and Shaver (1987) and Shaver, Hazan, and Bradshaw (1988), an entire field of "adult attachment" research and theory has emerged within the personality/social literature, as exemplified by the present volume. The central assumption of this burgeoning literature, following Bowlby (1969), is that the attachment system continues to operate from the cradle to the grave; specifically, it is assumed that the attachment system (in conjunction with caregiving and sex/reproduction systems) underlies many of the important dynamics and individual differences observed in adult romantic relationships. In this chapter I will challenge this assumption and offer an alternative (though closely related) model, drawing upon an evolutionary-psychological perspective and a variety of recent theoretical and empirical lines of research.

To summarize in advance, I will argue that the attachment system *qua* system may not be as centrally involved in adult romantic relationships as adult attachment researchers (including myself) have assumed. My analysis focuses on the evolutionary problems of mating and parental investment, building upon the bond-formation model recently proposed by Zeifman and Hazan (1997a, 1997b) but extending and deviating from this model in several ways. First, I argue that only the emotion we call love, and not the attachment system per se, has been co-opted by evolution in the service of maintaining pair-bonds; in making this argument I borrow from Frank's (1988) functional perspective on social emotions. Second, I argue that long-term pair-bonding is only one among the alternative reproductive strategies in the human repertoire, as articulated in *sexual strategies theory* (Buss & Schmitt, 1993) and *sociosexuality theory* (Gangestad & Simpson, 1990; Simpson & Gangestad, 1991). Third, I argue that individual differences in what we have been calling adult *attachment styles* may fundamentally reflect, at least in part, individual differences in reproductive strategies, which in turn are importantly related to childhood attachment experience, as demonstrated by Draper and Harpending (1982) and Belsky, Steinberg, and Draper (1991). Finally, I reexamine findings from several areas of adult attachment research in light of this revised perspective.

QUESTIONING THE STANDARD ADULT ATTACHMENT MODEL

A standard assumption of adult attachment theory is that the attachment system, as described by Bowlby (1969) in terms of systems control theory, continues to be operative across the life span and particularly within adult romantic relationships. While it is generally recognized that important differences exist between infant and adult attachment, the system is thought to operate according to the same general dynamics as in infancy. Rothbard and Shaver (1994) and Zeifman and Hazan (1997a), among others, provide literature reviews in support of this contention. Although adult attachment researchers readily admit to the existence of important differences between mother–infant and adult attachment, I believe these differences point to deeper theoretical problems than have been previously acknowledged.

If the attachment system is thought to be designed by natural selection to continue operating in adulthood as in infancy, one must ask what the adaptive *function* of attachment in adulthood might be (or, more precisely, might have been in ancestral environments). Bowlby (1969) argued cogently that the adaptive function attachment in infancy was the protection (and thus survival) of otherwise helpless infants. If the system is designed to continue operating beyond infancy, however, it presumably must serve (or have served) some adaptive function in adulthood as well. What function might this be? Previous writers have suggested two distinct possibilities.

Security/Protection

One possibility is that the attachment system continues to serve the same function in adulthood as it did in infancy: the provision of protection and security. Several theorists have argued this explicitly (e.g., West & Sheldon-Keller, 1994), although many others probably assume it implicitly. However, there are several reasons why this view seems implausible from an evolutionary perspective.

First, in contrast to infants, adults possess an extensive and differentiated repertoire for responding to different kinds of threats under different conditions. The attachment system is readily activated in infancy and overrides other systems because for an infant, the only available, adaptive response to virtually any form of danger is to increase proximity to one's attachment figure. Adults, however, must select from a diverse menu of behavioral options, including fighting in self-defense (including weapon use), fleeing/escaping, pooling defensive resources in coalitional alliances, and so forth. It would not be adaptive for an attachment system in adulthood—especially one targeting any particular individual—to be readily activated by environmental threats and thereby suppress activation of more adaptive responses.

Second, although some available responses to danger in adulthood involve turning to other people for assistance, it would not be adaptive for the spouse to be unique, or even primary, as the target of these efforts. A spouse—or for that matter, any single individual—would have offered little in the way of protection against adult-sized survival threats in ancestral environments. Predators and violent neighbors pose as much of a danger to one's spouse as to oneself, in stark contrast to mother–infant pairs, in which one member clearly possesses greater ability than the other to deal with threats. Relative to other alternatives, summoning one's spouse for comfort at the sight of a dangerous predator or a marauding band from a neighboring village simply is not an adaptive survival strategy.

Moreover, given the general size and strength difference between human males and females, seeking one's spouse for protection would seem a particularly maladaptive strategy for men, whose female partners would be especially ill equipped to offer physical protection against most dangerous environmental threats. Thus the assumption of a support/protection function of adult attachment leads to the expectation of sex differences in adult attachment, for which little if any evidence exists. (It is worth noting, however, that the limited research on behavioral [Simpson, Rholes, & Nelligan, 1992] and physiological [Carpenter & Kirkpatrick, 1996] responses to laboratory stressors in the presence of romantic partners has so far utilized only female participants, so it remains to be seen if sex differences do in fact exist in this context.)

Finally, it is crucial to note that the attachment system in infants is adaptive only because a complementary caregiving system in adults is responsive to attachment behavior. One's attachment figure must be motivated to provide protection and support at some cost (time, resources, exposure to danger) to him- or herself. The evolution of such *parental investment* mechanisms in parents is made possible by the genetic relatedness of the participants: Genes for protecting offspring lead to increased survival (and subsequent reproduction) of offspring, whose survival in turn promotes proliferation of those genes in the next generation (Trivers, 1974). Spouses, in contrast, are generally no more closely related genetically than any random pair of adults in a given population, and thus cannot be expected to be motivated to provide caregiving for each other at much cost to themselves. Providing assistance and support to another person, which invariably comes at some cost to the self, represents a form of altruism. From an evolutionary perspective, we should expect such altruism to be forthcoming from two groups of individuals: blood relatives (per kin-selection principles), and coalition partners (per reciprocal-altruism principles). Of course, pair-bonded adults do *share* genetic interests in the survival of offspring, and thus have some *indirect* interest in each others' welfare. At the same time, however, their genetic interests conflict in many ways as well, and the correlation of genetic interests is more fragile (Daly & Wilson, 1996). I will return to this issue in a subsequent section.

It might be objected that my exclusive focus on physical protection from environmental threats is unfair. In contemporary society, it might be argued, attachment relationships primarily provide psychological security and comfort rather than physical protection. However, it seems unlikely that the attachment system could be designed by natural selection for this function alone. Unless felt security somehow translated reliably into differential survival or reproductive success in ancestral environments, natural selection would have been blind to such purely psychological effects. This is not to say that romantic partners, as well as friends or other adult peers, cannot take on some of the qualities of attachment figures over the course of a long-term relationship. We simply should not expect nature to have designed the attachment system to operate in this way in adult romantic relationships. Instead, an evolutionary perspective suggests that although adult romantic relationships may involve a complex interplay of a variety of relationships processes and dynamics, they must be viewed first and foremost as *reproductive sexual relationships* that function largely in terms of mechanisms designed to enhance individuals' reproductive success. I outline such a perspective in the remainder of this chapter.

Pair-Bond Maintenance

Other theorists, particularly Zeifman and Hazan (1997a, 1997b), have argued that the attachment system remains intact across the life span but has been co-opted by evolution in the service of another function in adulthood: the maintenance of long-term pair-bond relationships. Following Konner (1982), Zeifman and Hazan argue that natural selection tends to be conservative and parsimonious, making use of existing mechanisms rather than inventing new ones wherever possible. A related view is suggested by Berman, Marcus, and Berman (1994), who argue that the function of adult attachment is "preservation of a dyadic family unit" (p. 214).[1]

Although the parsimony argument is compelling, it seems unlikely in principle that an entire *system*—particularly a complex control system such as that described by Bowlby—could be maintained intact despite a qualitative switch of function. For example, the kinds of situations that should activate the system, while perhaps partially overlapping, are certainly not isomorphic. It would not be adaptive, for example, for a pair-bond-maintenance mechanism to be activated by sickness, fatigue, or environmental threats. One cannot simply co-opt a radio to perform the functions of a television set: The complex interconnections among the parts are designed to receive radio waves and transduce them into sound, and cannot as a unit suddenly begin receiving television broadcasts and presenting them in a visual display.

On the other hand, if one started with a radio and wanted to build a television, one might well utilize some of the radio's important *components* to build a television set, and thus do so more efficiently than starting from scratch. Many of the necessary parts might be the same, but new parts need to be added, some old parts discarded, and the entire system reorganized. I believe that Zeifman and Hazan are basically correct to the extent that important *components* of mother–infant attachment (i.e., of the attachment and/or caregiving systems) have been co-opted by evolution in the service of maintaining long-term monogamous pair bonds. Specifically, I will argue that the crucial component shared by these systems is the emotional bond we call "love." In the next section I review both theoretical and empirical arguments for this view.

THE ROLE OF LOVE

To understand the pivotal role of love in parental caregiving, attachment, and adult pair-bonds, it is useful to ask what functional significance emotions serve in the first place. We perform actions every day that are essential for survival and reproduction with little or no emotional involvement; for example, we procure food, urinate, and build protective shelters. Why should caring for our children or maintaining a pair-bond relationship be any different?

Emotions as Commitment Devices

An intriguing perspective on this question is provided by Frank's (1988) theory of emotions as *commitment devices*. Frank offers the following simple example to illustrate the basic principle. Suppose that someone steals your $200 leather briefcase, and you know who the thief is. If you behave in an entirely rational manner you will be loath to spend hundreds or thousands of dollars, not to mention considerable time and energy, to recover the $200 briefcase. Even if you realize that it would be in your long-term interest to prosecute (i.e., to discourage more such behavior in the future), it would be very difficult to convince yourself to do this in light of the short-term costs incurred.

If a would-be thief knows all this as well, then what prevents him or her from stealing your briefcase with impunity? The answer is that if the thief steals your briefcase you likely will be become *outraged* and will not hesitate to do whatever is necessary to bring the thief to justice. This emotional response provides a mechanism that effectively commits you to a course of action—namely, exacting revenge—that overwhelms the rational analyses that otherwise would lead you to simply accept the loss. Moreover, and equally important, the thief knows of your capability for being outraged, and the more visible signs of this capability you display the less likely the thief is to try his luck. If you clearly are inclined to become incensed and consequently to behave "irrationally," it is no longer in the would-be thief's interest to steal the briefcase.

Love as a Commitment Device

According to Frank (1988), the emotion of love plays a comparable role in the establishment and maintenance of adult pair-bond relationships. The *commitment problem* to be solved is determining when to end the search for the "best" possible mate. No matter how long one searches and evaluates the mate market in choosing a partner, there is always the possibility of a more attractive alternative coming along later. Another analogy offered by Frank in this context is that of landlords and tenants, who are involved in a complex and costly search for the best available tenant and the best available apartment, respectively. At some point each must commit to a choice, or the former will continue to go on with an unrented apartment and the latter will continue to go homeless. In this case it is a *lease* that serves the role of a commitment device: With the potential benefits of a continued search removed (and/or costs increased), both parties are freed from the process and can get on with their lives. In the same way, a powerful emotional bond forming between two adults serves as a commitment device that frees them from the potentially interminable mate-selection process and permits them to get on with the business of childbearing and child rearing.

Although Frank does not discuss this case, it seems clear that parents' love for their offspring can be conceptualized along the same lines. In highly altricial species such as ours it certainly is adaptive, under most circumstances, for parents to invest heavily in offspring. However, it is not unusual for circumstances to arise in which withholding or withdrawal of investment provides an attractive alternative strategy, at least in the short term. Infanticide, as well as child abuse, neglect, and abandonment are not at all unusual in human societies and commonly occur under certain predictable (from an evolutionary perspective) conditions (Daly & Wilson, 1988). A strong emotional bond to one's offspring may, like a lease, function to enforce a "decision" to maintain high levels of parental investment despite immediate temptations to do otherwise. (See Mellen, 1981, for a related discussion.)

It is interesting from this perspective to note an even closer analogue to Frank's lease metaphor for love: *Marriage* is a pancultural human institution that "is everywhere intelligible as a socially recognized alliance between a woman and a man, instituted and acknowledged as a vehicle for producing and rearing children" (Daly & Wilson, 1996, p. 15). Such social contracts function as a kind of backup system to Nature's effective (but fallible) emotional-bond solution to the pair-bond commitment problem: It terminates the mate-selection game and permits the participants and those around them to get on with the business of childbearing and child rearing. The fact that a need exists for such cultural solutions to this problem is itself indicative that Nature's solution is not foolproof: Despite strong emotion mechanisms, pair-bonded adults and parents are nevertheless tempted occasionally to "break their leases" with partners and offspring. This in turn suggests the existence and operation of competing, alternative strategies, as I discuss in a subsequent section.[2]

The Process of Bond Formation

Zeifman and Hazan (1997a) have described a comprehensive model of "adult attachment formation," based on Bowlby's theorizing, that traces the stages of bond formation in adult romantic relationships. Drawing upon diverse lines of research, Zeifman and Hazan demonstrate persuasively the many parallels between this process and both mother–infant bonding and children's responses to separation and loss. Although the authors refer frequently (often only in passing) to the presumed role of security regulation and protection, their model seems at least as consistent with the simpler love-as-commitment-device hypothesis advanced here; it is not obvious why other elements of attachment, such as security regulation and protection, need be cast in central roles. That is, their model might better be described as a process of *bond formation* rather than *attachment* formation per se.

According to Zeifman and Hazan, the *preattachment* phase of initial attraction, flirtation, and courtship is a feeling-out stage in which individuals evaluate, and allow themselves to be evaluated by, each other. My interpretation of this stage diverges only slightly from Zeifman and Hazan's: I would argue that potential partners are being evaluated specifically with respect to their suitability as a long-term pair-bond partner and as a potential parent, rather than as a potential attachment figure per se.

The *attachment-in-the-making* stage is the process of "falling in love," in which the emotional bond becomes established. Several observations concerning to this stage are particularly striking from the perspective of the love-as-commitment-device perspective. For example, as noted by Zeifman and Hazan, infatuation is often characterized by idealization of partners (Brehm, 1988; Tennov, 1979), which might be interpreted as a cognitive manifestation of the process of shutting down the search for more attractive alternatives once a "commitment" has been made. Second, this stage is characterized by increased levels of self-disclosure, which Zeifman and Hazan (1997b) describe explicitly as a test of commitment. Third, Frank (1988) notes that once the relationship is well established, expression of an *exchange* orientation toward the relationship (e.g., keeping score of exchanged favors) is correlated *inversely* with marital satisfaction (Murstein, Cerreto, & MacDonald, 1977). Acknowledging the power of love as a commitment device, we want our partners to be motivated to stay in relationships with us because of love, not because of exchange considerations. The latter represents the very transitory, rational-choice strategy that love is designed to override in the first place.

Another intriguing aspect of the Zeifman–Hazan model is the postulated role of *sexual behavior* in promoting development of the emotional bond (Hazan & Zeifman, 1994; Zeifman & Hazan, 1997a). This idea, too, makes good sense in terms of the love-as-commitment perspective: Regular sex means that offspring are on the way; thus, it is time to commit to the relationship in preparation for parental investment 9 months down the road. It therefore seems reasonable to expect natural selection to have yoked emotional-bond formation to sexual behavior. Again, however, it is not clear how the attachment system per se is relevant or essential to the process.

The final stage of *clear-cut attachment* reflects life-as-usual once the emotional bond and long-term relationship commitment have been established. Zeifman and Hazan argue that it is only at this stage that all of the defining characteristics of true attachment, including safe haven and secure base functions, are found together. There is little doubt that long-term relationship partners can and do take on some of the characteristics of an attachment figure, such as providing comfort and support in difficult times, but this aspect of the relationship may reflect processes other than attachment. Zeifman and Hazan's (following Bowlby, 1969) description of the established relationship as a *goal-corrected partnership* seems apt in that any long-term relationship characterized by mutual trust has the makings of a *reciprocal alliance*. Thus, an alternative explanation for the apparent secure base and safe haven functions of established romantic relationships can be articulated in terms of principles of reciprocal altruism and coalition formation rather than attachment. I develop this point more fully in a subsequent section.

Interestingly, Daly and Wilson (1988) describe the formation of a mother's emotional bond toward her infant in terms nearly identical to Zeifman and Hazan's (1997b) description of attachment formation. After reviewing the controversial literature on this topic, Daly and Wilson (1988) conclude that the evidence does indeed support the importance of postpartum mother–infant contact for development of an emotional bond in the mother. Daly and Wilson describe a three-stage process beginning with an "assessment" stage, beginning immediately after birth, in which the mother assesses the quality of the infant and present circumstances. This stage frequently is characterized by an apparent emotional flatness or indifference on the mother's part. This phase is followed by "the establishment of an individualized love for the child" and finally a "gradual deepening of maternal love over the course of years" (p. 72). The parallels between this stage process and that described by Zeifman and Hazan should be obvious. In particular, both involve the "switching on" of a commitment device (love bond) following an appropriate evaluation and decision period.

In summary, Frank's model of social emotions provides a theoretical basis for a model of love as an evolved mechanism designed to commit adults to long-term pair-bond relationships (and parents to investment in offspring), freeing them from continued competition in the mate market and allowing them to get on with the business of childbearing and child rearing. The evidence and theory reviewed by Zeifman and Hazan (1997a, 1997b) with respect to pair-bond development and maintenance is completely consistent with this position.

Attachment, Caregiving, or Love?

Hazan and Shaver (1987; Shaver et al., 1988) and others have long argued that adult romantic relationships reflect the operation and integration of the *caregiving* system and the *sex/reproductive* system along with the attachment system. There is little doubt about the sex/reproductive component: From an evolutionary point of view, adult pair-bond relationships are first and foremost about reproduction. What I wish to argue here is that romantic relationships might involve neither the caregiving system nor the attachment system per se, but rather are organized around a single component shared by those systems: the emotional bond of love. In this section I offer some examples of how this perspective offers an alternative explanation for many of the research findings generally cited as evidence for attachment processes in romantic relationships.

It is clear that many aspects of adult romantic relationships resemble aspects of mother–infant relationships. What is not clear in many of these cases, however, is whether the observed phenomenon more closely parallels the attachment side of mother–infant relationships or the caregiving side. One such example was cited earlier, concerning the resemblance between the stages of bond formation in adult lovers (as described by Zeifman & Hazan, 1997a) and in mothers' bonding to their infants. In this section I briefly address three other examples in which adult love appears to be at least as closely related to adult caregiving as to infant attachment. Given this pattern of resemblances, it seems reasonable to postulate that neither the attachment system nor the caregiving system per se is involved in adult romantic relationships, but rather a component (love) shared by these two systems. Interestingly, this view converges (though for quite different theoretical reasons) with the suggestion by Berman and Sperling (1994) that attachment and caregiving be regarded, in adulthood, as a singular combined system rather than as two separate systems.

Responses to Separation and Loss

As summarized by Zeifman and Hazan (1997a), considerable evidence exists that "despite tremendous variation in associated customs, rituals, and attitudes, there is universal human response to the breaking of a pair-bond" (p. 246). Consistent with the notion of adult romantic relationships as attachments, it has been shown that (1) temporary separations of adults from their spouses, like infants' separations from their mothers, are at least mildly distressing as measured by self-reports (Vormbrock, 1993) and physiological reactivity (B. Feeney & Kirkpatrick, 1996), and (2) adults' responses to death of a spouse appear to follow a course parallel to children's responses to loss of their primary attachment figures (Bowlby, 1980).

An important problem with interpreting these data as evidence of attachment per se is that anxiety and grief are clearly not restricted to separations from or losses of attachment figures. An obvious and important counterexample is parents' responses to separation from or loss of a *child.* It is doubtful that anyone experiences greater anxiety than a parent who has temporarily lost track of his or her child, or that anyone experiences more intense and prolonged grief than a parent mourning the death of his or her child. Anxiety and grief as responses to separations and losses are thus not restricted to attachment figures per se. This also suggests that responses to separation and loss need not involve issues of security promotion or regulation in any way, as per the attachment interpretation. Instead, anxiety and grief appear to be responses to separations from and losses of persons with whom we have strong emotional (love) bonds more generally.

Love Behaviors

Many behaviors exhibited by adult lovers resemble behaviors of infants interacting with their primary caregivers. Adult lovers engage in kissing, cuddling, nuzzling, "baby talk," holding hands, and a variety of other behavior patterns commonly observed in mother–infant dyads (Shaver et al., 1988). Although these resemblances have been cited frequently as evidence of attachment in adult love relationships (e.g., Zeifman & Hazan, 1997a), it must be acknowledged that these behaviors resemble the behaviors of the *caregiver* in caregiver–infant dyads at least as much as they resemble the infant's behaviors. Some of the behaviors, such as putting one's arm around another, seem more obviously related to caregiving than to care receiving. Moreover, all of these behaviors clearly originate in caregivers long before infants' physical and cognitive development permits them to initiate or even mimic such behaviors. In short, the behavioral resemblances between adult lovers and mother–infant pairs suggest operation of a mechanism associated with caregiving at least as much as with attachment.

The Biology of Love

Third, Zeifman and Hazan (1997a) cite evidence for neurobiological similarities between adult pair-bond and mother–infant relationships. Specifically, they cite the work of Carter (1992) demonstrating that "oxytocin, a substance released during suckling–nursing interactions, and thought to induce maternal caregiving, is also released at sexual climax and has been implicated in the cuddling that often follows sexual intercourse" (in Zeifman & Hazan, 1997a, p. 249). Again, these data are consistent with the idea that oxytocin plays a role in the formation of both lovers' emotional bonds to each other and mothers' bonds to their infants—relationships in which I have argued love serves the role of a commitment device. Whether similar neurochemistry underlies infant attachment remains an open question.

In summary, various features of adult pair-bonding appear to involve a component shared by the attachment and caregiving systems and, if anything, more the latter than the former. The strong connections with *caregiving* should not be surprising, as it seems likely that adult romantic love is in evolutionary terms a more recent outgrowth of parental love toward offspring (Mellen, 1981). In adult pair-bond relationships, this emotional bond serves to commit individuals to a particular mate choice, enabling them to get on with the business of childbearing and child rearing, in much the same way as it commits parents to long-term investment in their offspring.

REPRODUCTIVE STRATEGIES AND ATTACHMENT

The discussion so far, consistent with Zeifman and Hazan (1997a, 1997b), has focused on a *normative* model of bond formation in adult love relationships (and in mother–infant pairs). The notion that this reproductive strategy—that is, long-term pair-bonding combined with high parental investment—reflects operation of a singular, species-universal mechanism, has been most fully developed by Miller and Fishkin (1997). In this section I take issue with this assumption. I draw upon several theories of human reproductive strategies to argue instead that (1) monogamous pair-bonding is not the only reproductive strategy in the human repertoire, and that (2) individual differences in these strategies are influenced importantly by childhood family environment variables, including attachment. Finally, I review data to support the hypothesis that (3) what we have been calling "adult attachment styles" may largely reflect differences in reproductive strategies rather than attachment per se.

Reproductive Strategies

According to Miller and Fishkin (1997), the combination of long-term monogamous mating combined with high parental investment represents a species-universal reproductive strategy. Individual deviations from this normative pattern are viewed as errors or aberrations—reflections of the process somehow going awry—resulting from modern conditions that differ from those in which the purportedly universal design features evolved. The authors amass a variety of arguments for the adaptive value of this strategy in human evolutionary history.

Bowlby (1969), with whom Miller and Fishkin (1997) explicitly align themselves on this point, was mistaken about this issue as well. Simpson (in press) explains a variety of aspects of evolutionary theory that were poorly understood by Bowlby, in many cases because his seminal work predated important theoretical advances in evolutionary biology such as Trivers's (1974) crucial insights regarding parental investment. Many theorists have questioned Bowlby's assumption that secure attachment represents *the* normative pattern, and insecure attachment a pathological or maladaptive deviation from this pattern (e.g., Hinde, 1982; Lamb, Thompson, Gardner, & Charnov, 1985). In Chisolm's (1996) words, "it is increasingly appreciated that the EEA [environment of evolutionary adaptedness] was neither as uniform nor as benign as Bowlby seems to have imagined" (p. 14). Neither long-term monogamous pair-bonding nor indiscriminately high parental investment is "normative" for humans; instead, humans appear to be equipped with alternative reproductive strategies as well (Buss & Greiling, in press; Kirkpatrick, in press-b).

Mating

It is obvious that individual differences in mating patterns abound. Some individuals fall in love more readily or frequently than others; some pursue relationships with multiple partners simultaneously or serially;

some commit to relationships for long periods of time and some do not. Moreover, it is clear from the anthropological data that monogamous pair-bonding is by no means a universal norm among human societies. For example, Buss and Schmitt (1993) cite sources documenting the widespread incidence across cultures of polygyny, high divorce rates, serial marriage, and adultery. According to Daly and Wilson (1996) "the ethnographic record reveals that men are ardent polygamists when the opportunity presents itself" (p. 13), particularly since the relatively recent advent of agriculture made possible the amassing of resources and thus increased variance in power and resource accrual by men. And while it is true that virtually all known societies prescribe marriage in some form or other, these relationships take a variety of different forms with respect to the nature of and amount of marital interaction (Draper & Harpending, 1982, 1988).

Other lines of evidence, as reviewed by Daly and Wilson (1988), suggest that humans fall somewhere along a continuum between the extremes of exclusive monogamy and polygamy. Degree of sexual dimorphism in body size, a strong correlate of polygynous mating across primates, places humans somewhere between the extremes anchored by our strongly monogamous and strongly polygynous primate cousins. The relative size of human testes, in comparison to other primates, suggests an evolutionary history characterized by moderately high levels of sperm competition (resulting, presumably, from a history of polyandrous mating). Similarly, the external location within the scrotum of testes in human males appears to be an adaptation "in those mammals who need to produce fertile ejaculates repeatedly in short order," which might be explained in terms of polygyny, sperm competition due to polyandrous matings, or both. Finally, the existence of other evolved mechanisms for male mate-guarding, sexual jealousy, and the like strongly suggest that extra-pair matings by sexual partners have always been something that needed to be guarded against.

In addition to these ethnographic and comparative data, a variety of theoretical arguments cast doubt on the possibility of a universal monogamous pair-bonding mechanism in humans. In reviewing the adaptive advantages of monogamous pair-bonding, Miller and Fishkin (1997) neglected to examine any of the adaptive *disadvantages* of this strategy or relative advantages of short-term mating strategies. Buss and Schmitt (1993) reviewed the evolutionary arguments and evidence on both sides of the ledger, examining the potential advantages and disadvantages for both short-term and long-term mating strategies in terms of potential reproductive success. Each strategy offers both costs and benefits, which in some cases (but not others) differ between the sexes. For example, males can sire a virtually unlimited number of offspring with multiple partners—a clear advantage in terms of reproductive fitness—whereas women may benefit by extra-pair matings with high quality males who will provide their offspring with similarly high quality characteristics. Such short-term mating strategies represent an alternative to long-term strategies against which the costs and benefits of long-term strategies must be weighed.

An informal game-theoretic analysis similar to the classic altruism problem (see Dawkins, 1976, for a discussion) can be used to illustrate the central issue. A population of pure monogamists, if it had somehow evolved, would be vulnerable to invasion by various "cheater" strategies. For example, males genetically endowed with an alternative mechanism designed to promote opportunistic, extra-pair matings would, by virtue of those pairings, leave more descendants, who in turn would enjoy relative reproductive success relative to the pure monogamists. The genes coding for the opportunistic strategy would spread at the expense of pure monogamy genes.

How this evolutionary game ends in a particular species is tricky to determine for a variety of reasons, including considerations of relative frequencies of the strategies in the population and of the various costs involved. My point here is merely to illustrate how modern evolutionary thinking casts doubt on the idea that humans possess a species-universal mechanism for pure monogamy. One possible outcome is a set of *frequency-dependent* strategies in which genes for both strategies are maintained in the population in some fixed relative proportion. Based on similar reasoning, Gangestad and Simpson (1990) have suggested that female individual differences in restricted versus unrestricted sociosexuality may be at least partly heritable. (Whether heritable individual differences in sociosexuality do exist is largely irrelevant to the present argument, and I will not pursue the matter further here.)

Parental Investment

Similarly, there exists considerable variation across and within cultures in the nature and level of parental investment in offspring (e.g., Whiting & Whiting, 1975). Draper and Harpending (1982) described cross-cultural differences in terms of whether *father-absence* or *father-presence* is normative. Draper and Harpending (1988) further distinguished societies in terms of whether children are raised primarily by parents or by peers and surrogates. Within cultures, attachment researchers have clearly demonstrated sufficient variability in quality and quantity of caregiving to produce measurable individual differences in infant attachment patterns. In the extreme, low quality caregiving can include various forms of abuse, neglect, abandonment, and even infanticide.

A universal strategy for indiscriminate parental investment, particularly among males, is unlikely to have evolved in humans for reasons similar to those discussed above vis-à-vis mating strategies. Parental investment is costly, and a potentially adaptive alternative would clearly involve "cheating" by leaving one's mate holding the bag. In fact, high levels of paternal care for offspring are rare among mammals, in part for this reason and in part because of the paternity-certainty problem faced by males in species characterized by internal fertilization and gestation (Daly & Wilson, 1996). From a reproductive-fitness point of view, males would "prefer" to avoid parental investment at all; the possibility of being cuckolded and investing in genetically unrelated offspring is even worse. Females, too, would "prefer" to avoid parental investment if possible, but given the biology of mammalian reproduction the female's reproductive efforts are typically "parasitized" by males (Daly & Wilson, 1996).

Life History Theory

As articulated in life history theory (e.g., Stearns, 1992), organisms possess a finite amount of resources (time, energy, etc.) to allocate across the various evolutionary problems of survival, growth, mating, and reproduction, which involve a variety of trade-offs. In infancy and childhood, the primary trade-offs involve the sometimes-conflicting goals of survival and growth/development, oscillations between which are reflected in the safe haven versus secure base functions of infant attachment (Chisolm, 1996). The relative partitioning of effort between growth/development and reproduction across the life span, in cross-species comparisons, is referred to as *r-* versus *K-selected* strategies (Pianka, 1970). K-selected organisms are characterized by lower fertility, delayed maturation, greater longevity, and high levels of parental investment, whereas r-selected species show the reverse pattern. *Homo sapiens* is clearly a K-selected species in this scheme. Nevertheless, although application of the concept of r- versus K-selection to *within*-species variation is controversial (see, e.g., Rushton, 1985, and Mealey, 1990, for opposing views), there is little doubt that human reproductive strategies vary along a related continuum. For example, in our own modern culture in which a low quantity/high investment strategy is at least nominally the norm, teenage childbearing in low income, inner city populations may reflect an "alternative life-course strategy" characterized by "an accelerated family timetable; the separation of reproduction and marriage; an age-condensed generational family structure; and a grandparental child-rearing system" (Burton, 1990, p. 123).

In adulthood, the *general life history problem* concerns allocation of resources between the production of offspring (*mating effort*) and the caring for and rearing of offspring (*parenting effort*)—that is, between current and future reproductive success (Stearns, 1992). This distinction underlies Belsky et al.'s (1991; also Belsky, 1997) conceptualization of *quantity* versus *quality* patterns of mating and rearing, Buss and Schmitt's (1993) *short-term* versus *long-term* mating strategies, and (with respect to sexual behavior specifically), Simpson and Gangestad's (1991) *unrestricted* versus *restricted* sociosexuality.

Childhood Experience and Reproductive Strategies

Drawing upon these lines of evidence and theory as well as others, a number of theorists have concluded that short-term versus long-term reproductive strategies represent *facultative* adaptations in humans; that is, humans possess the requisite mechanisms for carrying out both strategies in response to varying ecological conditions (e.g., Buss & Schmitt, 1993; Daly & Wilson, 1988). Moreover, several theorists have argued that crucial determinants of the path selected involve particular aspects of early family history. The human child needs to determine, in effect, whether he or she has been born into an environment in which a long-term reproductive strategy (i.e., long-term mating strategy, high parental investment) or a short-term reproductive strategy (short-term mating strategy, low parental investment) is more adaptive given local conditions.

Draper and Harpending (1982) have argued that one crucial cue is the pair-bond status of the mother. They (see also Draper & Belsky, 1990) draw upon diverse lines of evidence suggesting that children raised in father-absent versus father-present homes differ, in puberty and adolescence, in ways consistent with the pursuit of short-term versus long-term reproductive strategies. For example, adolescent boys from father-absent homes tend to show, relative to father-present adolescents, more antagonistic attitudes toward femininity and toward women, exaggerated masculinity, and a "relatively exploitative attitude toward females, with sexual contact appearing important as conquest and as a means of validating masculinity" (p. 257). Father-absent girls tend to show "precocious sexual interest, derogation of masculinity and males, and poor ability to maintain sexual and emotional adjustment with one male" (p. 258). Other studies show that girls from divorced households reach puberty earlier than those from intact households, and that children of divorce tend to marry earlier, have children sooner, and end their marriages more readily (see Draper & Belsky, 1990, and Belsky et al., 1991, for reviews).

More recently, Belsky et al. (1991) have extended this view into a more general theory in which father-absence is one of several important cues of "the availability and predictability of resources (broadly defined) in the environment, of the trustworthiness of others, and of the enduringness of close interpersonal relationships, all of which affect how the developing person apportions reproductive effort" (p. 650). In their model, various aspects of family context influence the quality and quantity of parenting experienced by the child, which in turn influence security of attachment, which in turn influences subsequent somatic and psychological development and, ultimately, adult reproductive strategy. Chisolm (1996) further elaborated the links between mother–infant attachment experience and the choice of reproductive strategies vis-à-vis life history theory, distinguishing avoidant and anxious–ambivalent attachment patterns as differential responses to perceptions of parents' *inability* (avoidant) versus *unwillingness* (anxious–ambivalent) to invest heavily in offspring. Alternatively, Belsky (1997) has speculated that parenting of resistant (anxious–ambivalent) children may be an adaptive strategy designed to foster helper-at-the-nest behavior with respect to siblings.

In summary, a variety of empirical and theoretical perspectives suggest that early family experience, including security of attachment, are crucial determinants of individual differences in adult reproductive strategies. Although direct evidence at present is confined to puberty and adolescence—the period during which such differences would be expected to first come into view—other indirect evidence reviewed in the next section suggests that individual differences in adult reproductive strategies are attributable at least in part to early attachment experience.

ADULT ATTACHMENT STYLES RECONSIDERED

In the first section of this chapter I argued that adult romantic relationships may not in fact reflect the attachment system per se, but rather co-opt from the caregiving and/or attachment system the emotional bond of love in the service of maintaining long-term pair-bonds. I then reviewed literature suggesting that (1) humans can and do pursue both short- and long-term reproductive strategies, and that (2) early family experience, including security of attachment, is a crucial determinant of individual differences in preference for these alternative strategies. With this background in place, I now turn to the issue of the nature and origin of individual differences in so-called *adult attachment styles*. I will argue, following the suggestion of Chisolm (1996), that these individual differences might not (at least principally) reflect attachment per se, but rather individual differences in adult reproductive strategies. (See also Belsky, 1997, for a related discussion.)

Measures of Adult Attachment Styles

The task of establishing parallels between mating strategies and adult attachment styles is made difficult by three measurement problems in the adult attachment literature: (1) the question of dimensions versus types, (2) the diversity of extant measures of attachment styles, and (3) the fact that adult attachment measures undoubtedly reflect something else (or multiple something elses) in addition to mating strategies. The first of these is not particularly problematic, because long- versus short-term mating strategies can themselves be conceptualized as either a continuous dimension or as "types" anchoring the extremes of the continuum (Buss & Schmitt, 1993). The other two complications require some additional discussion.

Although Hazan and Shaver (1987) measured attachment styles in terms of three distinct types, many subsequent researchers have come to conceptualize these individual differences in terms of two orthogonal dimensions (see Brennan, Clark, & Shaver, Chapter 3, this volume). Levy and Davis (1988) showed that ratings of the secure and avoidant styles are strongly inversely correlated and essentially orthogonal to ratings of the anxious–ambivalent scale. Studies by Collins and Read (1990), Simpson et al. (1992), and J. Feeney, Noller, and Callan (1994) all similarly converge on a two-dimensional framework characterized by a secure-versus-avoidant dimension and a second dimension related to anxiety. Brennan and Shaver (1995) confirmed the same structure in a factor analysis of seven multi-item attachment scales, labeling these two higher-order factors *insecurity* and *preoccupation with attachment*, respectively. I suggest that it is the avoidant-versus-secure or insecurity dimension that appears to reflect short- versus long-term mating strategies.

Bartholomew's (1990; Bartholomew & Horowitz, 1991) four-category conceptualization, resulting from the distinction between two avoidant styles, offers an alternative perspective. A two-dimensional framework underlies this 2 × 2 matrix of styles, in which the dimensions refer to the negative-versus-positive mental *model of self* and *model of others*, respectively. There are at least two possible interpretations of this framework in terms of the mating-strategies perspective. First, the model-of-others dimension may reflect the short-term/long-term strategy variable, with secure and preoccupied (akin to Hazan and Shaver's [1987] anxious–ambivalent style) styles corresponding to long-term mating and the two avoidant styles corresponding to short-term mating. Alternatively, Brennan and Shaver (1995; see also Brennan, Shaver, & Tobey, 1991) argue that a 45-degree rotation of this dimensional framework corresponds to their insecurity (secure vs. fearful) and preoccupation (preoccupied vs. dismissing) factors, in which case (as noted above) it is the former that appears to reflect individual differences in mating strategies.

In either case, however, the nature of the second dimension is less clear. In Bartholomew's (1990) conceptualization the model of self is related to self-esteem, particularly in the context of close relationships (i.e., the degree to which one sees oneself as lovable by others). In the framework proposed here, this dimension might be interpreted more specifically in terms of one's self-assessed mate value, that is, the degree to which one believes he or she is regarded by others as a desirable mate. For example, although both secure and preoccupied individuals desire long-term relationships, they may differ in the confidence they have in their ability to attract and maintain a long-term partner. This would explain why anxious–ambivalent (preoccupied) persons are so fearful of abandonment and demand such high levels of intimacy and closeness: They fear that their partners will fail to share their commitment and will instead continue searching for a more attractive mate.

An alternative measure of attachment in adulthood that has spawned a parallel (but, unfortunately, largely independent) line of research is the Adult Attachment Interview (AAI) developed by Main and her colleagues (e.g., Main, Kaplan, & Cassidy, 1985). This interview-based measure is based on a rather different conceptualization of attachment, as it is designed to measure current representations ("state of mind") of attachment among adults rather than orientations toward romantic relationships per se. Although the AAI classifies individuals into three primary categories (secure–autonomous, preoccupied, and dismissing–avoidant) that seem at least superficially to parallel the three Hazan–Shaver categories, the conceptual and empirical relationships between these measures is a matter of considerable controversy (see Bartholomew & Shaver, Chapter 2, this volume).

Conceptualization of adult attachment styles in terms of reproductive strategies offers an intriguing (though admittedly speculative) possibility for integrating the AAI line of research with the social-psychological literature. Recall that reproductive strategies involve two primary components—mating effort (i.e., short- versus long-term strategies) and parental investment (high vs. low)—that tend to be inversely related. I propose that in assessing one's current (adult) representations of attachment as experienced in childhood, the AAI may be measuring primarily one's conceptualization of *parental investment* (i.e., caregiving), whereas the social-psychological measures stemming from Hazan and Shaver (1987) represent one's orientation toward long-term versus short-term *mating*.

Although direct evidence is scarce, the proposed interpretation of adult attachment styles in terms of mating strategies is consistent with a broad array of findings from the extant literature on adult attachment. A comprehensive review of this literature is beyond the scope of the present chapter; however, illustrative findings from several important areas are summarized in the remainder of this chapter. (See Belsky, 1997, for a related discussion.)

Attachment and Sexuality

Despite the widely accepted assumption that romantic love involves the integration of attachment, sex, and caregiving (Shaver et al., 1988), surprisingly little empirical work has been done to examine the relationship between attachment and sexuality. However, the limited available data are consistent with the hypothesis that adult attachment styles reflect, at least in part, orientations toward long- versus short-term mating strategies.

Brennan and Shaver (1995) report significant correlations between various measures of secure-versus-avoidant attachment and *sociosexuality*, as measured by the Sociosexual Orientation Inventory (SOI; Simpson & Gangestad, 1991). The latter contrasts a *restricted* versus *unrestricted* sexual orientation, in which an unrestricted orientation involves having and expecting to have multiple sexual partners and one-night stands, frequent fantasizing about sex with someone other than one's current dating partner, belief that "sex without love is OK," being comfortable with and enjoying "casual" sex with different partners, and disagreeing that one has to be "closely attached" to someone in order to "fully enjoy having sex with him or her." This correlation between avoidance and unrestricted sociosexuality has been replicated in several unpublished studies by Simpson and colleagues (J. A. Simpson, personal communication, December 5, 1996). In another unpublished study utilizing the Bartholomew–Horowitz (1991) four-category measure of adult attachment, dismissing–avoidant respondents were the most likely to report preference for promiscuous sexual behavior (K. Brennan, personal communication, December 9, 1996).

Similarly, Miller and Fishkin (1997) found insecure men to desire a greater ideal number of partners than secure men over the next 30 years. Results from this study also showed that men reporting (retrospectively) cold, distant relationships with their fathers in childhood also reported a greater ideal number of sexual partners than did those reporting secure, warm relationships with their fathers. This latter finding is consistent with the Belsky et al. (1991) model linking childhood attachment and adult reproductive strategies. Similar but somewhat less clear results emerged with respect to maternal relationships, and all results were weaker for women (though it is not clear whether the weaker results for women are attributable to restricted variance in the ideal-partners variable).

Hazan, Zeifman, and Middleton (1994) investigated self-reports of a variety of sexual behaviors and interests in relation to attachment style. Consistent with the distinction between long- versus short-term mating strategies, secure respondents were the least likely to report involvement in one-night stands and sex outside established relationships, whereas avoidant respondents evinced the opposite pattern. Anxiety–ambivalence appeared to be related to unusual patterns of sexual interest. Interestingly, avoidant adults also preferred purely sexual contact (e.g., oral and anal sex) to more emotionally intimate sexual contact (kissing, cuddling), again consistent with the idea that they seek short-term sexual relationships without long-term commitment.

Continuity across the Life Span

One of the strongest lines of evidence for the idea of adult love as attachment comes from data suggesting that infant attachment styles have consequences for social development across the life span. There is considerable evidence that infant attachment classification is predictive of a host of social-behavioral, personality, and physiological (e.g., timing of menarche) variables through puberty and into adolescence—as far as current longitudinal data will take us. The literature reviewed by Belsky et al. (1991) in support of their model of reproductive strategies overlaps considerably with that reviewed by Rothbard and Shaver (1994) in support of their model of attachment continuity across the life span. The existing data appear consistent with both views of the nature of attachment sequelae.

Similarly, if adult attachment styles reflect adult reproductive strategies and the Belsky et al. (1991) model is correct, then childhood attachment experience should be related to adult attachment style classification—just as predicted by the continuity-of-attachment model. In data presented by Hazan and Shaver (1987), respondents reporting secure adult attachment styles described their mothers retrospectively as respectful, responsive, caring, accepting, confident, and undemanding—clearly consistent with having had a secure attachment to mother. Both insecure adult groups (avoidant and anxious–ambivalent) reported the opposite pattern. J. Feeney and Noller (1990) reported similar results in an Australian sample; in addition, they found avoidant adults to be more likely to report having experienced significant separations from their mothers during childhood.

This perspective also provides an alternative explanation for the *intergenerational transmission* of attachment patterns observed in many studies (e.g., Main et al., 1985; see Steele & Steele, 1994, for a review). If, as I suggested earlier, the AAI primarily reflects individual differences in parental investment (vs. mating) strategies, this would explain why mothers' classification on the AAI is predictive of (1) the provision of sensitive, responsive care to their children, and (2) their *children's* attachment classification in the Strange Situation (van IJzendoorn, 1995). Studies on intergenerational transmission of attachment patterns to date have been based on the AAI rather than social-psychological measures of adult attachment such as Hazan and Shaver's (1987). I would expect social-psychological measures, as measures of *mating* rather than *parental investment* strategies, to be somewhat less strongly predictive than the AAI of infant attachment classification. Consistent with this, Rholes, Simpson, Blakely, Lanigan, and Allen (in press) found recently that adults' avoidance (vs. security), as measured by a social-psychological attachment index, was significantly but only modestly predictive of a lesser desire to have children.

Conversely, a variety of variables related to adult relationship functioning (i.e., mating) would be expected to be more closely related to the social-psychological measures of adult attachment than to the AAI. Several such areas of research are reviewed in the following sections.

Internal Working Models

Many findings on the content of *internal working models* of attachment relationships are consistent with the view that adult attachment styles largely reflect short- versus long-term mating strategies. Rothbard and

Shaver (1994) summarize the attachment view by noting that "it would be expected that secure adults view others as trustworthy and dependable. . . . Avoidant adults would be expected to view others as generally untrustworthy and undependable . . . and relationships as either threatening to one's sense of control, not worth the effort, or both" (p. 61)—exactly what would be expected from the mating strategies perspective. In Hazan and Shaver's (1987) newspaper sample, self-classified avoidants "never produced the highest mean on a positive love-experience dimension" (p. 515). Secure persons scored highest on trust in love relationships, whereas avoidants evinced fear of closeness and intimacy. Secure lovers were most likely to agree that "in some relationships romantic love never fades," whereas avoidant lovers were most likely to say that "the kind of head-over-heels romantic love depicted in novels and movies does not exist in real life, romantic love seldom lasts, and it is rare to find a person one can really fall in love with" (p. 515). In their student sample, Hazan and Shaver (1987) reported that *none* of their avoidant respondents (compared to 15% of secures and 32% of anxious–ambivalent respondents) agreed with the item stating, "It's easy to fall in love. I feel myself beginning to fall in love often." Similarly, 80% of avoidants (vs. 41% of secures and 55% of anxious–ambivalent respondents) endorsed the item "It's rare to find someone you can really fall in love with." In short, avoidant adults are less likely than secure adults to believe in or, actually experience, the emotional bond of love or its correlates of trust, closeness, and intimacy.

Other aspects of mental models related to individual differences in adult attachment seem readily interpretable within the framework I propose as well. For example, Collins and Read (1990) found avoidants to view others as untrustworthy, to doubt the integrity and honesty of social role agents, such as parents, and to be generally suspicious of human nature and motives; secures reported the opposite pattern and were more likely to view people as generally well-intentioned and good-hearted. Hazan and Shaver (1990) suggested that avoidant adults may focus their energies on achievement in school, work, or career, rather than on close relationships. These correlates are all consistent with the suite of sequelae of father-absence in boys as described by Draper and Harpending (1982), which includes rejection of authority, exaggerated masculinity, denigration of females and femininity, greater interpersonal aggressiveness, increased risk of arrest and incarceration, a relatively exploitative attitude toward females, and a general lack of interest in developing "a durable, bonded relationship with a mate," all of which "would be appropriate in a courtship arena in which girls and women evaluate men by current appearance and status in the male hierarchy rather than by such traits as steadfastness or the ability to support a woman and children" (Draper & Belsky, 1990, p. 149). The experience of father absence and/or low parental investment serves as a signal that the environment is one of heightened intrasexual competition in which opportunistic, risky mating strategies are to be preferred over invested, long-term relationships.

Mate Preferences and Assortative Mating

A variety of studies suggest that avoidant adults, relative to secure adults, are less likely at a given point in time to be involved in a long-term relationship (Hazan & Shaver, 1987; Kirkpatrick & Hazan, 1994; Senchak & Leonard, 1992), which is of course what would be expected if secure persons are oriented toward long-term pair-bonding and avoidant persons are not. Kirkpatrick and Hazan (1994) found, in a 4-year prospective study, that persons classified as avoidant (vs. secure or anxious–ambivalent) at Time 1 were more likely at Time 2 to be "seeing more than one person" or to be "not seeing anyone and not looking"—the two primary alternatives to monogamous pair-bonding. Simpson (1990) similarly found avoidant respondents to report being simultaneously involved with multiple sex partners. Kirkpatrick and Hazan (1994) also found that anxious–ambivalent persons, in contrast, were most likely to indicate 4 years later that they were not seeing anyone but *were* looking—consistent with the idea that this group is oriented toward long-term mating but unsuccessful and/or unskilled at implementing the strategy in various ways.

If security of adult attachment largely reflects an orientation toward a long-term mating strategy, persons seeking a long-term mate should prefer partners who share this orientation. Several studies demonstrate that individuals of all adult attachment styles strongly prefer secure partners for long-term relationships, with avoidant partners the least preferred and anxious–ambivalent partners in between (e.g., Latty-Mann & Davis, 1996; Pietromonaco & Carnelley, 1994). Chappell and Davis (1996) confirmed the same sequence using Bartholomew's four-category attachment measure, with both avoidant styles (dismissing and fearful) the least preferred. These data are consistent with my interpretation of the security-versus-avoidance dimension, and of Bartholomew's model-of-others dimension, as reflecting long-term versus short-term mating strategies: Avoidants of both types are identified by others as short-term strategists to be avoided for long-term relationships. In addition, secures are more likely than insecures to display other desirable qualities of long-term (as compared to short-term) mates, such as kindness and understanding (Buss & Schmitt, 1993). Although Chappell and Davis (1996) and Latty-Mann and Davis (1996) interpreted these preferences in terms of a normative desire for partners who provide the best opportunity for forming a secure attachment, the findings are equally consistent with the view that "secure" partners are desirable simply because they are perceived to be oriented toward, and capable of maintaining, long-term pair bonds—independent of issues of comfort, security, and other aspects of attachment per se.[3]

Actual pairings of romantic partners, however, are complicated by other issues, as assortative mating is driven partly by preferences but also largely by the results of competition for preferred partners. Everyone prefers a secure partner for long-term relationships, but not everyone can have one (Latty-Mann & Davis, 1996). Several studies suggest that with respect to observed pairings, secure persons tend to be paired with other secures and insecures with insecures (Kirkpatrick & Davis, 1994; Senchak & Leonard, 1992). Along with Latty-Mann and Davis (1996), I suggest that this observed pattern of assortative mating is not a function of generalized similarity–attraction principles, but results instead from the fact that there are only so many secure (i.e., long-term–oriented) partners to go around— and other secure persons are most able to attract and keep them.

Relationship Satisfaction

If secure adult attachment reflects an orientation toward long-term mating strategies, one would expect individuals characterized by this style to find long-term relationships satisfying and enjoyable. Numerous studies support this hypothesis: Security of attachment is positively related to a variety of measures of relationship quality, satisfaction, happiness, and enjoyment (Collins & Read, 1990; J. Feeney & Noller, 1990; Hazan & Shaver, 1987; Kirkpatrick & Davis, 1994; Levy & Davis, 1988; Simpson, 1990).

On the other hand, several studies suggest that correlations between attachment style and one's *partner's* satisfaction may be moderated by gender: In general, partners' relationship dissatisfaction is more strongly related to men's *avoidance* and to women's *anxiety* (anxiety–ambivalence) than vice versa (Collins & Read, 1990; J. Feeney et al., 1994; Kirkpatrick & Davis, 1994; Simpson, 1990). It is not at all obvious from an orthodox attachment theory perspective why this should be so. The usual explanation for this pattern has drawn upon traditional sex-role stereotypes (Collins & Read, 1990; J. Feeney et al., 1994; Kirkpatrick & Davis, 1994). Given the stereotype of men as generally uncomfortable with intimacy and aloof in close relationships, men who do not conform to this stereotype should be highly valued and the source of considerable relationship satisfaction for their partners. Conversely, given the traditional male sex-role as independent and autonomous, a female partner's excessive clinginess and possessiveness should be strongly predictive of men's dissatisfaction.

Though consistent with the data, this sex-role explanation begs the question as to why such sex roles exist in the first place. Why isn't it women who tend to fear intimacy and seek autonomy? An evolutionary perspective on mating strategies provides a clear explanation for this cross-culturally universal pattern, as well as for the sex-differentiated relationships between attachment and relationship satisfaction. Although both men and women can (and do) pursue short-term as well as long-term mating strategies, separate consideration of the reproductive-success advantages and disadvantages for males and females clearly suggests that the ledger is differentially balanced: As a consequence of basic sex differences in mammalian reproductive physiology, males stand to gain considerably more on average (in terms of reproductive success) by pursuing short-term strategies than do females (Buss & Schmitt, 1993). From an evolutionary perspective, the greatest cost of long-term mating for men (but not for women) is the lost opportunity to mate with other females (thus increasing the number of genetic offspring in future generations). A partner who is unusually demanding of attention and intimacy, as well as highly jealous and possessive, makes these costs highly salient to men. On the other hand, the greatest benefit to females (but not males) of long-term mating is the provisioning of self and offspring by the male partner; correspondingly, the greatest problem faced by females is potential loss of the male's commitment to the provision of these resources. As a result, a male partner who displays aloofness, lack of commitment and self-disclosure, and so forth makes these problems highly salient to women. The logic behind these differences, then, is closely related to the logic of sex differences in mate selection preferences (Buss, 1992) and in sexual jealousy (Buss, Larsen, Westen, & Semmelroth, 1992). From an evolutionary point of view, an anxious–ambivalent partner is a male's worst nightmare, and an avoidant partner is a female's worst nightmare.[4]

Relationship Stability

Also consistent with the idea that adult attachment security reflects orientations toward long-versus short-term mating, secure adults have longer lasting relationships than avoidant adults (Kirkpatrick & Davis, 1994; Kirkpatrick & Hazan, 1994). Results for the anxious–ambivalent style are less clear. Kirkpatrick and Hazan (1994) found anxious–ambivalent respondents to be comparable to secure respondents in terms of being with the same relationship partner after a 4-year period, with avoidant respondents differing substantially from both. However, Kirkpatrick and Davis (1994) found this pattern only for women; among men, it was the anxious–ambivalent group that evinced the least stable relationships. This surprising result for men might be attributable to any number of methodological differences between the studies, and certainly warrants replication. In addition, it seems important to note that these attachment-style differences in relationship stability among men were considerably smaller at the second follow-up (30–36 months after initial testing) than at the first follow-up (12–14 months), whereas in the women's data the low stability of avoidants' relationships relative to the other two groups was *greater* at the second follow-up than at the first.

There are a variety of ways in which an avoidant person's short-term mating strategy may influence the course of their romantic relationships. First, as noted earlier, avoidant persons are the least likely to begin a committed relationship in the first place, either by avoiding close relationships entirely or by engaging in multiple (and, presumably, uncommitted) relationships simultaneously. However, some avoidant persons do find themselves in relationships for at least limited durations, and this should come as no surprise. Mating strategies fall along a continuum from short- to long-term (Buss & Schmitt, 1993), and while avoidant persons might (and do) engage in one-night stands, they might also be expected to become involved in serial or contemporaneous longer-term relationships of varying duration. Zeifman and Hazan (1997a) suggest that a crucial difference between avoidant and secure (i.e., short- and long-term strategists) may concern the likelihood of developing an emotional bond—a clear-cut *attachment*—that enables the relationship to grow into a long-term commitment (in their analysis, as mediated by differences in experienced physical contact).

Moreover, if avoidant persons fail to develop this bond and ensuing commitment over time, their partners may well perceive this and consequently initiate a break-up. Frank's (1988) model of emotions as commitment devices provides another useful insight into this process. In addition to committing individuals to a course of action that is adaptive in the long term (but not apparently so in the short term), a second crucial aspect of emotions is that they are *observable* and thus signal to others one's commitment to the emotion-driven course of action. In the stolen-briefcase scenario, the reason that the emotion of anger (and corresponding irrational desire for vengeance) serves as an effective deterrent to theft is the fact that the emotional expression of the emotion is publicly observable. Someone observed to be incapable of experiencing anger would be a tempting target for thieves. Similarly, an important aspect of love in pair-bonded relationships is that individuals can detect, through both verbal and nonverbal cues, whether their partners are truly "in love" with and committed to them. The emotional bond of love thus not only facilitates pair-bonding by committing one to the relationship; it simultaneously signals this commitment to the partner and thereby enhances the likelihood that the partner will remain committed to the relationship as well.

The fact that relationships of anxious–ambivalent persons are relatively stable (at least for women) is consistent with the idea that, like secure attachment, anxiety–ambivalence reflects in part an orientation toward long-term mating strategies. This view also provides a ready interpretation for the fact that the stability of these relationships (again, at least for women) is apparent despite low levels of satisfaction. As emphasized in Rusbult's (1980) *investment model,* satisfaction and enjoyment alone do not determine the fate of a relationship; instead, establishment of a *commitment* to the relationship—conceptualized here in terms of formation of an emotional bond—is crucial for cementing the relationship and making it resistant to dissolution in the face of attractive alternatives and temporary setbacks. Where these relationships fail, the problem is unlikely to be a lack of emotional bond but, perhaps, an inappropriately activated one: For example, anxious–ambivalent persons may drive their partners away with excessive demands for intimacy and their desire to "merge" with their partners (Hazan & Shaver, 1987). In diametric opposition to avoidant persons, these individuals may be showing signs of infatuation (signaling a shift from preattachment to attachment-in-the-making, per Zeifman & Hazan, 1997a) or of love (signaling clear-cut attachment) inappropriately early in the relationship. It is easy to see how a partner who falls further toward the short-term strategy end of the continuum might feel trapped by such rapid relationship development and head for the exit.

Conclusion

In this section I have argued, along with Chisolm (1996) and Belsky (1997), that individual differences in adult attachment styles principally reflect variation in reproductive strategies. The social-psychological measures of adult attachment derived from the work of Hazan and Shaver (1987) were interpreted in terms of short- versus long-term *mating* strategies; the AAI was interpreted in terms of orientations toward high versus low *parental investment.*

In doing so I have staked out a somewhat extreme position, but the argument could be made in either a strong or weak version. The strongest version would state that adult attachment styles are functionally reducible to mating strategies (or, in the case of the AAI, perceived parental investment). Clearly, the extant measures of these constructs are not isomorphic; the observed correlations between them (cited previously) suggest only a modest degree of shared variance. At least some of this nonoverlapping variance is probably attributable to the fact that the adult attachment measures are influenced by current relationship satisfaction, recent relationship experiences, and various sorts of self-report biases. The SOI undoubtedly suffers from its own (and perhaps different) self-report biases as well. In any case, the crucial empirical question to be addressed concerns the degree to which adult attachment styles are able to predict measures of relationship functioning (e.g., satisfaction and stability) above and beyond the variance predictable from individual differences in mating strategies (and from other non–attachment-related sources such as social desirability).

In its weakest form, the argument would state merely that mating strategies are *related to* adult attachment styles in one of several ways. For example, Hill, Young, and Nord (1994) have argued that adult attachment styles may *mediate* the relationship between early experience and adult reproductive strategies—in effect inserting an additional intermediate step to the Belsky et al. (1991) model. The addition of this extra step results in a less parsimonious model, however, and strong empirical evidence will be required to make a convincing case that the adult-attachment component is indispensable. Alternatively, mating strategies might influence self-reported attachment styles, or the two might be correlated simply by virtue of their shared causal basis in childhood experience. Should the strong version of the argument be empirically falsified, the next task would be to delineate the precise nature of the relationship between these constructs.

ADULT RELATIONSHIPS AND RESPONSES TO STRESS AND DISTRESS

In previous sections of this chapter I have tried to show that much of the evidence typically cited for attachment processes in adult love relationships is equally consistent with a simpler love-as-commitment-device model. For example, I argued that with respect to responses to separation and loss, intimate behaviors, and neurobiological processes, romantic love resembles both maternal caregiving and infant attachment, suggesting that adult love relationships involve a component (love) shared by those other systems rather than the systems per se. Next I argued that evidence for individual differences in adult attachment is consistent with an alternative interpretation in terms of individual differences in seeking or desiring to maintain long-term mating relationships. In these sections I have avoided what is perhaps the most important line of evidence cited in support of romantic relationships as attachments: that adults turn to their romantic partners for comfort and protection in response to stressful circumstances and psychological distress (Rothbard & Shaver, 1994; Zeifman & Hazan, 1997a). Although this observation seems particularly persuasive as evidence of attachment processes in adult love relationships, I offer in this section an alternative interpretation.

The most direct evidence for this dynamic comes from research by Simpson et al. (1992), in which female college students were led to anticipate a stressful experimental task and then were observed surreptitiously in interaction with their romantic partners while they awaited their fate. The results showed that among secure (as contrasted with avoidant) women, increased anxiety was associated with increased proximity seeking toward and comfort seeking from their partners, whereas avoidant women showed the opposite pattern (see Rholes, Simpson, & Grich Stevens, Chapter 7, this volume, for a more complete discussion).

Similarly, Mikulincer and colleagues (see Mikulincer & Florian, Chapter 6, this volume) have shown predictable differences among adult attachment styles with respect to coping strategies in response to missile attacks in Israel (Mikulincer, Florian, & Weller, 1993) and the demands of combat training among Israeli troops (Mikulincer & Florian, 1995); specifically, secure persons were more likely to seek social support in these circumstances, whereas avoidant persons tended to distance themselves from others.

More recently, Carpenter and Kirkpatrick (1996) examined college women's psychophysiological responses to stress in the presence versus absence of their romantic partners. Insecure women evinced greater physiological reactivity (relative to baseline) to introduction of the stressor in the presence than in the absence of their romantic partners; secure women, in contrast, showed little or no difference between these conditions. We interpreted these results as further evidence for attachment processes (and individual differences therein) in adult romantic relationships.

The problem with this interpretation is that a massive literature exists demonstrating that people turn to a variety of other persons for emotional (in addition to material) support in stressful situations. For example, the experimental designs employed by B. Feeney and Kirkpatrick (1996) and Carpenter and Kirkpatrick (1996) were borrowed from a series of prior studies of how physiological responses to stress are moderated by the presence of same-sex friends (Allen, Blascovich, Tomaka, & Kelsey, 1991; Edens, Larkin, & Abel, 1992; Kamarck, Manuck, & Jennings, 1990). One of these studies (Allen et al., 1991) even demonstrated that the presence of one's *pet dog* moderated physiological responses to stress relative to an alone condition! While it might be argued that close same-sex friends represent attachment figures (though this is a thorny theoretical issue in its own right), surely pet dogs cannot reasonably be construed in this manner.

Going back further into the social-psychological literature, classic studies by Schachter (1959) showed that people prefer to be with others, including complete strangers, when faced with threatening circumstances (in this case, anticipation of painful electric shocks). Although Schachter favored a social-comparison interpretation of his findings, others have interpreted these and other findings as also consistent with Schachter's "direct fear-reduction" hypothesis, according to which persons anticipating stressful situations are largely motivated to seek reassurance and comfort from others likely to be sympathetic to their plight (Kirkpatrick & Shaver, 1988; Shaver & Klinnert, 1980).

In short, if people turn to total strangers and pet dogs, as well as close friends and romantic relationship partners, for support in times of stress or distress, this raises serious questions about the viability and parsimony of an explanation based on attachment dynamics per se. Spouses and lovers might be somewhat more reliable, and thus somewhat more readily sought out in such cases, than other potential sources of social support, but there is no convincing evidence that this reflects a *qualitative* difference in underlying processes.

An Alternative View

As I argued at the beginning of this chapter, it seems unlikely that the attachment system would have evolved in such a way that romantic partners are adopted as attachment figures, *qua* attachment figures, in adulthood. The attachment mechanism in childhood biases the child toward seeking comfort and protection from primary caregivers, who are likely to be parents, specifically because parents can be counted on to provide these resources in light of their genetic interest in the child's welfare. Romantic partners cannot be so counted on. Provision of resources, including protection, is an act of *altruism* in the sense that it benefits the recipient at some cost to the provider. According to game-theoretical models in evolutionary biology, indiscriminate altruism is unlikely to have evolved because it is not an evolutionarily stable strategy; that is, a population of such altruists would easily be invaded and displaced by various forms of alternative "cheater" strategies (e.g., Dawkins, 1976). Instead, one can count on altruistic support and assistance from two general kinds of sources: genetic relatives, including (especially for children) parents and siblings, and coalition partners (i.e., those with whom one has established alliances based on reciprocal-altruism principles).

The mutual caregiving observed between romantic partners, like that between friends, may be largely interpretable in terms of these latter processes as well. Over the duration of a romantic relationship, as in a friendship, mutual trust develops as the two individuals demonstrate through repeated interaction their willingness and ability to share resources and help each other in various ways. This view, of course, is consistent with various theories concerning *equity* (e.g., Walster, Walster, & Berscheid, 1978) and *social exchange* in close relationships (e.g., Kelley & Thibaut, 1978), as well as with the conceptualization of established long-term relationships as "goal-corrected partnerships" (Zeifman & Hazan, 1997a). The important role of exchange considerations in such relationships is highlighted by the finding that perceived inequities in marital relationships are distressing, particularly to the underbenefitted party (Schafer & Keith, 1980).

Romantic relationships do, however, often seem to display characteristics of so-called *communal* relationships, which are distinguished by feelings of responsibility for the other's welfare rather than expectations of repayment (Clark & Mills, 1993). Clark and Mills (1993) cite close friendships and romantic relationships along with kin relationships as prototypical examples of communal (vs. *exchange*) relationships, but from an evolutionary point of view this classification seems dubious. Kin relationships are qualitatively different from nonkin relationships because, to varying extents depending on the degree of genetic relatedness, the welfare of collateral as well as descendent kin provides an alternative vehicle to a gene's survival and proliferation. Thus the theory of *kin selection* (Hamilton, 1964) provides a basis for altruistic caregiving behavior with respect to close kin, of which parental investment is a prime example.

In contrast, spouses and friends are genetically unrelated. These latter relationships may take on a communal appearance not because they are based on altruistic concern for the partner's welfare rather than exchange principles, but instead because the accounting is more flexible with respect to time frame and range of benefits (Batson, 1993). For example, the provision of physical protection (especially against other males) is a benefit males can offer to females in light of their greater size and strength (as evidenced by female preferences for physically strong mates, particularly in short-term mating contexts; Buss & Schmitt, 1993). Females may reciprocate by providing other forms of assistance and support along with other, qualitatively different kinds of benefits, such as sexual access.

On the other hand, parents certainly *share* genetic interests in the welfare of their offspring, rendering the spouse somewhat kin-like in the sense of correlated expected fitness. However, the strength of this link must be limited by virtue of its indirectness: Genetic interest in one's offspring is already limited by the fact that offspring share only 50% of one's genes, rendering weaker still the link to a partner who only partly contributes to the welfare of those offspring. In addition, because shared offspring represent only one component of each partner's potential reproductive fitness, marital partners also have a variety of conflicting fitness interests as well. For example, each spouse has interests in his or her own (different) kin, leading to potential conflicts over allocating resources to the respective families (thus the cross-culturally ubiquitous "in-law" problem), and a variety of temptations toward extrapair matings continues to exist for both partners. (See Daly & Wilson, 1996, for further discussion of evolutionary bases of marital conflict.)

In short, whereas parents can be counted on by children to go to extraordinary lengths to support and protect them, romantic partners cannot be expected to go nearly so far. Daly and Wilson (1988) conclude (with typical eloquence and flair) that

> although the overlap of interests between mates is analogous to that between genetic relatives, and although this overlap has the potential of surpassing that of even the closest kin (in the case of monogamists with minimal investment in collateral kin), the relationship between mates is nevertheless more easily betrayed. Blood is thicker than water

because the genetic fates of blood relatives are indissolubly linked, a consideration that favors forgiveness and reconciliation. Marital ties are thinner gruel: Because cuckolded males risk expending their lives unwittingly raising their rivals' children, the correlation between the expected fitnesses of mates can be abolished or reversed by infidelity. (p. 291)

Although a somewhat greater level of mutual caregiving and cooperation might be expected between spouses than between other genetically unrelated individuals, it is both limited and conditional in contrast to the caregiving in parent–child attachment relationships.

The most obvious implication of this view is that, from an evolutionary perspective, security regulation may not warrant a very central place in our thinking about romantic relationships. I am not the first to arrive at this conclusion, although my reasons differ from those of others. J. Feeney (Chapter 8, this volume), for example, argues that *relationship-centered* stressors—threats to the continuance of the relationship itself—may be more relevant to adult romantic relationships than are *environmental* stressors. Kobak and Duemmler (1994) similarly argue that goal conflicts within a relationship offer a better arena in which to study adult attachment than do responses to environmental stressors. In both cases the authors cite the fact that the attachment system is less readily activated in adulthood than in childhood—one of the principal differences generally cited between infant and adult attachment (e.g., Weiss, 1982). In this chapter I have tried to demonstrate why this is the case, and why the attachment system is unlikely to have evolved in such a way as to operate in adult romantic relationships in the same way as in childhood.

CONCLUSIONS AND IMPLICATIONS

In this chapter I have sketched a theoretical perspective on adult romantic relationships that in some ways is closely related to, and in other ways deviates radically from, the currently prevailing view of adult attachment. It is certainly radical in its proposition that adult romantic relationships may not, in fact, be attachments per se. However, it remains closely related to the attachment perspective in several respects: (1) It leaves essentially unchallenged Bowlby's (1969) view of attachment in childhood; (2) it retains the fundamental assumption that important individual differences in orientation toward and experience in adult relationships have their origins in early attachment experience; and (3) it suggests that a component of the infant attachment and/or parental caregiving systems plays a central organizing role in adult romantic relationships.

The framework sketched here can be seen as an extension and integration of recent theoretical developments in several areas related to adult attachment. It is very closely related to the model proposed recently by Hazan and Zeifman (1994; Zeifman & Hazan, 1997a, 1997b) in suggesting that the evolutionary function of adult "attachments" concerns the maintenance of long-term pair-bonds, and endorses their process model of bond formation. It differs from their view, however, in several ways. First, it questions the notion that security promotion and affect regulation are important components of adult pair-bonding, replacing "attachment system" with "love as a commitment device" based on Frank's (1988) model of emotions. It also deviates from Hazan and Zeifman, and particularly from Miller and Fishkin (1997), with respect to the nature of individual differences: It postulates that humans are not designed for universal monogamy, but rather possess at least two alternative, facultative reproductive strategies.

Where the model deviates from other attachment researchers on this point, however, it merges with other theories of differential reproductive strategies as articulated by Buss and Schmitt (1993) and Simpson and Gangestad (1991). It then links these views of reproductive strategies back to mother–infant attachment via the theoretical models of Draper and Harpending (1982), Belsky et al. (1991), and Chisolm (1996). However, it further extends these latter models by suggesting, along with Chisolm (1996) and Belsky (1997), that adult attachment styles as currently measured may largely *be* the differential reproductive strategies thought by these authors to develop from individual differences in early family experience.

Although the model proposed here is offered as an alternative to the prevailing adult attachment model, it should be clear that most of the evidence I have reviewed is consistent with both; I have noted just a few examples where the proposed perspective appears to fit the data better than an orthodox attachment orientation. No doubt other researchers will identify cases for which the reverse is true. Ultimately the issue must be decided on evidence, and critical studies that empirically test these models against each other will be difficult to devise. Until then I will suggest two reasons why this new framework should be regarded as a serious alternative to the adult attachment model.

First, I believe that, from an evolutionary perspective, it is a more parsimonious model. This may at first seem a dubious claim given that I suggest replacing a single-mechanism (attachment) model with one drawing upon several alternative mechanisms. However, the apparent parsimony of the adult attachment model is somewhat deceptive. For example, it, too, posits the importance of other processes (caregiving and sexual mating) in romantic relationships, and a fuller development of these components and their interrelationships undoubtedly will lead to a more complex whole. Second, attachment theorists (including myself; e.g., Kirkpatrick & Davis, 1994) have often resorted to other processes to explain experimental results such as sex differences in relationship stability and satisfaction. Thus, both models are comparably (non)parsimonious in this sense.

However, I submit that the model proposed here is the more parsimonious in the following specific way: From an evolutionary perspective, pair-bond relationships must be considered first and foremost as *reproductive* relationships. Theorizing about such relationships should therefore begin (as I have attempted to do here) with issues of reproduction and parental investment, and then add other mechanisms and components (such as attachment) only as necessary. Second, a complex mechanism or system should not be preferred when a simpler one will do. I have argued that an emotional bond co-opted from parental caregiving (and/or infant attachment) is sufficient to explain the maintenance of long-term pair bonds without hauling in the entire attachment system.[5] At the same time, I have offered a variety of arguments against the viability of attachment as a theoretical explanation for adult pair-bond relationship dynamics.

Finally, I would like to suggest that this model offers a potential basis for reconciling the social-psychological literature on adult attachment with two other literatures with which it currently has an unclear and uneasy relationship. As discussed in a previous section, it potentially integrates this literature with the parallel and competing attachment work of Main and others based on the AAI. I have argued that mating strategies and parental investment strategies—the two major components of reproductive strategies—may underlie these respective approaches. Although this account is highly speculative, it is currently the only viable hypothesis of which I am aware that links these two lines of research theoretically in a coherent way.

Second, the proposed framework provides grounds for integrating adult attachment work with another major, competing theory of adult love relationships with which the attachment approach has long had an unclear relationship: Rusbult's (1980) *investment model.* The notion of love as a commitment device, based on Frank's (1988) conceptualization, puts the emotion into "commitment" as defined and researched by Rusbult and colleagues. Once love-as-commitment-device is in place, the individual becomes highly motivated to stick with (is *committed* to) the relationship, despite transitory variations in satisfaction, availability and attractiveness of alternatives, and levels of investment. In the absence of such an emotional component, it is not at all clear why a rational decision maker would reach the stage of long-term commitment to the relationship. Moreover, the reconceptualization of adult attachment styles in terms of willingness and desire to become committed to a monogamous long-term relationship can easily be incorporated into the investment-model view. These suggestions are again speculative, but seem to provide fertile ground for linking these competing theoretical approaches.

Even if the model proposed here proves (at least largely) correct, would this mean that there is no role for attachment processes in adulthood? Although it is possible that, contrary to Bowlby (1969), the attachment system ceases to function as an integrated system in adulthood, a number of other possibilities remain. For example, the attachment system *qua* system might be activated by unusually severe threats to, if not in the day-to-day dynamics of, romantic relationships. Another possibility is that adult attachment styles continue to act as some kind of mediating variable between childhood attachment and adult reproductive strategy, as suggested by Hill et al. (1994). Third, the attachment system might function in domains of adult experience other than romantic relationships. I have argued elsewhere that belief in God may function as a true attachment, and that such beliefs are predictably related to early childhood experience and adult romantic relationships (see Kirkpatrick, in press-a, for a thorough discussion and review of empirical findings).

In any case, the theory sketched here awaits empirical testing, and ultimately the data must decide how it stands up against the traditional adult attachment model. Parts of it are probably wrong. Even if much of the theory proves incorrect, however, I hope that its introduction will provide a useful challenge to the adult attachment field. Although the resemblances between mother–infant attachment process and adult romantic relationships seem persuasive, the extant evidence for love-as-attachment is really largely circumstantial. It looks and quacks like a duck, so we have assumed that it is in fact a duck. Until now, adult attachment theory has enjoyed remarkable success in part (it seems to me) because it has gone largely unchallenged; there has been no other comparable model against which to test it. I hope the model described in this chapter will prove useful in this regard, and will serve to stimulate further empirical research and theory development that, in the end, will either enrich and strengthen adult attachment theory or facilitate its evolution into, or replacement by, an even more powerful theory of adult relationships.

ACKNOWLEDGMENTS

I am grateful to Jay Belsky, Kelly Brennan, David Buss, Cindy Hazan, Steve Rholes, Jeff Simpson, and Linda Zyzniewski for their helpful comments on an earlier draft of this chapter.

NOTES

1. Berman et al. (1994) do not spell out their evolutionary arguments in any detail, but their attribution of the adaptiveness of this mechanism to "species survival" (p. 214) is clearly inconsistent with modern evolutionary theory.

2. There is one important difference between these cultural and biological mechanisms, however: Biologically evolved mechanisms are adaptive to the extent they lead to proliferation of the genes that code for them, not to the extent

that they benefit groups, populations, or species (or even individuals; see Dawkins, 1976, for a brilliant exposition). The universality of marriage owes to the benefits that accrue to *groups* and the individuals living in them. Formal marriage agreements bring the possibility of peace within the group so that individuals can move beyond constant mate competition (which, undoubtedly, would be characterized by high levels of aggression and violence) to other life tasks. A society with no formal arrangements for resolving disputes over mates would be a dangerous and unpleasant place to live. In contrast, an evolved mechanism for pair-bond maintenance must have been adaptive in the inclusive-fitness sense, irrespective of its value to groups or societies. As discussed in a subsequent section, long-term pair-bonding does in fact confer certain reproductive benefits, at least under certain conditions, but it faces stiff competition from other competing mating strategies as well.

3. It may seem surprising that avoidant persons, who (from my perspective) are not oriented toward long-term relationships, also report a preference for secure rather than other avoidant partners in this research. It is important to note that this research, like most social-psychological research on mate preferences, focuses on individuals' preferences with respect to *long-term* relationship partners. Avoidant persons may not be interested in pursuing such long-term relationships, but this does not prevent them from realizing (and reporting) that a secure partner would be the best choice *if* they were to pursue such a relationship.

4. A couple of caveats may be in order. First, there is no assumption here concerning conscious awareness of the kinds of thought processes I have described. Instead, I merely assume that men's and women's evolved mechanisms for evaluating costs and benefits of different relationship types are differentially sensitive to various internal and external variables, and the "realization" (again, not in a conscious sense) that one is in a high cost/low benefit situation will be experienced (now consciously) as unpleasant. Second, it should of course be understood that this evolutionary explanation (or any other kind of scientific explanation, for that matter) should in no way be interpreted as an endorsement or justification of any particular pattern of behavior.

5. Note that this parsimony argument is *not* based on the questionable assumption that a theory based on fewer mechanisms is inherently superior to one based on a greater number of mechanisms. Evolutionary psychologists argue persuasively that our psychological architecture is comprised of numerous domain-specific mechanisms rather than a few domain-general ones, much as the rest of the body consists of numerous specialized organs (Buss, 1991; Tooby & Cosmides, 1992).

REFERENCES

Allen, K. M., Blascovich, J., Tomaka, J., & Kelsey, R.M. (1991). Presence of human friends and pet dogs as moderators of autonomic responses to stress in women. *Journal of Personality and Social Psychology, 61,* 582–589.

Bartholomew, K. (1990). Avoidance of intimacy: An attachment perspective. *Journal of Social and Personal Relationships, 7,* 147–178.

Bartholomew, K., & Horowitz, L. M. (1991). Attachment styles in young adults: A test of a four-category model. *Journal of Personality and Social Psychology, 61,* 226–244.

Batson, C. D. (1993). Communal and exchange relationships: What is the difference? *Personality and Social Psychology Bulletin, 19,* 677–683.

Belsky, J. (1997). *Attachment, mating, and parenting: An evolutionary interpretation.* Unpublished manuscript, Pennsylvania State University.

Belsky, J., Steinberg, L., & Draper, P. (1991). Childhood experience, interpersonal development, and reproductive strategies: An evolutionary theory of socialization. *Child Development, 62,* 647–670.

Berman, W. H., Marcus, L., & Berman, E. R. (1994). Attachment in marital relations. In M. B. Sperling & W. H. Berman (Eds.), *Attachment in adults: Clinical and developmental perspectives* (pp. 204–231). New York: Guilford Press.

Berman, W. H., & Sperling, M. B. (1994). The structure and function of adult attachment. In M. B. Sperling & W. H. Berman (Eds.), *Attachment in adults: Clinical and developmental perspectives* (pp. 1–28). New York: Guilford Press.

Bowlby, J. (1969). *Attachment and loss. Vol. 1. Attachment.* New York: Basic Books.

Bowlby, J. (1980). *Attachment and loss. Vol. 3. Loss.* New York: Basic Books.

Brehm, S. S. (1988). Passionate love. In R. J. Sternberg & M. L. Barnes (Eds.), *The psychology of love* (pp. 232–263). New Haven, CT: Yale University Pres.

Brennan, K. A., & Shaver, P. R. (1995). Dimensions of adult attachment, affect regulation, and romantic relationship functioning. *Personality and Social Psychology Bulletin, 21,* 267–283.

Brennan, K. A., Shaver, P. R., & Tobey, A. E. (1991). Attachment styles, gender and parental problem drinking. *Journal of Social and Personal Relationships, 8,* 451–466.

Burton, L. M. (1990). Teenage childbearing as an alternative life-course strategy in multigeneration black families. *Human Nature, 1,* 123–143.

Buss, D. M. (1991). Evolutionary personality psychology. *Annual Review of Psychology, 42,* 459–491.

Buss, D. M. (1992). Mate preference mechanisms: Consequences for partner choice and intrasexual competition. In J. H. Barkow, L. Cosmides, & J. Tooby (Eds.), *The adapted mind: Evolutionary psychology and the generation of culture* (pp. 249–266). New York: Oxford University Press.

Buss, D. M., & Greiling, H. (in press). Adaptive individual differences. *Journal of Personality.*

Buss, D. M., Larsen, R. J., Westen, D., & Semmelroth, J. (1992). Sex differences in jealousy: Evolution, physiology, and psychology. *Psychological Science, 3,* 251–255.

Buss, D. M., & Schmitt, D. P. (1993). Sexual strategies theory: An evolutionary perspective on human mating. *Psychological Review, 100,* 204–232.

Carpenter, E. M., & Kirkpatrick, L. A. (1996). Attachment style and presence of a romantic partner as moderators of psychophysiological responses to a stressful laboratory situation. *Personal Relationships, 3,* 351–367.

Carter, C. S. (1992). Oxytocin and sexual behavior. *Neuroscience and Biobehavioral Reviews, 16,* 131–144.

Chappell, K. D., & Davis, K. E. (1996). *Attachment, partner choice, and perception of romantic partners: An experimental test of the attachment-security hypothesis.* Unpublished manuscript, University of South Carolina.

Chisolm, J. S. (1996). The evolutionary ecology of attachment organization. *Human Nature, 7,* 1–38.

Clark, M. S., & Mills, J. (1993). The difference between communal and exchange relationships: What is and is not. *Personality and Social Psychology Bulletin, 19,* 684–691.

Collins, N. L., & Read, S. J. (1990). *Adult attachment, working models, and relationship quality in dating couples. Journal of Personality and Social Psychology, 58,* 644–663.

Daly, M., & Wilson, M. (1988). *Homicide.* New York: Aldine de Gruyter.

Daly, M., & Wilson, M. (1996). Evolutionary psychology and marital conflict. In D. M. Buss & N. M. Malamuth (Eds.), *Sex, power, conflict: Evolutionary and feminist perspectives* (pp. 9–28). New York: Oxford University Press.

Dawkins, R. (1976). *The selfish gene.* New York: Oxford University Press.

Draper, P., & Belsky, J. (1990). Personality development in evolutionary perspective. *Journal of Personality, 58,* 141–161.

Draper, P., & Harpending, H. (1982). Father absence and reproductive strategy: An evolutionary perspective. *Journal of Anthropological Research, 38,* 255–273.

Draper, P., & Harpending, H. (1988). A sociobiological perspective on the development of human reproductive strategies. In K. MacDonald (Ed.), *Sociobiological perspectives on human development* (pp. 340–372). New York: Springer-Verlag.

Edens, J. L., Larkin, K. T., & Abel, J. L. (1992). The effect of social support and physical touch on cardiovascular reactions to mental stress. *Journal of Psychosomatic Research, 36,* 371–382.

Feeney, B. C., & Kirkpatrick, L. A. (1996). The effects of adult attachment and presence of romantic partners on physiological responses to stress. *Journal of Personality and Social Psychology, 70,* 255–270.

Feeney, J. A., & Noller, P. (1990). Attachment style as a predictor of adult romantic relationships. *Journal of Personality and Social Psychology, 58,* 281–291.

Feeney, J. A., Noller, P., & Callan, V. J. (1994). Attachment style, communication and satisfaction in the early years of marriage. In D. Perlman & K. Bartholomew (Eds.), *Advances in personal relationships,* (Vol. 5, pp. 269–308). London: Jessica Kingsley.

Frank, R. H. (1988). *Passions within reason: The strategic role of the emotions.* New York: Norton.

Gangestad, S. W., & Simpson, J. A. (1990). Toward an evolutionary history of female sociosexual variation. *Journal of Personality, 58,* 69–96.

Hamilton, W. D. (1964). The genetical evolution of social behaviour. *Journal of Theoretical Biology, 7,* 1–52.

Hazan, C., & Shaver, P. (1987). Romantic love conceptualized as an attachment process. *Journal of Personality and Social Psychology, 52,* 511-524.

Hazan, C., & Shaver, P. (1990). Love and work: An attachment-theoretical perspective. *Journal of Personality and Social Psychology, 59,* 270–280.

Hazan, C., & Zeifman, D. (1994). Sex and the psychological tether. In D. Perlman & K. Bartholomew (Eds.), *Advances in personal relationships* (Vol. 5, pp. 151–177). London: Jessica Kingsley.

Hazan, C., Zeifman, D., & Middleton, K. (1994, July). *Attachment and sexuality.* Paper presented at the 7th International Conference on Personal Relationships, Groningen, The Netherlands.

Hill, E. M., Young, J. P., & Nord, J. L. (1994). Childhood adversity, attachment security, and adult relationships: A preliminary study. *Ethology and Sociobiology, 15,* 323–338.

Hinde, R. A. (1982). Attachment: Some conceptual and biological issues. In C. M. Parkes & J. Stevenson-Hinde (Eds.), *The place of attachment in human behavior* (pp. 60–76). New York: Basic Books.

Kamarck, T. W., Manuck, S. B., & Jennings, J. R. (1990). Social support reduces cardiovascular reactivity to psychological challenge: A laboratory model. *Psychosomatic Medicine, 52,* 42–58.

Kelley, H. H., & Thibaut, J. W. (1978). *Interpersonal relationships: A theory of interdependence.* New York: Wiley.

Kirkpatrick, L. A. (in press-a). Attachment and religious representations and behavior. In J. Cassidy & P. R. Shaver (Eds.), *Handbook of attachment theory and research.* New York: Guilford Press.

Kirkpatrick, L. A. (in press-b). On individual differences in attachment and reproductive strategies: Commentary on Buss & Greiling. *Journal of Personality.*

Kirkpatrick, L. A., & Davis, K. E. (1994). Attachment style, gender, and relationship stability: A longitudinal analysis. *Journal of Personality and Social Psychology, 66,* 502–512.

Kirkpatrick, L. A., & Hazan, C. (1994). Attachment styles and close relationships: A four-year prospective study. *Personal Relationships, 1,* 123–142.

Kirkpatrick, L. A., & Shaver, P. R. (1988). Fear and affiliation reconsidered from a stress and coping perspective: The importance of cognitive clarity and fear-reduction. *Journal of Social and Clinical Psychology, 7*(2/3), 214–233.

Kobak, R., & Duemmler, S. (1994). Attachment and conversation: Toward a discourse analysis of adolescent and adult security. In D. Perlman & K. Bartholomew (Eds.), *Advances in personal relationships* (Vol. 5, pp. 121–149). London: Jessica Kingsley.

Konner, M. (1982). *The tangled wing: Biological constraints on the human spirit.* New York: Holt, Reinhart & Winston.

Lamb, M., Thompson, R., Gardner, W., & Charnov, E. (1985). *Infant–mother attachment: The origins and developmental significance of individual differences in Strange Situation behavior.* Hillsdale, NJ: Erlbaum.

Latty-Mann, H., & Davis, K. E. (1996). Attachment theory and partner choice: Preference and actuality. *Journal of Social and Personal Relationships, 13,* 5–23.

Levy, M. B., & Davis, K. E. (1988). Lovestyles and attachment styles compared: Their relations to each other and to various relationship characteristics. *Journal of Social and Personal Relationships, 5,* 439–471.

Main, M., Kaplan, N., & Cassidy, J. (1985). Security in infancy, childhood, and adulthood: A move to the level of representation. In I. Bretherton & E. Waters (Eds.), Growing points of attachment theory and research. *Monographs of the Society for Research in Child Development, 50* (1–2, Serial No. 209), 66–104.

Mealey, L. (1990). Differential use of reproductive strategies by human groups? *Psychological Science, 1,* 385–387.

Mellen, S. L. W. (1981). *The evolution of love.* Oxford: Freeman.

Mikulincer, M., & Florian, V. (1995). Appraisal and coping with a real-life stressful situation: The contribution of attachment styles. *Personality and Social Psychology Bulletin, 21,* 406–414.

Mikulincer, M., Florian, V., & Weller, A. (1993). Attachment styles, coping strategies, and post-traumatic psychological distress: The impact of the Gulf War in Israel. *Journal of Personality and Social Psychology, 64,* 817–826.

Miller, L. C., & Fishkin, S. A. (1997). On the dynamics of human bonding and reproductive success: Seeking windows on the adapted-for human–environmental interface. In J. A. Simpson & D. Kenrick (Eds.), *Evolutionary social psychology* (pp. 197–235). Mahwah, NJ: Erlbaum.

Murstein, B. I., Cerreto, M., & MacDonald, M. (1977). A theory and investigation of the effect of exchange-orientation on marriage and friendship. *Journal of Marriage and the Family, 39,* 543–548.

Pianka, E. R. (1970). On r- and K-selection. *American Naturalist, 104,* 592–597.

Pietromonaco, P., & Carnelley, K. (1994). Gender and working models of attachment: Consequences for perception of self and romantic partners. *Personal Relationships, 1,* 63–82.

Rholes, W. S., Simpson, J. A., Blakely, B. S., Lanigan, L., & Allen, E. A. (in press). Adult attachment styles, the desire to have children, and working models of parenthood. *Journal of Personality.*

Rothbard, J. C., & Shaver, P. R. (1994). Continuity of attachment across the life span. In M. B. Sperling & W. H. Berman (Eds.), *Attachment in adults: Clinical and developmental perspectives* (pp. 31–71). New York: Guilford Press.

Rusbult, C. E. (1980). Commitment and satisfaction in romantic associations: A test of the investment model. *Journal of Experimental Social Psychology, 16,* 172–186.

Rushton, J. P. (1985). Differential K theory: The sociobiology of individual and group differences. *Personality and Individual Differences, 6,* 441–452.

Schachter, S. (1959). *The psychology of affiliation.* Stanford, CA: Stanford University Press.

Schafer, R. B., & Keith, P. M. (1980). Equity and depression among married couples. *Social Psychology Quarterly, 43,* 430–435.

Senchak, M., & Leonard, K. E. (1992). Attachment styles and marital adjustment among newlywed couples. *Journal of Social and Personal Relationships, 9,* 51–64.

Shaver, P. R., Hazan, C., & Bradshaw, D. (1988). Love as attachment: The integration of three behavioral systems. In R. J. Sternberg & M. Barnes (Eds.), *The anatomy of love* (pp. 68–99). New Haven, CT: Yale University Press.

Shaver, P. R., & Klinnert, M. (1980). Schachter's theories of affiliation and emotion: Implications of developmental research. In L. Wheeler (Ed.), *Review of personality and social psychology* (Vol. 3, pp. 37–71. Beverly Hills, CA: Sage.

Simpson, J. A. (1990). Influence of attachment styles on romantic relationships. *Journal of Personality and Social Psychology, 59,* 971–980.

Simpson, J. A. (in press). Attachment theory in modern evolutionary perspective. In J. Cassidy & P. R. Shaver (Eds.), *Handbook of attachment theory and research.* New York: Guilford Press.

Simpson, J. A., & Gangestad, S. W. (1991). Individual differences in sociosexuality: Evidence for convergent and discriminant validity. *Journal of Personality and Social Psychology, 60,* 870–883.

Simpson, J. A., Rholes, W. S., & Nelligan, J. S. (1992). Support seeking and support giving within couples in an anxiety-provoking situation: The role of attachment styles. *Journal of Personality and Social Psychology, 62,* 434–446.

Stearns, S. (1992). *The evolution of life histories.* New York: Oxford University Press.

Steele, H., & Steele, M. (1994). Intergenerational patterns of attachment. In D.

Perlman & K. Bartholomew (Eds.), *Advances in personal relationships* (Vol. 5, pp. 93–120). London: Jessica Kingsley.

Tennov, D. (1979). *Love and limerance: The experience of being in love*. New York: Stein & Day.

Tooby, J., & Cosmides, L. (1992). The psychological foundations of culture. In J. H. Barkow, L. Cosmides, & J. Tooby (Eds.), *The adapted mind* (pp. 19–136). New York: Oxford University Press.

Trivers, R. L. (1974). Parent–offspring conflict. *American Zoologist, 14,* 249–265.

van IJzendoorn, M. (1995). Adult attachment representations, parental responsiveness, and infant attachment: A meta-analysis of the predictive validity of the Adult Attachment Interview. *Psychological Bulletin, 117,* 387–403.

Vormbrock, J. K. (1993). Attachment theory as applied to war-time and job-related marital separation. *Psychological Bulletin, 114,* 122–144.

Walster, E., Walster, G. W., & Berscheid, E. (1978). *Equity: Theory and research.* Boston: Allyn & Bacon.

Weiss, R. S. (1982). Attachment in adults. In C. M. Parkes & J. Stevenson-Hinde (Eds.), *The place of attachment in human behavior* (pp. 171–184). New York: Basic Books.

West, M. L., & Sheldon-Keller, A. E. (1994). *Patterns of relating: An adult attachment perspective.* New York: Guilford Press.

Whiting, J. W. M., & Whiting, B. B. (1975). Aloofness and intimacy of human husbands and wives: A cross-cultural study. *Ethos, 3,* 183–207.

Zeifman, D., & Hazan, C. (1997a). Attachment: The bond in pair-bonds. In J. A. Simpson & D. Kenrick (Eds.), *Evolutionary social psychology* (pp. 237–263). Mahwah, NJ: Erlbaum.

Zeifman, D., & Hazan, C. (1997b). A process model of adult attachment formation. In S. Duck & W. Ickes (Eds.), *Handbook of personal relationships* (2nd ed., pp. 179–195). Chichester, England: Wiley.

14

Adult Romantic Attachment and Individual Differences in Attitudes toward Physical Contact in the Context of Adult Romantic Relationships

KELLY A. BRENNAN
SHEY WU
JENNIFER LOEV

The current volume describes the past decade of research on adult romantic attachment, spearheaded by Cindy Hazan and Phillip Shaver (Hazan & Shaver, 1987; Shaver & Hazan, 1993). Much of this work has focused on comparisons of infant and adult attachment (Shaver, Hazan, & Bradshaw, 1988; see also Kirkpatrick, Chapter 13, this volume); measurement of individual differences in adult attachment styles (see Bartholomew & Shaver, Chapter 2; Brennan, Clark, & Shaver, Chapter 3; Fraley & Waller, Chapter 4; and Klohnen & John, Chapter 5, this volume); attachment and romantic relationship functioning (Collins & Read, 1990; Noller & Feeney, 1993; Simpson, 1990; Roberts & Noller, Chapter 12, this volume); therapeutic relationship functioning (Dozier & Tyrrell, Chapter 9, this volume); caregiving (Kunce & Shaver, 1994); sexuality (Hazan & Zeifman, 1994; Hazan, Zeifman, & Middleton, 1994); personality (Shaver

& Brennan, 1992; Fraley, Davis, & Shaver, Chapter 10, this volume); working models (Collins & Read, 1990; Pietromonaco & Carnelley, 1994); intergenerational transmission of working models (Henry & Holmes, Chapter 11, this volume; Rothbard & Shaver, 1994); working models and affect regulation (Simpson, Rholes, & Nelligan, 1992; see also Mikulincer & Florian, Chapter 6; Rholes, Simpson, & Grich Stevens, Chapter 7; and Feeney, Chapter 8, this volume); as well as other issues relevant to validation of the attachment construct. The lion's share of this research has focused on individual differences in the quality of attachment, as opposed to the conditions that contribute to the formation or maintenance of adult attachment.

In this chapter, we take a different tack—by taking seriously the idea that attachment formation in adulthood parallels the processes of attachment formation in infancy using the communication channel of touch, or physical-contact seeking. That is, touch appears to be an effective means of regulating arousal in mother–infant relationships and may also be important for understanding the formation and mainte- nance of affectional bonds in later life. In adult romantic relationships, touch is integral to three major behavioral systems combined in "love": attachment, caregiving, and sexuality (Shaver et al., 1988). Thus, al- though the relationship between attachment and touch has been docu- mented in the primate and infant literatures, it is relatively unexplored in the literature on adult pair-bonds. In order to explore this topic, we have designed a set of measures to assess attitudes toward touch in the context of adult romantic relationships. Such attitudes ought to covary reliably with factors associated with relationship development and func- tioning. Before introducing the measures and describing the research from which they were derived, we will first provide an overview of theoretical and empirical approaches to the study of touch. We will convey the general flavor of the wide array of research on touch and explain its relevance to adult relationship phenomena, placing particular emphasis on developmental processes related to the formation of attach- ment in adulthood.

A GENERAL OVERVIEW OF APPROACHES
TO THE STUDY OF TOUCH

Touch has been described as the most powerful, yet least understood form of nonverbal communication. In line with this observation, much of the research and theorizing about touch in the communication and social psychology literature has concentrated on attitudes toward and responses to touch outside the context of close relationships. For example, re- searchers have focused on the meaning of touch (Heslin, Nguyen, & Nguyen, 1983; Jones, 1985; Knapp, 1978; Monsour, 1992). There is functional or professional touch, such as that of a masseur or a doctor; there is social or polite touch, such as that which occurs between casual acquaintances or strangers; and then there is touch that, when used appropriately, engenders warm and loving feelings (Knapp, 1978). Using observational methods, researchers have studied how people use touch to convey emotions in social settings (e.g., Trussoni, O'Malley, & Barton, 1988); establish or reinforce social dominance hierarchies (e.g., Henley, 1977); enhance liking, trust, and persuasion (e.g., Wycoff & Holley, 1990); and how touch, especially self-touching (interpreted as "self-soothing" behavior), may reflect cognitive processing and one's state of mind (e.g., Barroso & Feld, 1986; Goldberg & Rosenthal, 1986). Experimental studies in which touch is manipulated have demonstrated clear physiological benefits from being touched during or after stressful experiences in the laboratory (Dreschner & Gantt, 1979; Dreschner, Whitehead, Morrill-Corbin, & Cataldo, 1985). Other research has shown that manipulated touch from a stranger or professional caregiver may increase the effectiveness of medical care and counseling (Bacorn & Dixon, 1984; Driscoll, Newman, & Seals, 1988; Willison & Masson, 1986; Wilson, 1982; Woodmansey, 1988). Touch has also been demonstrated to increase compliance (e.g., Goldman, Kiyohara, & Pfannensteil, 1984; Patterson, Powell, & Lenihan, 1986) and prosocial behavior (Goldman & Fordyce, 1983).

Nearly every society has evolved a set of carefully defined, though largely unspoken, rules about touch. In addition to these normative rules, there are individual differences that determine how comfortable people are with touching and being touched. Previous research has focused on these differences, particularly with regard to (1) sex differences in patterns of touching and being touched by same- versus opposite-sex persons (e.g., Fisher, Rytting, & Heslin, 1976; Hall & Veccia, 1990; Major, Schmidlin, & Williams, 1990) and (2) personality traits associated with patterns of comfort with touching and being touched (e.g., Andersen et al., 1987; Fromme et al., 1989). Most of this research has focused on the construct of *touch avoidance*—the tendency to approach or avoid tactile communication, which appears to be a stable individual differences construct.

With regard to sex differences, Andersen and Leibowitz (1978) found that men were more uncomfortable with same-sex touch, whereas women were more uncomfortable with opposite-sex touch. Andersen and Leibowitz (1978) attributed their findings to gender stereotyping, or socialization, and to homophobic attitudes. That is, because touch often implies intimacy and self-disclosure, same-sex touching (e.g., hugging, kissing on the cheeks, or hand holding) between heterosexual men is considered inappropriate, not to mention unmasculine in American culture. Women, on the other hand, have always been allowed more latitude in emotional expression via same-sex touch in American culture, although casual opposite-sex touching is still not encouraged. This interpretation fits with other research suggesting that gender differences in touch behaviors may reflect sociohistorical status differences (e.g., Derlega, Lewis, Harrison, Winstead, & Costanza, 1989; Major, 1981; Roese, Olson, Borenstein, Martin, & Shores, 1992).

In addition, these gender differences may interact with relational stage, such that women may be less open to touch during courting but more open to touch after an intimate relationship has been established (Heslin & Alper, 1983; Heslin et al., 1983; M. Nguyen, Heslin, & Nguyen, 1976; T. Nguyen, Heslin, & Nguyen, 1975). Guerrero and Andersen (1991) tested this idea by coding unobtrusively observed touch behavior of couples in a public setting (in line at the movies or the zoo). Afterwards, couples were independently asked to complete a questionnaire about the status of their relationship to determine their "relational stage": early (i.e., first date or "dating casually"), intermediate (i.e., dating seriously or "marriage bound"), or stable (i.e., married). No gender differences were found: Both males and females touched most during intermediate relationship stages. Guerrero and Andersen, following Morris (1977), interpreted their results in light of the idea that public displays of commitment (also called "tie-signs") fall off after an intimate relationship has been established. The lack of gender differences, which contrasts with the work of Heslin and colleagues, may be due to differences in observations of *public* touch behavior (Guerrero & Andersen, 1991) versus reports of *private* (including sexually oriented) touch behavior (Heslin et al., 1983).

Guerrero and Andersen (1991) also assessed couple members' touch avoidance scores. Touch avoidance scores retrodicted observations of early and intermediate couples' touch behavior but not the behavior of those in stable relationships. Guerrero and Andersen concluded that the impact of touch avoidance lessened as the relationship deepened and couple members became more acquainted, more sure of each other (i.e., with less need for public displays), and more likely to express their physical contact needs in the bedroom. It is also plausible, given the research described later in this chapter, that "touch avoiders," who appear akin to persons with avoidant attachment styles, may not stick around long enough to reach the stable stage.

With regard to traits, touch avoidance has been associated with neuroticism, poor interpersonal skills, and lower self-perceived negative social image (Andersen, Andersen, & Lustig, 1987; Andersen & Leibowitz, 1978; Andersen & Sull, 1985; Deethardt & Hines, 1983). Touch avoidance has also been associated with lower interpersonal evaluations (Sorensen & Beatty, 1988), dissatisfaction with life, lack of assertiveness, and poor problem-solving styles (Fromme et al., 1989). In a their national survey, Andersen and Leibowitz (1978) also found that both same- and opposite-sex touch avoidance were positively related to communication apprehension and negatively related to self-disclosure. In other words, someone who is averse to touch may be apprehensive about interpersonal communication and unlikely to reveal his or her emotions. Additional research (e.g., Fromme et al., 1989), including that of Andersen and his colleagues (e.g., Andersen et al., 1987), revealed that touch avoidance is also related to self-esteem. Specifically, people with higher self-esteem have more favorable attitudes toward touch in general, are more likely to initiate touching in various social situations, and report higher levels of satisfaction with their lives, themselves, and their childhood.

DEVELOPMENTAL CONSIDERATIONS

With minor exceptions, researchers who study touch in adulthood have ignored possible developmental factors in the formation of individual differences in attitudes toward touch. Deethardt and Hines (1983), theorizing about the role of tactile communication in personality development, suggested that patterns of physical contact with parents should be related to later patterns of seeking physical contact with people outside the family. Schutte, Malouff, and Adams (1988), in a small sample, discovered connections between frequency of current touch behavior in adulthood and ratings of frequency of touch in the family of origin.

In contrast to researchers studying touch in adulthood, developmental researchers have had much to say about childhood origins of individual differences in physical–contact seeking. Normative investigations of early adult-infant social interaction confirm the important role of touch. For example, Stack and Muir (1992) reported that, during face-to-face interactions with adults, 5-month-old infants smiled and gazed more when they were actively touched. Furthermore, this effect persisted even if adults posed a neutral expression (a condition that previously had decreased infant smiling and gazing) or made their hands invisible to the infants. Beyond facilitating social development, touch may affect infants' physical and cognitive development in the first year of life (Field, 1995; Korner, 1990). Historically important observational research by Rene Spitz (1946) showed the importance of touch for the growth and well-being of neonates. Infants provided with sufficient nutrition in hygienic foundling homes often failed to thrive, compared to infants reared by their "delinquent" young mothers in a penal institution. In his famous "surrogate mother" experiments on neonatal macaque monkeys, Harlow (1958) demonstrated that "contact comfort," a component of mother–infant bonding, is of utmost importance to the primate infant's growth and development. Indeed, when the attachment system was activated by the presence of a frightening toy or when young monkeys were placed in an unfamiliar environment, they preferred to cling to a soft, warm but nonlactating inanimate "mother" rather than a lactating surrogate wire "mother," which was in all other respects the same as the cloth-covered one.

Attachment theory provides an ideally suited framework for understanding developmental antecedents of individual differences in physical-contact seeking. Touch appears not only important but crucial in the formation of attachments in infancy. Writing from an evolutionary-ethological perspective based partly on Harlow's experiments, Bowlby (1969/1982, 1973, 1980) argued that infants possess an innate "attachment plan" (e.g., crying and protesting when parents are not within reaching distance) designed to ensure close proximity with their primary caregivers. Physical contact with an attachment figure serves as the infant's most tangible, concrete indicator of safety. As such, establishing physical contact is the ultimate form of "proximity seeking," a central concept in attachment theory. Proximity- or contact-seeking behavior enhances the infant's chances for survival (and hence eventual reproduction), thus furthering the parents' reproductive success. Echoing Bowlby's view, Montagu (1986) also suggested that touch is the most fundamental means by which mothers express love for their newborns, and that satisfaction with physical contact during infancy and childhood often determines the nature of the attachment relationship and the child's subsequent social development.

Although it seems indisputable that all infants have an innate need to stay close to and have physical contact with their caregivers, and that this proximity-seeking behavior is beneficial to both the infant and its caregiver, at some point, near the end of the infant's first year of life, individual differences begin to emerge. As is well known by now, Ainsworth and her colleagues (Ainsworth, Bell, & Stayton, 1971; Ainsworth, Blehar, Waters, & Wall, 1978; Bell & Ainsworth, 1972) observed notable differences in mother–infant dyads in both laboratory and home environments. The Strange Situation laboratory assessment is a 20-minute procedure during which the mother (or other primary caregiver) and infant go through a series of increasingly stressful episodes, including two separations. In the first separation, the infant is left with a stranger; in the second, the infant is left alone. Based on coded observations of the infants' reactions to both reunions (particularly the second, more stressful one), Ainsworth et al. (1978) identified three major groups of mother–infant dyads: those involving secure infants, anxious–ambivalent (or anxious–resistant) infants, and anxious–avoidant infants. Analyses of in-home observations (made in the months prior to the laboratory interaction procedure) showed that mothers of secure infants behaved in a more contingently responsive way to their infants compared to mothers of infants classified as insecure. That is, mothers of secure infants responded consistently and promptly to their infant's signals. Mothers of the avoidant infants, in contrast, appeared rejecting of their infants, responding to their cries reluctantly or angrily, if at all. Mothers of anxious–resistant infants appeared inept or at a loss concerning what to do with their infants: They exhibited a variety of both positive and negative maternal behavior, but not in a consistent pattern. As a result, their infants reacted in either a distraught or anxious manner typical of someone who does not know what to expect from the external environment.

Home observational studies conducted in the first months of life show that variations in patterns of physical contact between mothers and infants reliably covary with attachment styles assessed in the laboratory Strange Situation at the end of the infant's first year (Ainsworth et al., 1978). Secure attachment at 1 year is associated with earlier observations of maternal handling of the infant described as "affectionate." In contrast to mothers of babies later rated as secure, mothers who picked up their infants in an "abrupt or interfering" way in the first months of life were more likely to have avoidantly attached babies. Mothers of avoidant children were also more likely to have been coded as providing their infants with "unpleasant experiences in the context of bodily contact" (Ainsworth et al., 1978, p. 300). In addition, "inept" pickups were more characteristic of mothers of avoidant and, especially, anxious–resistant infants, compared to mothers of secure infants. Mothers of secure infants were more likely to be rated as being "tender and careful" when they held their infants, compared to mothers of anxious–resistant infants. Ainsworth et al. (1971) reported that infants scored as avoidant in the Strange Situation were earlier coded by observers in the home as being either averse to physical contact with the mother or ambivalent about such contact. In fact, Ainsworth et al. (1978) summed up their description of the avoidant infants mainly in terms of maternal "rejection communicated through aberrant reactions to close bodily contact" (p. 152). In describing anxious–resistant babies, Ainsworth et al. (1978, p. 300) noted that these infants' mothers were not averse to close bodily contact, yet they failed to provide affectionate physical contact, "instead using holding time largely for routines" (i.e., routine infant care, such as feeding or bathing). This research indicates that it is not the overall quantity of physical contact but rather the quality of such contact that is important for the formation of secure attachments.

An experimental test has demonstrated the importance of physical contact for the formation of attachment security (Anisfeld, Casper, Nozyce, & Cunningham, 1990). Anisfeld et al. (1990) reported that increased physical contact between mothers and their infants promoted secure attachment. In their study, a group of low socioeconomic status (SES) mothers were randomly assigned to carry their newborns in either soft baby carriers, which fostered physical contact, or hard infant seats, which precluded physical contact. Observations made at 3½ and 13 months showed that mothers who had been randomly assigned to use the soft baby carriers were significantly more responsive to their infants than mothers in the other group. For instance, mothers assigned to use the soft carriers were more likely to initiate and engage in vocal interchange with their infants, and they also responded to their infants' needs and wants more promptly. The increased time spent by the mother–infant dyads in close contact also had an effect on certain infant behaviors, such as crying. Anisfeld et al. (1990) suggested that infants carried in soft carriers cried significantly less because they had less need to protest unresponsiveness on the part of their mothers. As mentioned, according to Bowlby (1969/1982), during the first years of life infants have a programmed need for proximity to their attachment figures. Maternal responsiveness and sensitivity to this need, argued Anisfeld et al. (1990), is essential in promoting secure mother–infant attachment.

It is not surprising that the quality of physical contact plays an important role in determining attachment security or that individuals differing in attachment security differ in their comfort with touching and being touched by attachment figures. Ainsworth et al. (1978) postulated that the quality of the early mother–infant relationship has serious consequences for the infant's development and subsequent social behavior. Consistent with this interpretation, a host of investigators have corroborated Ainsworth's findings (e.g., Sroufe, Carlson, & Shulman, 1993). Relevant to the current analysis of touch is Main's (1990) work demonstrating cross-generational continuity in aversion to physical contact. By the end of the first year, infants whose mothers were rejecting of infant initiated contact seemed to have "taken on" the maternal pattern. That is, these infants ceased to desire physical contact with their mothers—even when in a stressful situation. Main (1990) also found that parental aversion to physical contact was positively related to the parent's felt rejection by his or her own parents during childhood. It seems very likely, then, that stable individual differences in aversion to physical contact would affect the formation and maintenance of adult romantic relationships, a topic discussed in detail next.

TOUCH AND THE FORMATION OF ADULT PAIR-BONDS

We believe it is important to study touch in adult relationships, particularly attachment relationships. Touch researchers generally agree that touch ought to play an important role in the maintenance of close relationships (Andersen & Leibowitz, 1978; Burgoon, Buller, Hale, & deTurck, 1984; Guerrero & Andersen, 1991; Johnson & Edwards, 1991; Pisano, Wall, & Foster, 1986; Willis & Briggs, 1992). Touch promotes physical as well as psychological intimacy. As mentioned, most of the research on touch in romantic relationships has focused on touch as a function of relational stage and commitment (e.g., Guerrero & Andersen, 1991; Johnson & Edwards, 1991), gender and age differences (e.g., Willis & Briggs, 1992), and individuals' level of touch avoidance (e.g., Guerrero & Andersen, 1991). There is, however, one study relevant to both touch and attachment in adult romantic relationships. Simpson et al. (1992)

videotaped spontaneous interactions between dating couples minutes before the female member of the dyad was supposed to participate in an "anxiety-provoking" experiment. Simpson et al. (1992) predicted and found theoretically important attachment-style differences in support seeking and support giving behavior under stress. Specifically, as level of anxiety rose, women scoring high in avoidance showed more resistance to touch from their partners; in contrast, women scoring high in security reacted with more reciprocal facial touching and kissing. Simpson et al.'s (1992) study was important for revealing couple-members' observable attachment behaviors in response to stressful conditions. Soliciting and providing physical contact comfort under stressful conditions is likely to be a major purpose of the attachment behavioral system in adulthood as well as in infancy.

As mentioned, little is known about the process of becoming attached. Shaver et al. (1988) have cogently argued that falling in love in adulthood involves some of the same variables as the formation of bonds between infants and parents, except that in adulthood caregiving is more mutual and there is a sexual component. While not everyone agrees with Shaver et al. (cf. Kirkpatrick, Chapter 13, this volume), nearly all theorists agree that both types of bonds share the common emotion of love.[1] Regardless, two individuals' heightened sensitivity and responsiveness to each other's needs is likely to promote falling in love and feelings of intimacy (Reis & Shaver, 1988). The initial phase of falling in love is accompanied by escalating levels of intimate touch, leading to sexual behavior. Sexual behavior, in turn, may be the "sexual tether" contributing to increasing levels of psychological intimacy and security (Hazan & Zeifman, 1994). Once an attachment bond is formed, it may be maintained in large part through the nonverbal channel of touch—and not just with regard to sexual behavior. Other behaviors are relevant to touch in relationships, such as caregiving, nonverbal signs of commitment (by signaling to outsiders with public displays of their affection for each other), and general affectionate touching. Such affectionate touching includes but is not limited to proximity seeking during separations and reunions. Understanding the role of touch in the formation and maintenance of attachment bonds in adulthood would be facilitated by measures designed to assess variation in attitudes toward touch in the context of adult romantic relationships.

CURRENT MEASURES OF INDIVIDUAL DIFFERENCES IN TOUCH ATTITUDES AND BEHAVIOR

The studies reviewed in the previous sections demonstrate the importance of studying touch in close relationships, particularly in attachment relationships. A reliable and valid set of relationship-relevant touch measures would greatly contribute to such research. Although several self-report instruments assessing attitudes toward touch already exist, their usefulness for assessing touch in the context of romantic attachment relationships appears limited. Each measure will be described briefly before we turn to a consideration of the constructs we had in mind when developing our touch scales.

Jourard (1966) created a self-report measure to assess adults' experiences of being touched by others. Specifically, he asked respondents to say whether, in the past year, they had touched or been touched on various parts of their bodies by their mothers, fathers, and same- or opposite-sex friends. This measurement was insufficiently validated but set a precedent for asking subjects to report about both touching and being touched by opposite- and same-sex persons.

Andersen and Leibowitz (1978) were the first to develop a self-report instrument assessing individual differences in comfort with touch. Their measure includes 18 items comprising two dimensions: same-sex touch avoidance (e.g., "I find it difficult to be touched by a member of my own sex") and opposite-sex touch avoidance (e.g., "I think it is vulgar when members of the opposite sex touch me"). The two-factor structure has been replicated by others (e.g., Remland & Jones, 1988), and both factor-based scales show high internal consistency and test–retest reliability (e.g., Andersen et al., 1987).

Deethardt and Hines (1983) developed a 15-item measure of individual differences in attitudes toward touch. Reasoning that "tactile behavior [is] a cognitively experienced, communicative event more important to the actor than informative to the outside observer" (p. 155), Deethardt and Hines asked 70 students in a communication class to generate statements about their touch behaviors. Analytic reduction of the resulting pool of 162 items initially revealed three factors, one of which was very similar to Andersen and colleagues' measure of same-sex touch avoidance.[2] Deethardt and Hines distinguished between two kinds of opposite-sex touch attitudes: one concerning romantic partners and the other, opposite-sex acquaintances. It is interesting, from our perspective, that some of their (spontaneously generated) items clearly indicated attachment concerns relevant to proximity seeking and/or expressing affection: "I enjoy touching my girlfriend/boyfriend when greeting that person"; "When I am with my girlfriend/boyfriend I really like to touch that person to show affection." For other items, it is not clear whether the item assesses attitudes relevant to attachment: "I enjoy my girlfriend/boyfriend touching me when watching T.V. at home." Some of the items seemed oddly worded (e.g., "When I tell a same-sex intimate friend I have just gotten a divorce, I want that person to touch me"), perhaps because the initial item pool was generated by the research participants themselves. The self-generated item set probably explains the lack of items regarding use of touch for clearly sexual or aggressive purposes, which people may either fail to recognize consciously or be unwilling to describe for the benefit of science.

Building on Jourard's (1966) work, Schutte et al. (1988) devised a 54-cell grid instrument to assess the frequency of specific types of touch (e.g., kissing on the cheek, kissing on the lips, handshake, touching on the arm or shoulder) in relationships with various same- or opposite-sex targets (i.e., close friend, parent, acquaintance, stranger, spouse, boyfriend/girlfriend). Despite Schutte et al.'s small sample size, their unidimensional touch-frequency scale demonstrated high reliability and was correlated with frequency of touching in one's family of origin as well as with outsiders' (friends', romantic partners', family members') reports of the frequency of the subjects' touch behavior assessed with the same measure.

In a similar, small-scale survey of participants in a personal growth program (20 males and 16 females), Edwards (1984) constructed a questionnaire focused on the experience of touching and being touched by nonspecific others. Respondents were asked to rate the frequency and intensity of the 26 experiences. Factor analysis revealed five factors: (1) openness to touch as a means of exploration and self-expression, (2) perceptions of being touched as threatening, (3) touch as sexually arousing, (4) perceptions of touch as serious and caring, and (5) perceptions of being threatening when touching others. Although Edwards's items have a high degree of face validity, to our knowledge his five-factor structure has not been replicated.

Fromme et al. (1989) devised a 12-item Touch Test to assess one's level of comfort giving and receiving touch from same- or opposite-sex strangers, friends, and parents. The measure was developed as part of a class in which volunteers were solicited to participate in a study on hugging. The Touch Test showed a high degree of predictive validity: Subjects high in reported comfort with touch were more likely to volunteer for and enjoy the hugging study. Nonetheless, the scale had problems. Some of its items were very similar to Andersen and Leibowitz's items, whereas others were poorly written (i.e., multiple-barreled) or odd in other ways (e.g., "How comfortable would your mother [or stepmother, etc.] be in kissing you at a party?" "How comfortable would you feel hugging a same-sex person who was homely?").

Of the measures just described, the most widely used is Andersen and Leibowitz's (1978) 8-item opposite-sex Touch Avoidance Measure, which has undergone by far the best psychometric validation. This scale is largely nonspecific and unsuited for use in studies of romantic relationships, however. Thus, despite their usefulness in studies of interpersonal communication, the measures devised by Andersen and Leibowitz (1978) and by other researchers (Deethardt & Hines, 1983; Edwards, 1984;

Fromme et al., 1989; Schutte et al., 1988) have insufficient content validity to assess aspects of touch that are theoretically relevant to the formation of adult romantic attachment bonds.

In constructing a measure of relationship touch, we made the assumption that touch is relevant to the study of close relationships in general and to attachment relationships in particular. We reasoned that individuals with a history of warm, loving, and responsive attachment relationships (i.e., securely attached people) would view touch as comforting and as a means of communicating affection; in seeking proximity, such individuals would be neither overly clingy nor averse to touch. Insecurely attached individuals, on the other hand, are likely to view touch in a negative light. For instance, they may see touch as a way to control or dominate their partners; use touch to express anger and resentment; and experience a high degree of either touch deprivation (or "skin hunger," to use Montagu's [1986] terminology) or touch aversion. That is, attitudes toward touch probably reflect existing attachment dynamics in relationships.

Thus, a measure of attitudes toward touch in the context of adult romantic relationships should include items that assess both touch aversion and craving for more touch. Both constructs are likely to turn on developmental experiences of psychological and physical rejection in childhood. Such a measure should also include aspects of touch related to public displays of commitment. The tendency to interpret touch as sexual and to use touch to communicate sexual intent is also of paramount importance for the study of touch in romantic relationships. From an attachment perspective, safe haven behavior, or the extent to which individuals use touch to provide and solicit care from partners, is central. In addition, affectionate touching may be related to the formation of attachment bonds as well as the maintenance of such bonds (independent of sexual behavior). Other factors, such as using touch to communicate aggression, and general ambivalence, or confusion, about the meaning of touch are also likely to be related to attachment insecurity.

OVERVIEW OF THE CURRENT RESEARCH

In the research summarized here, our primary goal was to construct a new measure to adequately assess individual differences in attitudes toward touch in the context of romantic relationships. In creating items, we drew on previous research on touch avoidance, but also wrote items to assess constructs relevant to attachment behavior, sexual behavior, caregiving, relationship aggression, and attitudes about touching in public. We included items to assess differences in both *touching* (e.g., "I often touch my partner as a way to express my feelings for him or her") and *being touched* by partners (e.g., "My partner often touches me as a way to express his or her feelings for me"), although research shows that the two modes of touch correlate very highly (Deethardt & Hines, 1983). In all, we created items with the following constructs in mind: (1) comfort touching and being touched by partners in front of others (possibly an indicator of commitment); (2) comfort with the amount of touch in one's romantic relationship (i.e., degree of "touch deprivation"); (3) general aversion to a partner's touch, as well as more specific anger, aggression, ambivalence, or confusion about touch in romantic relationships; (4) the use of touch to alleviate stress or anxiety in self or partner (i.e., caregiving, or "safe haven" touch); (5) the use of touch to convey affection; and (6) and the use and interpretation of touch to communicate sexual intent or express sexuality.

PHASE I

In Phase I, our pool of touch items, Andersen and Leibowitz's (1978) Touch Avoidance Measure, and a measure of affect sensitivity were administered in mass-testing sessions. In conducting this initial "pilot" study, we had two goals in mind. First, we sought to discriminate our new touch scales from Andersen and Leibowitz's measure (the most widely used and best validated touch measure). We expected our touch items to overlap to some extent with the preexisting touch measures, especially with regard to generalized aversion to touching and being touched. We expected our scales to diverge with the preexisting touch measures to the extent to which our scales tap experiences specific to touching and being touched by romantic relationship partners, not just generalized "others."

Second, we included a measure of "affect sensitivity" as a way to obtain convergent validity, and to clarify the meaning of the touch factors that emerged. The measure of affect sensitivity we included was the Trait Meta-Mood Scale, designed to assess the construct of *emotional intelligence* (Salovey, Mayer, Goldman, & Palfai, 1992)—the capacity to understand, articulate, and regulate emotions. Patterns of sensitivity to one's own and others' emotions has been associated with attachment styles (Sroufe et al., 1993) and with the general ability to communicate and relate to others (Salovey et al., 1992). We expected that affect sensitivity would be related to relationship touch aversion in a theoretically meaningful way. That is, because a major function of touch in the formation of adult attachment bonds should be the communication of emotions, we expected that individuals who attend to their feelings, understand their feelings, and are able to regulate their feelings would be comfortable with touching and being touched by romantic partners in a variety of contexts and for a variety of purposes (e.g., caregiving, sex, giving and receiving affection).

Method

Participants and Procedure

A total of 564 undergraduate students (242 males and 322 females) enrolled in Introductory Psychology courses at the University of Texas at Austin participated in this study. At the time of testing, 214 (37.9%) of them reported that they were not dating, 87 (15.4%) were dating several people casually, 222 (39.4%) were dating one person seriously, 19 (3.4%) were living with someone or married, and 22 (3.9%) did not specify their status. Those who were dating, living with, or married to someone reported relationship lengths ranging from 7 days to 9 years, with a median length of 12.5 months. Participants were tested in groups of up to 50 in classrooms around campus. Upon arrival, participants were told the nature of the study and then given a packet of questionnaires to complete. The packet consisted of a consent form and several measures, as described in the next section.

Materials

Relationship Touch Measure. A total of 95 Likert-type items were constructed to tap dimensions relevant to touch in the context of romantic relationships. Nine of the 95 items were taken from Edwards's (1984) touch questionnaire and reworded to be appropriate to the context of romantic relationships. Respondents were asked to respond to the items with their current or most important romantic relationship in mind. Items were scaled along a 7-point continuum ranging from 1, "not at all like me," to 7, "very much like me."

Touch Avoidance. The Touch Avoidance Measure (Andersen & Leibowitz, 1978) consists of 10 Likert-type items that measure touch avoidance with same-sex persons and 8 items measuring touch avoidance with opposite-sex persons. Examples of same-sex touch avoidance items (alpha = .82) are: "I often put my arm around friends of the same sex (reverse-scored, or R)"; "Touching a friend of the same sex does not make me uncomfortable (R)", and "I dislike kissing relatives of the same sex." Some items from the opposite-sex scale (alpha = .81) are "I like it when members of the opposite sex touch me (R)"; "I'd enjoy giving a massage to an opposite sex friend (R)"; and "I think it is vulgar when members of the opposite sex touch me."

Affect Sensitivity. The Trait Meta-Mood Scale (TMMS; Salovey et al., 1992) consists of 31 Likert-type items assessing individual differences in emotional intelligence, which is conceptualized as a combination of three factors: *Attention to Feelings* (e.g., "I pay a lot of attention to how I feel"),

Clarity of Feelings (e.g., "I am usually very clear about my feelings"), and *Mood Repair* (e.g., "Although I am sometimes sad, I have a mostly optimistic outlook"). In the present sample, Cronbach's alphas for the Attention to Feelings, Clarity of Feelings, and Mood Repair were .86, .87, and .84, respectively.

Results

Scores on the 95 relationship touch items were subjected to a principal components analysis followed by an oblique rotation. An initial analysis extracted 20 factors with eigenvalues greater than one, accounting for 62.6% of the total variance. Judging from the eigenvalues plot, four to seven factors could be included. The seven-factor solution appeared fairly clean but resulted in two factors that included only three or four items. In the end, a five-factor solution was deemed optimal. Once the factors were extracted, items corresponding to each factor were unit-weighed and averaged to form five relationship touch subscales.

The first factor-based scale was labeled *Safe Haven Touch* (alpha = .90). Its two highest loading items were "When my partner is stressed or anxious, I want to touch him or her," and "When I am not feeling well, I really need to be touched by my partner." This scale appears to be about caregiving or, more accurately, careseeking, since *most* of its items concern using one's partner as a haven of safety—not providing a haven for one's partner. The second scale, *Desires More Touch* (alpha = .87), includes items about desiring more touch in public (e.g., "Sometimes I wish my partner were more comfortable touching in public"), along with other, less specific items about desiring more touch (e.g., "I sometimes wish my partner would touch me more"). The third factor, *Sexual Touch* (alpha = .86), as its name implies, included items dealing with interpretation of touch as sexual and with using touch to communicate sexual intimacy ("I usually become sexually aroused when my partner touches me" and "I use touch as a means to initiate sexual interaction with my partner"). The fourth factor, which we initially named *Negativity about Touch* (alpha = .81), included a combination of several negative constructs. Some items dealt with finding touch threatening (e.g., "I sometimes feel as if I am being threatened when my partner touches me"), whereas others reflected ambivalence or confusion about touch (e.g., "Sometimes I like my partner to touch me but at other times I don't want my partner to touch me at all—even in the same situation"), and still others were about problems ensuing in the relationship because of a mismatch of touch preferences (e.g., "My partner continually complains that I don't touch him or her enough"). The fifth factor was called *Affectionate Proximity* (alpha = .85) and included items assessing the use of touch to communicate affection (e.g., "I like to hold my partner's hand to demonstrate my affection for him or her").

Table 14.1 contains the intercorrelations among the five relationship

TABLE 14.1. Correlations among the Five Relationship Touch Scales (Phase I)

Scale	I	II	III	IV	V
I. Safe Haven Touch	—	.09[*]	.35[***]	−.41[***]	.62[***]
II. Desires More Touch		—	.22[***]	.03	−.03
III. Sexual Touch			—	−.31[***]	.34[***]
IV. Negativity about Touch				—	−.51[***]
V. Affectionate Proximity					—

[*]$p < .05$; [***]$p < .001$.

touch scales. The Safe Haven Touch scale is moderately related to the scales measuring sexual touch and negativity about touch, and is highly correlated with the scale measuring affectionate touch. Negativity about touch is negatively associated with sexual touch and affectionate proximity. Sexual and affectionate touch are moderately correlated. The scale assessing a desire for more touch is associated weakly with safe haven and sexual touch but not significantly with negative or affectionate touch.

Table 14.2 displays correlations of the five relationship touch scales with the same- and opposite-sex subscales of Andersen and Leibowitz's (1978) Touch Avoidance Measure. With one exception, the new scales were all significantly associated with both touch avoidance scales. The Sexual Touch scale was significantly associated with the opposite-sex scale but not the same-sex scale. The other new touch measures appear to be more strongly associated with Andersen and Leibowitz's opposite-sex scale than with their same-sex scale, but for some (Safe Haven and Affectionate Proximity), the discrimination appears negligible.

Three pairs of regression analyses were conducted to predict the three emotional intelligence scales (Attention to Feelings, Clarity of Feelings, and Mood Repair) from the five relationship touch scales and the two touch avoidance scales. For each pair of analyses, scores on Andersen and Leibowitz's (1978) Touch scales were entered in a block in Step 1; in Step 2, scores on the relationship touch scales were entered. This procedure was then repeated, with scores on the relationship touch scales entered first, followed by the touch avoidance measures. (Tables 14.3 and 14.4 list

TABLE 14.2. Correlations between Two Touch Avoidance Scales and the Five Relationship Touch Scales (Phase I)

Relationship touch scale	Same-sex touch avoidance	Opposite-sex touch avoidance
Safe Haven Touch	−.21[***]	−.24[***]
Desires More Touch	.12[**]	−.18[***]
Sexual Touch	−.03	−.42[***]
Negativity about Touch	.13[**]	.35[***]
Affectionate Proximity	−.20[***]	−.28[***]

[**]$p < .01$; [***]$p < .001$.

TABLE 14.3. Correlations between the Five Relationship Touch Scales, Two Touch Avoidance Measures, and Three Emotional Intelligence Scales (Phase I)

Scales	Attention to Feelings	Clarity of Feelings	Mood Repair
Safe Haven Touch	.28***	.07	−.11**
Desires More Touch	.08*	−.15***	−.11**
Sexual Touch	.18***	.09*	.03
Negativity about Touch	−.29***	−.32***	−.19***
Affectionate Proximity	.37***	.16***	.18***
Same-sex touch avoidance	−.14**	−.12**	−.05
Opposite-sex touch avoidance	−.25***	−.16***	−.16***

$^*p < .05$; $^{**}p < .01$; $^{***}p < .001$.

the bivariate correlations and standardized regression weights for predicting the emotional intelligence scales from the touch measures.)

In predicting Attention to Feelings, the new touch scales outpredicted the old measures by a wide margin. As can be seen in Table 14.4, Affectionate Proximity accounted for the most variance in the final equation. Those who use touch to express affection report paying more attention to their feelings. Andersen and Leibowitz's scales accounted for a small but still significant portion of variance in attention to feelings, as evidenced by its beta in the final equation. Those avoidant of same-sex touch reported less attention to feelings. Similar results were obtained in predicting Clarity of Feelings. That is, the new scales accounted for more variance than did the old scales, but the old touch scales nonetheless contributed to the final equation. Those with more negative attitudes toward touch appeared less likely to understand their own feelings. Those craving more touch as well as those low in opposite-sex touch avoidance also appeared less likely to understand their own feelings. In predicting

TABLE 14.4. Standardized Regression Weights Predicting Three Emotional Intelligence Scales' Correlations with the Five Relationship Touch Scales, Two Touch Avoidance Scales, and Three Emotional Intelligence Scales (Phase I)

Scales	Attention to Feelings	Clarity of Feelings	Mood Repair
Safe Haven Touch	.07	−.09	.02
Desires More Touch	.03	−.13**	−.13**
Sexual Touch	−.04	.03	−.07
Negativity about Touch	−.07	−.32***	−.11*
Affectionate Proximity	.31***	−.04	.09
Same-sex touch avoidance	−.13**	−.05	.00
Opposite-sex touch avoidance	−.05	−.10*	−.13*
Multiple R	.44***	.37***	.27***

$^*p < .05$; $^{**}p < .01$; $^{***}p < .001$.

Mood Repair, the Desires More Touch scale and the Andersen and Leibowitz opposite-sex Touch Avoidance Measure shared equally in their contribution, followed by the Negativity about Touch scale. Thus, those low in desire for more touch, opposite-sex touch avoidance, and negativity about touch all reported being better able to repair their moods.

Summary of Findings

With one exception, all five of the new touch scales were associated with both Andersen and Leibowitz (1978) touch avoidance scales. (Using touch to express sexuality was unrelated to same-sex touch avoidance.) Our new scales were associated more with opposite- than with same-sex touch avoidance. Given the pattern of intercorrelation of the new scales, along with their association with Andersen and Leibowitz's opposite-sex Touch Avoidance Measure, it seems reasonable to suspect the new scales' common variance overlaps to a large degree with the already established touch avoidance construct. That is, touch avoidance is a more abstract construct that, when assessed in relation to our scales, appears to obscure several more distinct components related to sexuality, affection, caregiving, touch deprivation, and general negativity about touch.

Both new and old touch measures correlated moderately with three aspects of affect sensitivity included under the rubric of "emotional intelligence": attention to feelings, clarity of feelings, and the ability to repair one's mood. These correlations were not as high as to suggest that we have merely invented another way to assess patterns of emotion regulation. Simultaneous regression analyses showed that the new touch measures outperformed the old touch measures with regard to attention to feelings and clarity of feelings. Mood repair was not strongly predicted by either set of measures. Thus, attitudes about touch appear to be associated more with attention to and clarity of emotions than with ability to improve one's mood. The tendency to pay attention to feelings was most associated with the use of touch to convey affection. Said another way, individuals open to feelings are more apt to use touch as a means to establish proximity and emotional closeness. Clarity of feelings was most associated with a lack of negativity about touch in relationships. Individuals unsure of what emotion they are experiencing are more likely to report a host of negative reactions to touching. Although these findings are generally compatible with an attachment-style interpretation of individual differences in attitudes toward touch, it seems parsimonious to consider that current relationship satisfaction may be a stronger, more proximal source of attitudes toward touch in romantic relationships. Of course, longitudinal research is necessary to resolve this issue. In the meantime, the next phase of our research entailed strengthening our measures and testing their association with self-perceived relationship quality.

PHASE II

In Phase I, we created a set of measures to assess attitudes toward touch in romantic relationships. There were problems with the factor structure, in that two of the scales (Negativity about Touch and Desires More Touch) included more than one construct. Negativity about Touch comprised a host of negative items, including some designed to assess confusion about touch, ambivalence about touch, touch aversion, and the use of touch to display dominance. Desires More Touch included both general items and items specifically aimed at desiring more physical contact with partners in public.

In Phase II, we had three goals in mind. First, we sought to improve the new touch measures by creating additional items to elaborate the constructs incompletely assessed in Phase I: Negativity about Touch and Desires More Touch. Hence, we wrote enough additional items to distinguish touch aversion from the use of touch to achieve dominance or control. We also wrote items to distinguish general touch deprivation from the desire for more touch from partners in public. Second, we again included Andersen and Leibowitz's Touch Avoidance Measure for purposes of obtaining discriminant validity. Third, we included indices of self-perceived relationship quality to test its association with the new and old touch measures. We assessed participants' relationships using quantitative measures of satisfaction/distress as well as qualitative measures of relational stages. We expected that positive relationship evaluations would be associated with favorable interpretations and uses of touch in the context of romantic relationships.

As for relational stage, our goals were more modest and exploratory because our sample did not include enough stably involved (i.e., married) individuals to enable the same comparisons made by Guerrero and Andersen (1991). We created four levels of relational stage, depending on whether participants described themselves as feeling committed, in love, both, or neither. Those merely committed may be similar in some respects to the "stable" couples Guerrero and Andersen studied—or as similar as our sample allowed. Those uncommitted but in love are similar to the "early" stage couples. Those both committed and in love are akin to the "intermediate" stage couples. (Those neither in love nor committed may not have been included in Guerrero and Andersen's sample, or were included in the "early" stage group—those on a first date or dating casually.)

Our primary reason for looking at relational stages was to examine whether comfort with levels of touching in public would covary as found in the observational research by Guerrero and Andersen. We expected to find that those both in love and committed ("intermediate" stage) would report the most comfort touching and being touched by partners in public. In addition, we had a number of ancillary hypotheses. We expected that individuals who called themselves "committed" ("stable" stage) or "in love" ("early" stage) ought to describe themselves as more touch deprived than those in the "intermediate" relationship stage of being both in love and committed.

Method

Participants and Procedure

A total of 322 subjects participated in Phase II. All were enrolled in Introductory Psychology courses at the University of Texas at Austin. About half the sample was male (174) and half female (148). At the time of testing, 122 (37.9%) of them reported that they were not dating, 45 (14.0%) were dating several people casually, 36 (11.2%) were dating one person casually, 97 (30.1%) were dating one person seriously, 12 (3.7%) were living with a partner or married, and 10 (3.1%) did not identify their dating status. The people who were dating or in a relationship reported a median relationship length of 9 months. Participants were tested in groups of up to 50 in classrooms around campus. Upon arrival, they were told that the study concerned personality differences and how they relate to touch. The experimenter then asked each subject to complete a packet of questionnaires, including demographic questions, touch items, and relationship measures.

Materials

Touch Measures. We included Andersen and Leibowitz's (1978) same-sex (alpha = .84) and opposite-sex (alpha = .79) touch avoidance scales, described in Phase I, along with a supplemental set of relationship touch items (80 items total).

Relationship Assessments. Subjects were asked to rate (using 7-point Likert-type scales) the degree to which their current or most important romantic relationship could be characterized by a set of 23 adjectives. Principal components analysis revealed two orthogonal factors underlying responses to these items, accounting for 51.2% of the total variance. The highest loading items on each factor were unit-weighted and averaged. The first factor-based scale, Intimacy (alpha = .90), includes the following adjectives: loving, close, in love, giving, invested, magical, and committed. The second factor-based scale, Distress (alpha = .83), contains the following items: unhappy, troubled, strained, tense, argumentative, cruel, and violent. In addition, subjects were asked to report their relationship status, and, if in a relationship, the degree to which they felt committed to their current relationship as well as the length of time in that relationship. Both scales have been associated with the satisfaction scale of Spanier's (1976) Dyadic Adjustment Scale, a widely used measure of marital distress, but are only modestly correlated with each other ($r = -.44$), indicating the utility of empirically distinguishing positive and negative evaluations. An additional advantage of these adjective-based scales is that they can be used to assess the quality of dating as well as marital relationships.

Results

Ratings on the 80 relationship touch items were subjected to a principal components analysis followed by an oblique rotation. An initial analysis extracted 20 factors with eigenvalues greater than one, accounting for 66.4% of the total variance. The seven-factor solution was chosen, based on the pattern of eigenvalues and distribution of factor loadings. Items corresponding to each factor were unit-weighted and averaged to form the following subscales.

The first factor-based scale was named *Desires More Touch*. This eight-item scale consisted solely of items about desiring more touch from partners, without any of the "public touch" items that combined with touch-deprivation items in Phase I. The second factor-based scale was called *Affectionate Proximity* and included nine items, which concern using touch to communicate affection and achieve emotional closeness. The third factor-based scale was *Sexual Touch*, which included the same seven items as in Phase I, which concern interpreting touch as sexual and using touch to communicate sexual intimacy. The fourth factor-based scale, *Touch Aversion*, included eight items assessing general disdain for touching, and interpretation of touch as threatening, intrusive, or simply annoying (e.g., "I often have to remind my partner to stop touching me"). The fifth scale assesses *Discomfort with Public Touch*, and includes five items concerning comfort with touching and being touched by partners in public (e.g., "I don't think displays of physical affection are appropriate in public.") The sixth scale assesses the use of touch to exert control. We named this six-item scale *Coercive Control*, because it includes items to assess aggression, dominance, and general use of touch to control partners (e.g., "I often touch my partner to assert my feelings of contol.") The seventh and last scale was the same eight-item *Safe Haven* touch scale that emerged in Phase I. (See Appendix 14.1 for scale items and alphas.)

The intercorrelations of the seven relationship touch scales are shown in Table 14.5. Safe Haven touch, Touch Aversion, and Affectionate Proximity were all intercorrelated (all $rs > .50$). In addition, Aversion and Discomfort with Public Touch were correlated with each other ($r = .48$).

These patterns of uneven correlations suggest that there is a deeper structure underlying the touch subscales. To test this idea, a principal components analysis was conducted on the scale scores. Two factors

TABLE 14.5. Correlations among the Seven Relationship Touch Scales (Phase II)

Scale	I	II	III	IV	V	VI	VII
I. Desires More Touch	—	.17**	.07	.21***	.10	.24***	.00
II. Affectionate Proximity		—	.25***	-.53***	-.38***	-.12*	.55***
III. Sexual Touch			—	-.22***	-.12*	.12*	.28***
IV. Touch Aversion				—	.48***	.25***	-.52***
V. Discomfort with Public Touch					—	.06	-.35***
VI. Coercive Control						—	-.02
VII. Safe Haven Touch							—

*$p < .05$; **$p < .01$; ***$p < .001$.

emerged with eigenvalues greater than one, together accounting for 56.4% of the variance. The two factors were rotated using an oblique procedure. The first factor was associated with *high* scores on Touch Aversion ($r = .79$) and Discomfort with Public Touch ($r = .64$), and *low* scores on Safe Haven ($r = -.80$), Affectionate Proximity ($r = -.79$), and Sexual Touch ($r = -.49$). The second factor consisted of *high* scores on Coercive Control ($r = .74$), Desires More Touch ($r = .70$), and Sexual Touch ($r = .49$).

Table 14.6 displays the correlations between the seven new relationship touch scales and Andersen and Leibowitz's (1978) Touch Avoidance Measure. Only a handful of correlations were significant, and none of the correlations exceeded .30. Same-sex touch avoidance was negatively associated with Affectionate Proximity and Safe Haven scales, and positively associated with the Discomfort with Public Touch and Desires More Touch scales. Opposite-sex touch avoidance was associated with high scores on Discomfort with Public Touch and low scores on the Sexual Touch and Safe Haven scales.

Table 14.7 lists correlations between the touch scales, on the one hand, and the two relationship functioning scales, on the other hand. Note that the Andersen and Leibowitz's touch avoidance scales were not significantly associated with either aspect of relationship functioning. Several associations emerged, however, between the new touch measures and

TABLE 14.6. Correlations between Two Touch Avoidance Scales and the Seven Relationship Touch Scales (Phase II)

Relationship touch scale	Same-sex touch avoidance	Opposite-sex touch avoidance
Desires More Touch	.13*	-.09
Affectionate Proximity	-.28***	-.10
Sexual Touch	.11	-.24***
Touch Aversion	.04	.18**
Discomfort with Public Touch	.18**	.25***
Coercive Control	-.09	-.01
Safe Haven Touch	-.16**	-.16**

*$p < .05$; **$p < .01$; ***$p < .001$.

TABLE 14.7. Correlations between the Five Relationship Touch Scales, Two Touch Avoidance Scales, and Two Relationship Functioning Scales (Phase II)

Scales	Intimacy	Distress
Desires More Touch	−.32[***]	.35[***]
Affectionate Proximity	.43[***]	−.21[***]
Sexual Touch	.24[***]	−.03
Touch Aversion	−.44[***]	.35[***]
Discomfort with Public Touch	−.22[***]	.20[***]
Coercive Control	−.09	.27[***]
Safe Haven Touch	.37[***]	−.17[**]
Same-sex touch avoidance	−.10	.06
Opposite-sex touch avoidance	.06	.03

[**]$p < .01$; [***]$p < .001$.

relationship functioning. Relationship Intimacy was associated with a high degree of Affectionate, Safe Haven, and Sexual Touch, and with a low degree of Touch Aversion, Desires More Touch, and Discomfort with Public Touch. Coercive Control was unrelated to Relationship Intimacy, but was associated with Relationship Distress. Relationship Distress was also positively associated with Touch Aversion, Desires More Touch, Discomfort with Public Touch, and low degrees of Affectionate and Safe Haven touch. Sexual Touch was unrelated to the Relationship Distress scale.

Next, an analysis was performed to explore the connections between touch attitudes and a new variable created to reflect relational stage. First, we conducted a median split of the sample currently in a relationship into high and low commitment groups; next, we divided subjects according to whether they had or had not reported being "in love" at the time of testing (regardless of whether they reported being in a relationship). Thus, Group 1 comprised individuals who were neither in love nor committed; Group 2, those who were in love but not committed; Group 3, those who were committed but not in love; and Group 4, those who were both in love and committed. The resulting group means for the relationship and touch avoidance scales are shown in Table 14.8. An analysis of variance was computed on the means. As can be seen in Table 14.8, neither of Andersen and Leibowitz's (1978) touch avoidance scales was associated with relational stage. Interestingly, discomfort with touching and being touched by partners in public appeared unrelated to relational stage, indicating that this construct may not have much to do with public displays of commitment. Respondents who reported being both committed and in love (Group 4) scored higher on affectionate and safe haven touch, and lower in craving for more touch from partners, compared to those committed but not in love (Group 3) and those neither committed nor in love (Group 1). Group 4 also scored lowest in touch aversion compared to the other

TABLE 14.8. Scores on Seven Relationship Touch Scales and Two Touch Avoidance Scales as a Function of Relational Stage (Phase II)

| | Relational stage | | | | |
	Group 1 Neither	Group 2 In love	Group 3 Committed	Group 4 Both	$F(3, 317)$
Desires More Touch	2.53_b	2.48_{ab}	2.52_b	2.11_a	8.72^{***}
Affectionate Proximity	4.06_a	4.21_{ab}	4.24_a	4.47_b	13.08^{***}
Sexual Touch	3.50_a	3.48_{ab}	3.70_{ab}	3.74_b	2.65^{*}
Touch Aversion	2.23_b	2.17_b	2.03_b	1.80_a	11.19^{***}
Discomfort with Public Touch	3.78	2.60	2.71	2.62	1.25
Coercive Control	1.98	2.15	1.92	1.87	1.31
Safe Haven Touch	3.40_a	3.47_{ab}	3.38_a	3.76_b	8.90^{***}
Same-sex touch avoidance	2.98	2.88	3.02	2.88	.75
Opposite-sex touch avoidance	1.59	1.62	1.67	1.72	1.80

Note. Within each row, means whose subscripts differ are significantly different at $p < .05$.
$^{*}p < .05$, $^{***}p < .001$.

groups. The use of touch to express sexuality distinguished between Groups 1 and 4, with the latter group reporting a higher tendency to use touch to express sexuality.

Summary of Findings

In this second study, the touch measures were revised by adding items to assess more differentiated facets subsumed by the general touch aversion and touch deprivation constructs assessed imperfectly in the first study. Seven factors emerged. As expected, three factors again emerged in Phase II: Safe Haven Touch, Sexual Touch, and Affectionate Proximity. Both Negativity about Touch and Desires More Touch from the first study split into two scales each with the addition of more items in the second study. Negativity about Touch split into Touch Aversion and Coercive Control. Desires More Touch split into a general factor concerned with feeling touch deprived (which we also named "Desires More Touch") and a specific factor concerning Discomfort with Public Touch. The new touch measures were only modestly associated with Andersen and Leibowitz's (1978) touch avoidance scales, and were more strongly correlated with relationship functioning. Andersen and Leibowitz's touch avoidance scales were uncorrelated with either relationship intimacy or distress, and were also unrelated to relationship "stage." As mentioned earlier, Guerrero and Andersen (1991) found that touch avoidance was associated with variation in public touch behavior according to relational stages: Touch avoidance was important in early or intermediate stages, but not in later, more stable stages (i.e., marriage). Several of the new relationship touch scales were associated with our version of "relational stage." Those both committed and in love appeared to use touch in a more secure manner relative to those merely committed or neither committed nor in love. Those committed and in love reported being less touch deprived as well as less averse to touch, and had a greater tendency to use touch to express affection and as a haven of safety. Compared to those neither in love nor committed, those committed and in love scored higher in the use and interpretation of touch in romantic relationships as sexual. (Dis)comfort with public display of affection was originally thought to be associated with relationship stage, but there was no association in this sample.

GENERAL DISCUSSION

Research on touch is fairly new, as is adult romantic attachment research. In this chapter we have summarized literature on touch and individual differences in touch attitudes and behavior in the context of relationships from infancy to adulthood. Touch is an important component of mother–infant attachment and may be useful for understanding adult romantic attachment as well. In examining how touch in relationships fits within an attachment theory framework, we sought to avoid examining individual differences in attachment quality. Instead, we focused on how the normative process of becoming and staying attached implicates close bodily contact. Human skin has been described variously as the largest sense organ, encompassing a total area of about 18 square feet; one's sense of touch, or tactility, cannot be "switched off" or "lost," as can other senses, such as vision or hearing. Prior to the development of other senses, physical contact is parents' primary means of communicating with their infants. Indeed, it is the sense of touch that enables us to understand the very boundaries of our selves (Walsh, 1991). The formation of a sense of ourselves as separate from others begins, in the most literal sense, with touch. Individual differences in the experience of touching and being touched appear to stem from our developmental histories, encompassing the influence of both early and later relationship experience as well as cultural influences.

It was our intent to provide researchers studying touch and the contribution of touch to the formation and maintenance of attachment bonds with a set of theoretically relevant measures to assess individual differences in attitudes toward touch in close relationships. We developed seven new scales with an eye toward improving on the most widely used touch measure, Andersen and Leibowitz's (1978) Touch Avoidance Measure. The Touch Avoidance Measure includes both same- and opposite-sex touch subscales, which assess one's tendency to touch or be touched by others. We reasoned that, at the behavioral level, people may avoid touch for many different reasons, some of which may be associated with lack of opportunity, cultural differences, family-of-origin differences, and gender, but also with a host of relationship factors—from one's relationship stage to the comfort with touch displayed by one's partner. Most of all, we chose to focus on how the process of becoming attached and maintaining attachment in adults might be related to the use of touch, as is the case with infant attachment.

Although our relationship touch scales were developed independently of their association with particular attachment styles, subsequent research points to theoretically meaningful associations of the new touch measures with attachment styles. Chapter 3 in this volume, by Brennan et al., displays attachment style differences in four of the seven touch scales (see Table 3.7). Secure and preoccupied groups scored similarly high in the use of touch to express affection. Both avoidant groups scored lower, particularly the dismissing group. Both avoidant groups scored similarly high in touch aversion, followed by the preoccupied group, which scored higher than the secure group. Fearful and preoccupied groups scored similarly high in the desire for more touch, or touch deprivation; the secure group scored lowest on this scale, and the dismissing group scored intermediately. The use of touch for a haven of safety separated all four groups in the following order: Preoccupieds were highest, followed by secures, fearfuls, and dismissings, who were least likely to engage in this kind of (primarily careseeking) touch.

Brennan et al. did not list attachment style results for the other three touch scales—Discomfort with Public Touch, Sexual Touch, and Coercive Control, so we will briefly describe them here. In the same data set, the following attachment style differences emerged. Secure and preoccupied groups scored similarly low on discomfort with public touch, compared to fearful and dismissing groups, who did not differ from each other. Secure and preoccupied groups scored similarly high on the scale measuring use of touch to express sexuality, compared to the two avoidant groups, who again did not differ from each other. Fearful and preoccupied groups scored similarly high on the scale measuring the use of touch for coercive control, relative to dismissings, who scored higher than secures.

The picture painted by this research showed theoretically expected patterns of touch as a function of attachment style category. To better understand these associations, a discriminant function analysis was conducted by Kelly Brennan (using the same data set) to predict attachment style categories from the seven touch scales. The analysis produced two highly significant functions. The first function was associated with low scores on the Affectionate Proximity and Safe Haven touch scales, and with high scores on the Touch Aversion scale. This function, akin to *Avoidance*, separated dismissing and fearful individuals from secure and preoccupied individuals. The second function was associated with high scores on the Desires More Touch and Coercive Control scales. This function, akin to *Anxiety*, separated fearful and preoccupied individuals from secure and dismissing individuals. (Public Touch and Sexual Touch formed a third discriminant function that did not significantly contribute to the prediction of attachment category membership.)

Whereas the Touch Avoidance Measure is nonspecific with regard to the type of relationship, our scales were created to reflect individual differences in how touch is used in romantic relationships. Despite this difference, both kinds of measures are to some extent tapping a similar construct—but at different levels of analysis. The Touch Avoidance Measure is relatively abstract, whereas our scales include concrete items conveying information about the function of touch. That is, the Andersen and Leibowitz's (1978) touch avoidance items tend to obscure the underlying meaning of the particular touch behavior described. For example, the item "I enjoy touching members of the opposite sex" could have a number of different meanings related to sexuality, touch aversion, expression of affection, body consciousness, and so on. The pattern of associations of the opposite-sex touch avoidance measure with our new scales allows more insight into the construct that Andersen and Leibowitz measured. Opposite-sex touch avoidance was associated with not using touch to express one's sexuality, not using touch to give and receive support under stress, and discomfort touching and being touched by partners (in public or private). Because of their greater specificity, our measures were associated with patterns of emotional intimacy and distress in relationships, whereas the Andersen and Leibowitz's measure was unrelated to these aspects of relationship functioning or to other aspects of relationship quality (i.e., feeling committed or in love). When our new touch scales were examined in connection with affect sensitivity, they outperformed Andersen and Leibowitz's measure, particularly with regard to their association with attending to and understanding one's feelings, aspects of affect sensitivity relevant to attachment formation. Although preliminary, these results support the usefulness of distinguishing among different types of touch and the ways in which touch is used in relationships, as opposed to focusing solely on the behavioral tendency of touch avoidance.

Several limitations of the current approach merit comment. First, studies must be conducted to assess the behavioral correlates of self-reported attitudes toward touch in the context of relationships. Second, it is important to conduct longitudinal research to test the contribution of physical-contact seeking to relationship formation in general, and to the growth and maintenance of attachment in particular. Feelings of love, attraction, and attachment, in turn, are likely to lead to predictable increases and variations in the use of touch, suggesting reciprocal causation. Such research would provide a better understanding of touch patterns as both cause and consequence of *relational stages*—as opposed to *personality differences*—that may affect the quality of (as well as manner of describing) one's relationships. Third, it is appropriate to note that our touch measures are highly associated with gender, although we did not provide information about gender in the current chapter. For example, males were more likely to use touch to express sexuality and more likely to interpret touch as sexual, whereas females were more likely to use touch to express affection. These differences may be important in elucidating gender differences in relationship functioning. Fourth, the constructs assessed by our measures may be culture- or generation-specific. Attitudes toward public displays of affection, as well as touch aversion and deprivation, coercive control, and perceptions of touch as sexual are likely to vary across cultures and, within cultures, across generations or life stages. The use of touch to express affection or provide a haven of safety, however, are likely to be culturally universal to the extent that they are associated with attachment processes.

Much research has been conducted to explore the benefit of touch in human development, yet, until relatively recently, touch has been ignored in the study of adult pair-bonds. Most of the traditional research on touch in adulthood is relevant to a social psychology of the relatively meaningless interpersonal interactions of strangers. Researchers interested in mapping the terrain of touch have examined the personality construct of *touch avoidance*, but are largely silent with regard to the developmental origins of touch avoidance. Attachment theory provides insight about who is likely to be touch avoidant, in addition to how touch may contribute to the formation and maintenance of romantic relationships. Until now, there were no measures specifically designed to aid research on individual differences in the use of touch in romantic relationships. We believe our scales are more suited than existing measures for this purpose.

In sum, touch is an important component of mother–infant attachment, and is likely to be useful in understanding adult pair-bonds as well as other kinds of close relationships in adulthood. We invite researchers to consider relationship touch as an important topic worthy of study in the next decade of research on adult romantic attachment.

Appendix 14.1

SEVEN TOUCH SCALES, PHASE II

DESIRES MORE TOUCH (alpha = .86)

1. I wish my partner were as receptive to my touch as I am to his or her touch.
8. Sometimes I wish my partner were more comfortable with being touched by me.
15. Sometimes I am not very happy with the level of touch in my relationship.

22. Even in private, I can't get my partner to touch me enough.
29. Sometimes my partner goes out of the way to avoid being touched by me.
36. I sometimes wish my partner would touch me more.
43. It makes me sad that my partner won't or can't touch me the way I'd like to be touched.
51. I have considered ending my relationship because of my partner's discomfort with touching and being touched.

AFFECTIONATE PROXIMITY (alpha = .83)

2. Sometimes, for no particular reason, I love to just hold my partner.
9. I wish my partner would just hold me for hours.
16. I like my partner to hold my hand to demonstrate his or her affection for me.
23. I like to hold my partner's hand to demonstrate affection for him or her.
30. After a sexual interaction, I really enjoy being held by my partner.
37. If my partner were willing, I could just caress him or her for hours on end.
44. My partner's touch makes me feel loved.
48. I usually hug my partner to show how happy I am to see him or her.
50. I often touch my partner as a way to express my feelings for him or her.

SEXUAL TOUCH (alpha = .86)

3. I usually become sexually aroused when touching my partner.
10. I usually become sexually aroused when my partner touches me.
17. My partner's touch almost always makes me feel aroused.
24. Most of the time I find being touched by my partner very arousing.
31. Just being touched by my partner is usually enough to arouse me sexually.
38. I use touch as a means to initiate sexual interaction with my partner.
45. My partner uses touch as a means to initiate sexual closeness with me.

TOUCH AVERSION (alpha = .82)

4. My partner continually complains that I don't touch him or her enough.
11. I often have to remind my partner to stop touching me.
18. I generally don't like my partner to touch me.
25. My partner often complains that I don't touch him or her enough.
32. I am not always sure when I want my partner to touch me.
39. I am always glad to have my partner touch me. (R)
42. I sometimes find my partner's touch intolerable.
46. Sometimes I find my partner's touch really annoying.
49. If my partner and I have been apart, it often takes me awhile to get used to his or her touch.

DISCOMFORT WITH PUBLIC TOUCH (alpha = .72)

7. My partner and I don't feel inhibited touching each other in front of others. (R)
14. I don't think that displays of physical affection are appropriate in public.
21. I like touching and being touched by my partner, especially when others are around to see. (R)
28. It feels very natural for my partner and I to touch each other, even when others are around. (R)
35. I think it is embarrassing when my partner touches me in public.

COERCIVE CONTROL (alpha = .71)

6. I use touch to convey my hostility or resentment toward my partner.
13. I often touch my partner to assert my feelings of control.
20. Sometimes the only way I can express negative feelings toward my partner is by using touch to get attention.
27. When I'm angry with my partner, I sometimes feel like hitting him or her.
34. Often without thinking first, I have slapped or hit my partner when we disagreed.
41. My partner often touches me to assert his or her feelings of control.

SAFE HAVEN TOUCH (alpha = .79)

5. When I'm not feeling well, I really need to be touched by my partner.
12. When I'm distressed or ill, I prefer not to be touched by my partner. (R)
19. Even when angry with my partner, I still want to be touched by him or her.
26. I avoid touching my partner when he or she is distressed or ill. (R)
33. When I'm upset with my partner, I still need physical reassurance from him or her.
40. When I am facing a difficult situation, I like being touched by my partner.
47. When my partner is feeling under the weather, my first reaction is to touch him or her.

Note. "R" indicates reverse-scored items. For each item, respondents are asked to describe themselves using a Likert-type scale, ranging from 1 ("not at all like me") to 7 ("very much like me"). Subscales are scored by reversing the appropriate items, then averaging the scores for each scale.

ACKNOWLEDGMENTS

We are most grateful to Deborah Jacobvitz and Phillip Shaver for their helpful comments on a previous draft.

NOTES

1. According to Kirkpatrick (Chapter 13, this volume), although both types of relationships include love, from an evolutionary standpoint that is where the similarity ends. The primary function of the caregiver–infant relationship is the protection and care of the infant, whereas the primary function of adult pair-bonds is reproduction. Caregiving may or may not be present in adult pair-bonds and is certainly not necessary. Kirkpatrick argues provocatively that adult pair-bonds may be less relevant to the attachment system than to the sexual behavior system. That is, adult romantic "attachment" styles may actually be *mating* styles composed of the following two dimensions: (1) one's adoption of short- versus long-term mating strategies, and (2) one's self-assessment of "mate value," akin to relational self-esteem.

2. Other research (i.e., Berryhill, 1982, cited in Deethardt & Hines, 1983) failed to replicate the three dimensions and found only one, very similar to general touch aversion.

REFERENCES

Ainsworth, M. D. S., Bell, S. M., & Stayton, D. J. (1971). Individual differences in Strange Situation behavior of one-year-olds. In H. R. Schaffer (Ed.), *The origins of human social relations* (pp. 17–57). London: Academic Press.

Ainsworth, M. D. S., Blehar, M., Waters, E., & Wall, S. (1978). *Patterns of attachment: A psychological study of the Strange Situation.* Hillsdale, NJ: Erlbaum.

Andersen, J. F., Andersen, P. A., & Lustig, M. W. (1987). Opposite sex touch avoidance: A national replication and extension. *Journal of Nonverbal Behavior, 11,* 89–109.

Andersen, P. A., & Leibowitz, K. (1978). The development and nature of the construct touch avoidance. *Environmental Psychology and Nonverbal Behavior, 3,* 89–106.

Andersen, P. A., & Sull, K. K. (1985). Out of touch, out of reach: Tactile predispositions as predictors of interpersonal distance. *Western Journal of Speech Communication, 49,* 57–72.

Anisfeld, E., Casper, V., Nozyce, M., & Cunningham, N. (1990). Does infant carrying promote attachment?: An experimental study of the effects of increased physical contact on the development of attachment. *Child Development, 61,* 1617–1627.

Bacorn, C. N., & Dixon, D. N. (1984). The effects of touch on depressed and vocationally undecided clients. *Journal of Counseling Psychology, 31,* 488–496.

Barroso, F., & Feld, J. K. (1986). Self-touching and attentional processes: The role of task difficulty, selection stage, and sex differences. *Journal of Nonverbal Behavior, 10,* 51–65.

Bell, S. M., & Ainsworth, M. D. S. (1972). Infant crying and maternal responsiveness. *Child Development, 43,* 1171–1190.

Berryhill, N. (1982). *The influence of age, sex, family size, and community size on attitude toward tactile communication.* Unpublished master's thesis, Texas Tech University.

Bowlby, J. (1973). *Attachment and loss: Vol. 2. Separation: Anxiety and anger.* New York: Basic Books.

Bowlby, J. (1980). *Attachment and loss: Vol. 3. Loss: Sadness and depression.* New York: Basic Books.

Bowlby, J. (1982). *Attachment and loss: Vol. 1. Attachment* (2nd ed.). New York: Basic Books. (Original work published 1969)

Burgoon, J. K., Buller, D. B., Hale, J. L., & de Turck, M. A. (1984). Relational messages associated with nonverbal behavior. *Human Communication Research, 10,* 351–378.

Collins, N. L., & Read, S. J. (1990). Adult attachment, working models, and relationship quality in dating couples. *Journal of Personality and Social Psychology, 58,* 644–663.

Deethardt, J. F., & Hines, D. G. (1983). Tactile communication and personality differences. *Journal of Nonverbal Behavior, 8,* 143–156.

Derlega, V. J., Lewis, R. J., Harrison, S., Winstead, B. A., & Costanza, R. (1989). Gender differences in the initiation and attribution of tactile intimacy. *Journal of Nonverbal Behavior, 13,* 83–96.

Dreschner, V., & Gantt, W. (1979). Tactile stimulation of several body areas (effect of person). *Pavlovian Journal of Biological Sciences, 14,* 2.

Dreschner, V., Whitehead, W., Morrill-Corbin, E., & Cataldo, F. (1985). Physiological and subjective reactions to being touched. *Psychophysiology, 22,* 96–100.

Driscoll, M. S., Newman, D. L., & Seals, J. M. (1988). The effect of touch on perception of counselors. *Counselor Education and Supervision, 27,* 344–354.

Edwards, D. J. (1984). The experience of interpersonal touch during a personal growth program: A factor analytic approach. *Human Relations, 37,* 769–780.

Field, T. M. (Ed.). (1995). *Touch in early development.* Mahwah, NJ: Erlbaum.

Fisher, J. D., Rytting, M., & Heslin, R. (1976). Hands touching hands: Affective and evaluative effects of an interpersonal touch. *Sociometry, 39*(4), 416–421.

Fromme, D. K., Jaynes, W. E., Taylor, D. K., Hanold, E. G., Daniell, J., Rountree, J. R., & Fromme, M. L. (1989). Nonverbal behavior and attitudes toward touch. *Journal of Nonverbal Behavior, 13,* 3–14.

Goldberg, S., & Rosenthal, R. (1986). Self-touching behavior in the job interview: Antecedents and consequences. *Journal of Nonverbal Communication, 10*(1), 65–80.

Goldman, M., & Fordyce, J. (1983). Prosocial behavior as affected by eye contact, touch, and voice expression. *Journal of Social Psychology, 121,* 125–129.

Goldman, M., Kiyohara, O., & Pfannensteil, D. A. (1984). Interpersonal touch, social labeling, and the foot-in-the-door effect. *Journal of Social Psychology, 125*(2), 143–147.

Guerrero, L. K., & Andersen, P. A. (1991). The waxing and waning of relational intimacy: Touch as a function of relational stage, gender and touch avoidance. *Journal of Social and Personal Relationships, 8,* 147–165.

Hall, J. A., & Veccia, E. M. (1990). More "touching" observations: New insights on men, women, and interpersonal touch. *Journal of Personality and Social Psychology, 59,* 1155–1162.

Harlow, H. F. (1958). The nature of love. *American Psychologist, 13,* 673–685.

Hazan, C., & Shaver, P. R. (1987). Romantic love conceptualized as an attachment process. *Journal of Personality and Social Psychology, 52,* 511–524.

Hazan, C., & Zeifman, D. (1994). Sex and the psychological tether. In D. Perlman & K. Bartholomew (Eds.), *Advances in personal relationships* (Vol. 5, pp. 151–177). London: Jessica Kingsley.

Hazan, C., Zeifman, D., & Middleton, K. (1994, July). *Adult romantic attachment, affection, and sex.* Paper presented at the 7th International Conference on Personal Relationships, Groningen, The Netherlands.

Henley, N. (1977). *Body politics: Power, sex, and nonverbal communication.* Englewood Cliffs, NJ: Prentice-Hall.

Heslin, R., & Alper, T. (1983). Touch: A bonding gesture. In J. M. Wiemann & R. Harrison (Eds.), *Nonverbal interaction* (pp. 47–75). Beverly Hills, CA: Sage.

Heslin, R., Nguyen, T. D., & Nguyen, M. L. (1983). Meaning of touch: The case of touch from a stranger or same sex person. *Journal of Nonverbal Behavior, 7,* 147–158.

Johnson, K. L., & Edwards, R. (1991). The effects of gender and type of romantic touch on perceptions of relational commitment. *Journal of Nonverbal Behavior, 15,* 43–55.

Jones, S. E. (1985). A naturalistic study of the meanings of touch. *Communication Monographs, 52,* 19–56.

Jourard, S. M. (1966). An exploratory study of body-accessibility. *British Journal of Social and Clinical Psychology, 5,* 221–231.

Knapp, M. L. (1978). *Nonverbal communication in human interaction* (2nd ed.). New York: Holt, Rinehart & Winston.

Korner, A. F. (1990). The many faces of touch. In K. E. Barnard & T. B. Brazelton (Eds.), *Touch: The foundation of experience* (pp. 269–297). Madison, CT: International Universities Press.

Kunce, L., & Shaver, P. R. (1994). An attachment-theoretical approach to caregiving in romantic relationships. In D. Perlman & K. Bartholomew (Eds.), *Advances in personal relationships* (Vol. 5, pp. 205–237). London: Jessica Kingsley.

Main, M. (1990). Parental aversion to infant-initiated contact is correlated with the parent's own rejection during childhood: The effects of experience on signals of security with respect to attachment. In K. E. Barnard & T. B. Brazelton (Eds.), *Touch: The foundation of experience* (pp. 461–495). Madison, CT: International Universities Press.

Major, B. (1981). Gender patterns in touching behavior. In C. Mayo & N. M. Henley (Eds.), *Gender and nonverbal behavior* (pp. 15–37). New York: Springer-Verlag.

Major, B., Schmidlin, A. M., & Williams, L. (1990). Gender patterns in social touch: The impact of setting and age. *Journal of Personality and Social Psychology, 58,* 634–643.

Monsour, M. (1992). Meanings of intimacy in cross- and same-sex friendships. *Journal of Social and Personal Relationships, 9*(2), 277–295.

Montagu, A. (1986). *Touching: The human significance of the skin* (3rd ed.). New York: Harper & Row.

Morris, D. (1977). *Manwatching: A field guide to human behavior.* New York: Abrams.

Nguyen, M. L., Heslin, R., & Nguyen, T. (1976). The meaning of touch: Sex and marital status differences. *Representative Research in Social Psychology, 7,* 13–18.

Nguyen, T., Heslin, R., & Nguyen, M. L. (1975). The meaning of touch: Sex differences. *Journal of Communication, 25,* 92–103.

Noller, P., & Feeney, J. A. (1993, August). *Relationship satisfaction, attachment, and nonverbal decoding in early marriage.* Paper presented at the annual conference of the American Psychological Association, Toronto.

Patterson, M. L., Powell, J. L., & Lenihan, M. G. (1986). Touch, compliance, and interpersonal space. *Journal of Nonverbal Behavior, 10*(1), 41–49.

Pietromonaco, P., & Carnelley, K. (1994). Gender and working models of attachment: Consequences for perceptions of self and romantic partners. *Personal Relationships, 1,* 63–82.

Pisano, M. D., Wall, S. M., & Foster, A. (1986). Perceptions of nonreciprocal touch in romantic relationships. *Journal of Nonverbal Behavior, 10*(1), 29–40.

Reis, H. T., & Shaver, P. R. (1988). Intimacy as an interpersonal process. In S. Duck (Ed.), *Handbook of personal relationships: Theory, research, and interventions* (pp. 367–389). Chichester, UK: Wiley.

Remland, M. S., & Jones, T. S. (1988). Cultural and sex differences in touch avoidance. *Perceptual and Motor Skills, 67,* 544–546.

Roese, N. J., Olson, J. M., Borenstein, M. N., Martin, A., & Shores, A. L. (1992). Same-sex touching behavior: The moderating role of homophobic attitudes. *Journal of Nonverbal Behavior, 16,* 249–259.

Rothbard, J. C., & Shaver, P. R. (1994). Continuity of attachment across the life span. In M. B. Sperling & W. H. Berman (Eds.), *Attachment in adults: Clinical and developmental perspectives* (pp. 31–71). New York: Guilford Press.

Salovey, P., Mayer, J. D., Goldman, S. L., & Palfai, T. P. (1992, July). *The Trait Meta-Mood Scale and emotional intelligence: Measuring attention to, clarity, and repair of mood.* Paper presented at the annual meeting of the European Society for Experimental Social Psychology, Leuven/Louvain-la-Neuve, Belgium.

Schutte, N. S., Malouff, J. M., & Adams, C. J. (1988). A self-report measure of touching behavior. *Journal of Social Psychology, 128*(5), 597–604.

Shaver, P. R., & Brennan, K. A. (1992). Attachment styles and the "Big Five" personality traits: Their connections with each other and with romantic relationship outcomes. *Personality and Social Psychology Bulletin, 18,* 536–545.

Shaver, P. R., & Hazan, C. (1993). Adult romantic attachment: Theory and evidence. In D. Perlman & W. Jones (Eds.), *Advances in personal relationships* (pp. 29–70). London: Jessica Kingsley.

Shaver, P. R., Hazan, C., & Bradshaw, D. (1988). Love as attachment: The integration of three behavioral systems. In R. J. Sternberg & M. Barnes (Eds.), *The anatomy of love* (pp. 68–99). New Haven, CT: Yale University Press.

Simpson, J. A. (1990). Influence of attachment styles on romantic relationships. *Journal of Personality and Social Psychology, 59,* 971–980.

Simpson, J. A., Rholes, W. S., & Nelligan, J. S. (1992). Support seeking and support giving within couples in an anxiety-provoking situation: The role of attachment styles. *Journal of Personality and Social Psychology, 62,* 434–446.

Sorensen, G., & Beatty, M. J. (1988). The interactive effects of touch and touch avoidance on interpersonal evaluations. *Communication Research Reports, 5*(1), 84–90.

Spanier, G. B. (1976). Measuring dyadic adjustment: New scales for assessing the quality of marriages and similar dyads. *Journal of Marriage and the Family, 38,* 15–28.

Spitz, R. (1946). Anaclitic depression. *Psychoanalytic Study of the Child, 2,* 313–342.

Sroufe, L. A., Carlson, E., & Shulman, S. (1993). Individuals in relationships:

Development from infancy through adolescence. In D. C. Funder, R. D. Parke, C. Tomlinson-Keasey, & K. Widaman (Eds.), *Studying lives through time: Personality and development* (pp. 315–342). Washington, DC: American Psychological Association.

Stack, D. M., & Muir, D. W. (1992). Adult tactile stimulation during face-to-face interactions modulates five-month-olds' affect and attention. *Child Development, 63,* 1509–1525.

Trussoni, S. J., O'Malley, A., & Barton, A. (1988). Human emotion communication by touch: A modified replication of an experiment by Manfred Clynes. *Perceptual and Motor Skills, 66,* 419–424.

Walsh, A. (1991). *The science of love: Understanding love and its effects on mind and body.* Buffalo, NY: Prometheus Books.

Willis, F. N., Jr., & Briggs, L. F. (1992). Relationship and touch in public settings. *Journal of Nonverbal Behavior, 16,* 55–63.

Willison, B. G., & Masson, R. L. (1986). The role of touch in therapy: An adjunct to communication. *Journal of Counseling and Development, 64,* 497–500.

Wilson, J. M. (1982). The value of touch in psychotherapy. *American Journal of Orthopsychiatry, 52*(1), 65–72.

Woodmansey, A. C. (1988). Are psychotherapists out of touch? *British Journal of Psychotherapy, 5*(1), 57–65.

Wycoff, E. B., & Holley, J. D. (1990). Effects of flight attendants' touch upon airline passengers' perceptions of the attendant and the airline. *Perceptual and Motor Skills, 71,* 932–934.

Index